ROYAL
POXES &
POTIONS

ROYAL DOCTORS
& THEIR SECRETS

RAYMOND LAMONT-BROWN

Cover illustration: detail from The Death of HRH Albert, Prince Consort
by Oakley (Wellcome Institute Library, London)

First published in 2001
This edition first published in 2009

The History Press
The Mill, Brimscombe Port
Stroud, Gloucestershire, GL5 2QG
www.thehistorypress.co.uk

British Library Cataloguing in Publication Data.
A catalogue record for this book is available from the British Library.

ISBN 978 0 7524 5469 6

Typesetting and origination by The History Press
Printed in Great Britain

CONTENTS

CHRONOLOGY OF COURT MEDICAL PRACTITIONERS

3200–2980 BC	Ancient Egyptian rulers begin to have personal physicians.
2563–2423 BC	Women royal doctors at Ancient Egyptian courts.
460–355 BC	Hippocrates of Cos leads the custom of having physicians at Greek courts.
46 BC	Medical men employed on ad hoc basis in the cadres of Imperial Rome.
131–200 AD	Galen court physician to Emperor Marcus Aurelius; court physicians now have distinctive roles.
766–809	Abbasid Caliph Harun Al-Rachid promotes court physicians.
1042–66	Baldwin, Abbot of Bury St Edmunds, first physician mentioned at court of Edward the Confessor.
1066–87	Brother Nigel; first mention of court physician on a payroll of William the Conqueror.
1216–72	Court rolls began to detail rights, duties and status of royal physicians.
	First knighthoods recorded for medical court service.
	Henry III establishes a separate medical household for his queen.
1272–1307	Edward I encourages royal doctors to take an interest in military medicine.
1461	Pool of doctors at Edward IV's court, covering many nationalities.
(1462	Barber-surgeons of London granted a charter.)
1474	New Ordinances established, defining duties of royal doctors at English court.

1500s	Andreas Vesalius and Ambroise Paré role-models for court physicians.
(1506	Guild of Surgeons and Barbers, at Edinburgh, incorporated by town council and ratified by James IV.)
	James IV encourages royal doctors in Scotland to give care to patients outside the court, thus forming a prototype of a national health service.
(1518	Henry VIII grants charter for the foundation of the Royal College of Physicians of London.)
	A new generation of physicians and surgeons join royal court.
(1540	Surgeons join with Barbers to form United Company of Barber-Surgeons.)
	First Master of the United Company of Barber-Surgeons is Thomas Vicary, promoted to sergeant-surgeon at royal court.
1544	Antoine Brisset first Scottish court doctor to be mentioned as military surgeon.
1560s	Dr John Dee vacillates at Queen Elizabeth I's court; he is dubbed 'Queen Elizabeth's Merlin'.
1587	Royal doctors benefit from will of executed Mary, Queen of Scots; a rare public record.
1594	Royal physician Roderigo López executed at Tyburn for plotting Queen Elizabeth I's assassination.
(1599	Faculty of Physicians and Surgeons of Glasgow chartered.)
(1617	Worshipful Society of Apothecaries of London chartered by James VI & I.)
1628	Physician-in-extraordinary William Harvey demonstrates circulation of the blood.
(1657	Fraternity of Apothecaries founded at Edinburgh.)
1660	Richard Wiseman, 'the Father of English Surgery', appointed surgeon-in-ordinary to Charles II. Describes the 'King's Evil' (scrofula).

(1667	Royal College of Physicians founded in Ireland.)
(1681	Royal College of Physicians of Edinburgh chartered.)
1685	Charles II is purported to have been murdered by royal doctors in a case of 'iatrogenic regicide'.
(1694	College of Surgeons of Edinburgh chartered.)
1714	Sir David Hamilton accused by fellow royal physicians of hastening the death of Queen Anne.
1735	Sir Caesar Hawkins becomes sergeant-surgeon to George II. Dubbed quintessential eccentric court physician.
1753	Royal doctor Archibald Cameron executed at Tyburn, the last Jacobite to be hanged, drawn and quartered.
(1778	Royal College of Surgeons of Edinburgh chartered.)
1788	Onset of George III's descent to madness and the unprecedented domestic and political prominence of royal doctors at court. Dr Francis Willis, for the first time ever, breaks royal protocol to treat the monarch.
1819	Queen Victoria vaccinated against smallpox; the first member of the royal family to be so treated.
1822	George IV's physician Sir William Knighton dubbed 'the king's spy'.
(1832	Foundation of the British Medical Association.)
1837	Accusations abound that royal doctors' bulletins on William IV's last days were 'manipulated' for electoral advantage by Viscount Melbourne, Liberal prime minister.
1839	Royal doctor Sir James Clark and Queen Victoria involved in the 'Lady Florence Hastings case'.
1844	The office of HM First Physician in Scotland lapses.

1853   Sir James Clark invites Dr John Snow to give Queen Victoria chloroform at the birth of Prince Leopold.

1861   Erstwhile foreign secretary, George William Frederick Villiers, 4th Earl of Clarendon, publicly criticises royal doctors for death of Prince Albert.

1871   Joseph Lister operates for the first time on Queen Victoria. The queen witnesses Lister's innovative expertise. He had introduced antiseptic surgery in 1867.

1896   Chicago medical practitioner Dr Howard avers royal doctor Sir William Gull is 'Jack the Ripper'.

1899   Queen Victoria draws up new 'Regulations' of service for married royal doctors.

1901   Sir James Reid carries out Queen Victoria's 'secret' funerary instructions. He hides John Brown artefacts in the royal coffin.

1902   Sir Frederick Treves operates on Edward VII for appendicitis.
                Sir James Reid negotiates 'blackmail' letters concerning John Brown and Queen Victoria from royal physician Dr Profeit's son George.

1928   George V undergoes operation on the chest by surgeon-in-ordinary Sir Hugh Ripley. A further operation is carried out by Wilfred Batten Lewis Trotter.

(1929   Foundation of the (Royal) College of Obstetricians and Gynaecologists.)

(1948   National Health Service comes into operation.)

1949   Sir James Paterson Ross performs a right lumbar sympathectomy of George VI.

1951   A pneumonectomy performed on George VI at Buckingham Palace by royal surgeon Sir Clement Price-Thomas.

(1952   Foundation of the (Royal) College of General Practitioners.)

1953   Queen Elizabeth the Queen Mother elected to

	Honorary Fellowship of the Royal College of Physicians of Edinburgh.
1961	Effective hip replacement operations become common; Queen Elizabeth the Queen Mother has hip replacements at set times.
(1962	New Designation: Royal College of Physicians and Surgeons of Glasgow.)
1964	Queen Elizabeth the Queen Mother attends the King Edward VII Hospital for Officers for appendix operation.
1966	Queen Elizabeth the Queen Mother has emergency abdominal operation. Details not announced, leading to lurid speculations.
(1967	Opening of Lister Institute, Edinburgh.)
(1971	Royal College of Surgeons reports cigarette smoking kills some 27,500 people a year in Britain. Historians dub lung cancer 'royal killer'.)
1972	Prince Philip incapacitated by yellow jaundice; attended by royal doctors Sir John Weir and Sir Harold Evans.
(1978	Smallpox is declared eradicated.)
1984	National press agog when Queen Elizabeth the Queen Mother has surgery under general anaesthetic for removal of fishbone from throat.
1986	Report in press that euthanasia was carried out on George V by royal physician Lord Dawson of Penn.
2000	The late Queen Elizabeth the Queen Mother breaks collar-bone in 100th year.
2001	The late Princess Margaret admitted to King Edward VII's Hospital for Officers for observation.
9 Feb 2002	Princess Margaret, Countess of Snowdon (b.1930) died following cardiac problems at King Edward VII Hospital, London.
30 March 2002	Queen Elizabeth the Queen Mother died at Royal Lodge in her 102th year.

February 2004   Appointment of Dr Timothy Evans as a royal physician causing 'quite a stir' because of his practises of 'alternative medicine'. He replaced Sir Nigel Southward who retired after 28 years of service.

29 April 2007   Death of Sir George Pinker (b.1924), Surgeon Gynaecologist to Queen Elizabeth II. He supervised nine royal births.

2008   Professor John Cunningham, Head of the Medical Household and Physician to Queen Elizabeth II, receives CVO.

THE KING IS DEAD, LONG LIVE HIS DOCTORS

Some said it was the most cynical act ever in the history of the British monarchy. Others declared it was royal murder. A few opined that the reported act of euthanasia had preserved the dignity of the sovereign. Today the evidence surrounding the last hours of the life of King George V is conflicting. Dictionaries of quotations contain the moving words written in first draft by physician-in-ordinary Bertrand Edward, Viscount Dawson of Penn (1864–1945), on a menu card in the royal household dining-room at Sandringham House, where the king lay dying. The simple message read: 'The King's life is moving peacefully towards its close.'[1]

Yet cynicism dripped from the words for some when they were told that King George's death had been hastened for the convenience of the assembled media. It was considered undignified in the royal household for the monarch's death to be first carried in the lightweight evening tabloids. So, the truth came out that Lord Dawson had chemically shortened the monarch's life by a few hours so that the heavyweight papers like *The Times* would be first to carry the king's obituary. A lethal dose of morphia and cocaine was administered into the jugular vein and George V died at 11.55 p.m. on Monday, 20 January 1936.

The revelation about the king's accelerated demise was first given a public airing in 1986 by Francis Watson, biographer of Lord Dawson. The consequent publicity surrounding the disclosure brought to the public eye once more the profoundly secret role of the royal doctor. While the *Independent* raised the question in the headline 'Was George V's death treason?', others began to realise that the consultations of a royal physician must go further than matters that are strictly concerned with physical or mental illness, or with medical matters in general. After all, the royal physician's patient is unique to the day and the hour. Historically, royal doctors may have been known to push a bad or senile monarch into eternity to fulfil the political need for a more suitable successor to the throne. But in modern terms the royal doctor's role has added more facets, including contributing where possible to the enduring dignity of the monarchy. Yet there are others who believe that royal doctors have always been employed for more sinister roles.

In recent times, for example, crime historians have opined that George V was 'murdered' to seal secrets that would, as Christabel, Lady Aberconway, vouchsafed to writer Michael Thornton, 'still cause the Throne to totter'.[2] In the research for his book *The Ripper and The Royals*, Melvyn Fairclough noted how Bernard Fitzalan-Howard, 16th Duke of Norfolk, Earl Marshal of England, and Hugh Montague, 1st Viscount Trenchard, Commissioner for the Metropolitan Police from 1931 to 1935, had separately and independently told influential artist Walter Sickert that George V's death had been hastened to silence him.[3]

The reason had been known for years by royal doctors who had colluded, averred courtiers, in a startling and hardly believable secret. For years certain royal biographers have suggested that King George V's elder brother, the mentally unstable Prince Albert Victor, Duke of Clarence and Avondale, was a key player in the 'Jack the Ripper' murders, and that he had not died of pneumonia in 1892, but had survived until 1933 to be 'incarcerated at Glamis [castle]'.[4] Thus the prince's funeral and elaborate tomb by Sir Alfred Gilbert in the Albert Chapel at Windsor Castle remain an elaborate sham. George V had thus reigned unconstitutionally – and his remorse for his brother's illegal detention had been feverishly shouted out from his deathbed while he was mortally ill. To prevent the royal secret from spreading, Lord Dawson was used as the instrument of silence. As with many such rumours, its very implausibility has led to its durability.

Rather than be privy to burdensome royal secrets and responsibilities, and despite the glittering prizes to be garnered from such service, several prominent medics have declined royal preferment – often for extremely idiosyncratic reasons.

The distinguished physician and Gulstonian lecturer Baldwin Hamey Jr (1600–76) turned down the post of royal physician (and a knighthood) because he did not approve of King Charles II's morals.[5] Another physician, Erasmus Darwin (1731–1802), refused George III's blandishments, telling the monarch that he was intent on putting all his non-professional efforts into pursuing a rich widow who was already being wooed by others.[6] Sir Henry Wentworth Acland (1815–1900), on the other hand, refused twice to be Queen Victoria's physician because he thought he could do better for himself (and humanity) in academe.[7]

In the lengthy and still-evolving history of royal doctors, many have given loyal service, others have feathered their own nests, while some have been out and out mountebanks. One of the latter was John Radcliffe (1652–1714).[8] A Fellow of Lincoln College, Oxford, Radcliffe practised medicine in that city and then transferred to London, where his expertise earned him 'twenty guineas a day', an incredible amount for that era.[9] His irascibility and undiplomatic outbursts made him many enemies. At the early age of 36, he was appointed physician to Princess Anne Sophia of Denmark (daughter of King Frederick III of Denmark), but was subsequently dismissed as he failed to turn up when she summoned him for consultations. Radcliffe was called to minister to Queen Mary II when she developed smallpox – and many blamed his supposed negligence for the queen's death on 28 December 1694.

King William III called in Radcliffe when he developed oedema of the legs, but was aghast at the physician's insulting behaviour to his condition. Radcliffe was never called to his court again. When Queen Anne fell ill, however, for the last time in 1714, Radcliffe refused to attend her and was much criticised for his attitude. In mitigation Radcliffe was ill himself – he died some three months after Queen Anne – but his name was in bad odour at court for many years.[10]

Other doctors, in contrast, were to win the serious respect, confidence and affection of their sovereigns. For instance, King George IV, while Prince of Wales, was moved to write to his physician-in-ordinary, Sir Walter Farquhar (1738–1819), in 1800, from Carlton House, 'I place my whole and entire confidence in you'.[11] Similarly, in a note accompanying a silver epergne (ornamental table centrepiece), George wrote: 'Let me entreat your acceptance of the case which accompanies this note as a testimony of the true and high regard of your very sincere friend.'[12]

Queen Victoria saw the comings and goings of many physicians and surgeons during her long life and reign. Honours were bestowed and presents given to a multitude of medics. More favoured doctors were given a wide range of gifts by members of the royal family and Sir James Reid (1849–1923), who had been appointed resident medical attendant to Queen Victoria in 1881, reported in his journal in 1889 'a pretty good haul this Christmas'.[13] Sir James Clark (1788–1870), physician-in-ordinary to Queen Victoria and Prince Albert, did even better. Clark had been resident physician to the Duchess of Kent, Queen Victoria's mother, since 1835, and on his retirement in 1860 the queen gifted him the Tudor-Gothic house of Bagshot Park in Surrey, erstwhile home of her cousin Prince William Frederick, Duke of Gloucester and Edinburgh. The queen often visited this 'grace and favour residence', which gave the old physician much pleasure; he lived there until his death.[14]

In more modern times, King George VI hurried to the bedside of his dying physician Sir Maurice Cassidy (1880–1949) to bid him farewell, thank him for past devotion and confer on him the insignia of the Knight Grand Cross of the Victorian Order.[15]

As with any other royal appointment that of royal physician brought its frustrations, embarrassments and confusions – and in some cases the premature death of the appointee through stress. This was the fate of the famous royal *accoucheur* Sir Richard Croft (1762–1818). On 2 May 1816 Princess Charlotte Augusta of Wales, born at Carlton House on 7 January 1796, the only child of George, Prince of Wales, and Princess Caroline of Brunswick, married Prince Leopold George Frederick of Saxe-Coburg-Saalfeld, Duke of Saxony. Following two miscarriages the princess fell pregnant again and a child was expected any time after 19 October 1817. The court and people awaited the birth with interest but as the days passed and no baby appeared Croft and his colleague Matthew Baillie (1766–1823), former physician to George III, adopted the quite new procedure of issuing an official statement on the royal health:

Claremont, 22 October: Her Royal Highness has occasionally suffered a little from headache, for which it has been necessary, at different times, to extract blood. On one occasion Her Royal Highness submitted to four incisions in the arm without effect in consequence of the veins being deeply buried. On a consultation of the Physicians and Surgeons, it was deemed improper to make any further attempts, and the blood was ordered to be drawn from a vein at the back of the hand, where the operation has several times been successfully performed . . . with great relief to Her Royal Highness.[16]

At last Charlotte went into labour on 3 November and the distinguished personages, from Viscount Sidmouth, the home secretary, to Earl Bathurst, the secretary for war, who were required to attend the birth were assembled. Croft announced that proceedings were 'in every way in as much forwardness as he would desire it'. Because of uterine inertia a still-born prince was produced. Within six hours of her delivery the princess herself was dead; modern medical thought avers that she died because of complications exacerbated by inherited porphyria.

Henry Brougham, 1st Lord Brougham and Vaux, the Whig lawyer and MP, reported that the whole kingdom had 'feelings of the deepest sorrow'.[17] Indeed the sense of loss was constitutionally shattering; Princess Charlotte was the only direct legitimate heir apparent to the throne. The medical profession was also shocked and perplexed at the event; it was the first time that a royal lady had been delivered by an *accoucheur*, and many sought a scapegoat. Sir Richard Croft was blamed for the tragedy with the accusation of 'negligence and of mismanaging the confinement'; professional voices averred that he should have called in Dr John Sims, the third of the princess's physicians, much earlier. The Prince of Wales considered that Croft was seriously maligned over the death and wrote:

His Royal Highness's acknowledgement of the zealous care, and indefatigable attention manifest by Sir Richard Croft towards his beloved daughter during her late and eventful confinement; and to express His Royal Highness's entire confidence in the medical skill and ability which he displayed, during the arduous and protracted labour, whereof the issue, under the will of Divine Providence has overwhelmed His Royal Highness with such deep affliction.[18]

As the months went by following the princess's burial at St George's Chapel, Windsor, Croft became more anxious and depressed. He was called out to a patient, one Mrs Thackeray, at 86 Wimpole Street, London, who was a cousin-in-law to the writer William Makepeace Thackeray. A female infant was safely delivered – but alas Mrs Thackeray died in labour. Now deeply depressed by the outcome at Wimpole Street and re-living the traumas of Princess Charlotte's deathbed, Croft excused himself, retired to a small bedroom that had been set aside for his use, and shot himself.[19]

By and large the appointment of royal doctors has been achieved by the personal recommendation of senior doctors, either to the monarchs directly or to their advisers. An example of the former procedure is seen in the appointment of Dr Joseph Lister (1827–1912). On 2 July 1870 Sir William Jenner (1815–98), president of the Royal College of Physicians and physician-in-ordinary to Queen Victoria, wrote to her thus:

Under all the conditions I am sure Your Majesty will do well as Your Majesty says to appoint an Edinburgh Surgeon. – There is a surgeon of the highest reputation in Edinburgh who succeeded (James) Syme (1799–1870) in his professorship (Mr. Lister formerly of Glasgow).[20]

From the reign of George III appointments of royal doctors were made with the agreement of government ministers, although at this date selection was considered a 'family matter'. From Edward VII's first court, suitable candidates have been selected by the current physician-in-ordinary. Today a certain reserve shrouds new appointments. A representative of the Lord Chamberlain's office commented recently: 'We do have our own selection procedure . . . and although not maintained in a document as such, is a matter of policy not made generally available.'[21]

To the historian, royal doctors of the twenty-first century are far less colourful than their predecessors. Formerly many ranked as spies, assassins, mountebanks, political shysters or money-grubbing non-entities. Over the centuries, such men formed an idiosyncratic and colourful branch of the medical profession. As royal illnesses frequently triggered political crises, actions by royal doctors had considerable effects on the nation. Their story is thus an important and largely untold one. It is a story that unfolds from the very early days of kingship.

MAGIC, SIN AND SARACENS

Medical science as we have come to recognise it began in the Egypt of the pharaohs. Although influenced by the superstitions of magic in antiquity, the physicians and surgeons of Ancient Egypt achieved an international fame that was recognised by such as the Greek physician Hippocrates of Cos, who fathered modern medicine in the fifth century BC. The extent of the Ancient Egyptian doctors' knowledge of medicine is set out in two docutments, the New Kingdom, Eighteenth Dynasty (c. 1570 BC) *Edwin Smith Surgical Papyrus*[1] and the contemporary *Ebers Medical Papyrus*,[2] wherein cases of injury are discussed and anatomy is mixed with prescribed treatments and speculative medical philosophy. The skills of the Ancient Egyptian doctors gave them important positions in the courts of the pharaohs, and clay tablets found at Tell el Amarna recount how the courts of Syria, Assyria and Persia employed royal doctors from Egypt.

The importance of royal doctors grew out of the need to keep a sovereign well, so that his realm or empire could be properly governed and kept in good discipline. There were always plenty of candidates for the throne if a monarch were incapacitated by disease or mental illness, so the position of trusted, loyal royal doctors became an important court prerogative.

The concept of a ruler having a personal physician dates back to around the Archaic Period of Ancient Egypt, within the era of the First Dynasty (3200–2980 BC). One so identified is Sekhet'enanach.[3] Among his tomb hieroglyphics the physician appears dressed in leopard skins and carrying two sceptres. The text records that 'he healed the king's nostrils', and had his work immortalised in a sculpture of the healed royal patient.[4]

Among medical historians a better known royal physician's name is that of Imhotep. As magic extended to all aspects of daily life in Ancient Egypt, Imhotep became the prototype Magician-Physician of the ancient world.[5] He began to be

COURT DOCTORS OF THE PHARAOHS

The stela set up as a false door in the tomb of Ir-en-akhty of the 1st Intermediate Period (2280–2050 BC) shows the number of royal doctors the Ancient Egyptian court of the period supported. The hieroglyphs and transliterations of some of the doctors (*swnw*) can be set out thus:

swnw per aa: court physician

sehedj swnw per aa: inspector of court physicians

swnw irty per aa: court opthalmologist

swnw khet per aa: court gastroenterologist

neru phuyt: proctologist, a practitioner dealing with the diseases of the anus

aaa mu m-khenu netetet: interpreter of liquids

It may be noted that there were women royal doctors at court, an example being the Lady Peseshet of the Fifth–Sixth Dynasty (2563–2423 BC), described as 'overseer of the female physicians'.

Examples of hieroglyphs as used by court doctors on prescriptions, requisitions, or instructions:

	to smear, or anoint with medicinal unguents		a migraine
	ointment		human flesh
	bandage		medicinal snake
	[doctor as] magician		chloride of sodium [common salt]
	surgical knife		

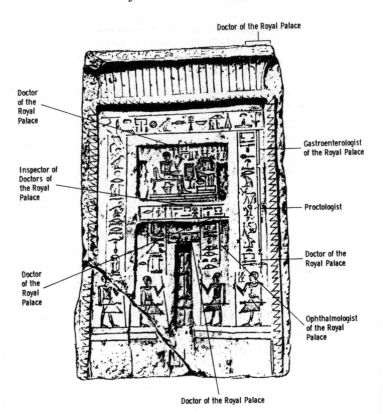

Doctor of the Royal Palace

Doctor of the Royal Palace

Doctor of the Royal Palace

Inspector of Doctors of the Royal Palace

Doctor of the Royal Palace

Gastroenterologist of the Royal Palace

Proctologist

Doctor of the Royal Palace

Ophthalmologist of the Royal Palace

Doctor of the Royal Palace

worshipped as a god around 2850 BC.[6] As Imonthes, the Greeks identified Imhotep as equal to their own Aesculapius, whose cult was established by 850 BC.[7] By the time Aesculapius's cult had been absorbed into the culture of Ancient Rome, in the third century BC,[8] Imhotep had become 'Patron/Tutelary Deity of Medicine' to Aesculapius's 'Emblemetic Deity of Medicine'.[9] We know that Imhotep served also as Grand Vizier to King Djoser of the Third Dynasty (2778–2680 BC), for whom he designed the great 200ft high Step Pyramid at Saqqara, some 14 miles south of Cairo.[10] Three temples are known to have been built in honour of Imhotep's skills, at Memphis, Thebes and Philae,[11] where his amulets could be bought to fight off disease and his cures sought by incubation (a sleep-over at the temple).

Far from Egypt, medicine in China's royal circles began at about the same time with Emperor Shen Nung, who flourished both as a pharmacist and as a medical amateur. Astonishingly, his famous *Pen Tsao* (Great Herbal) remained in print until 1911. The tradition of emperors as doctors was carried on by Hwang Ti (2650 BC), believed to be the author of the volume *Nei Ching* (Book of Medicines), which contains remarkable comments on the circulation of the blood – years before the English physician William Harvey (1578–1657) made his discoveries known in 1628.[12] Thereafter Chinese emperors employed doctors within their courts, although medical practice remained steeped in magic and sorcery for centuries. By the eighteenth century the Chinese imperial court was a great fount of medical knowledge. During 1744 the Ch'ing Emperor Ch'ien-lung (r. 1736–96) became patron of the forty-volume standard encyclopedia of Chinese medicine, *The Golden Mirror of Medicine*.

The practice of medicine in Japan followed tenets derived directly from China. Early Japanese doctors were skilled in the treatment of sword wounds, in consequence of the activities of both retained and itinerant *samurai* (warriors) within the Japanese feudal state. Contact with western doctors at the Dutch enclave at Nagasaki from the seventeenth century enhanced their knowledge of surgery and anatomy, and gave them an insight into general western medical techniques. Many of Japan's leaders in the field of medicine were trained in Germany by the beginning of the twentieth century. Magic played an important role in Japan when medical attention was required at court. As the bodies of the imperial family were deemed sacrosanct, no doctor could touch them, let alone give them injections.[13] Full medical treatment was not allowed in the imperial Japanese household until 1928 when at the age of 2 Princess Sachiko, second daughter of the Emperor Hirohito and Empress Nagako, developed a mortal illness.[14]

It was Hippocrates of Cos (460–355 BC), the most celebrated physician of the ancient world, who helped to separate magic from medicine and stimulated scientific enquiry into the practice of medicine. Since the days of Croesus, last King of Lydia, court physicians had communed with the gods to perform 'miracles of healing, even restoring the dead to life' with the intervention of Aesculapius.[15] Hippocrates extracted the medical facts from the superstitions these physicians uttered at the Delphic Oracle, and new medical protocols were evolved and written up in the *Corpus Hippocratium*.

The spirit of Hippocrates and his immediate followers was passed on to doctors within the empires of Alexander and Rome. Alexander III 'the Great' (356–323 BC), King of Macedonia, maintained the Greek custom of having personal physicians at court, and in 332 BC there was established the medical school of Alexandria, led by Herophilus the anatomist and Erasistratus the physiologist. By a gradual process of infiltration the medical system of Greece was transferred to the Roman Empire. Up to 46 BC, when Julius Caesar granted physicians full rights of Roman citizenship, medical men, most of whom were Greek, were of low degree, many being slaves in Roman households. Within the imperial cadres of Rome, doctors were employed only on an *ad hoc* basis.[16]

One physician who certainly won Roman imperial favour was Galen (*c.* AD 131–200), whose expertise laid the foundations of experimental physiology and dominated medical thought for some 1,200 years. Galen studied medicine at Alexandria and became a court physician to Emperor Marcus Aurelius. Thereafter court physicians began to be mentioned within a distinctive role; one such was the Byzantine scholar Oribasius, physician to Emperor Julian the Apostate.

As Christianity developed as a theological dogma, medicine went into decline, with disease now being looked on as a divine punishment for sin. Bigoted early Christians regarded miracles as the only true healing agent, and disregarded medical practice. Furthermore, as the body was deemed sacred, and dissection of it anathema, the study of anatomy and physiology could not be pursued practically, but only in the volumes of Galen. Although this attitude was to change within the medieval Church, the dawn of Arabian medicine added greatly to the expansion of therapeutic knowledge in the Middle Ages. The courts of Syria and Persia pioneered the use of court physicians skilled in medical practice, their knowledge gleaned from the old Greek texts, now translated into Arabic. Soon, too, court physicians became famous for their expertise, like the Syrian-Christian

Jibra-il-Bukht-Yishu, personal physician to Harun Al-Raschid, the famed Abbasid Caliph of the *Arabian Nights*.

Encouraged by the intense activity within the Arab world, court physicians flourished and the works of such men as the ninth-century Egyptian-Jew Isaac Judaeus, physician to the rulers of Tunisia, remained in print until the seventeenth century. The youngest known court physician of the era was the Persian Abu Ali Hussein ibn Sina, by-named Avicenna (980–1037), whose book *Canon of Medicine* was set reading up to modern times.[17]

As the western Caliphate (including Spain) achieved its own political importance, by the twelfth century Arabian physicians were influential in Europe; one such, the Cordova-born Moses bin Maimon, known as Maimonides (1135–1204), became court physician to the sultan of Egypt and Syria, the celebrated Saladin (1137–93). In 1191 a great army of crusaders, headed by the monarchs of France and England, captured the city of Acre on the Bay of Haifa, and Richard I (1157–99), King of England, is said to have invited Maimonides to be his royal physician, although he declined. Yet Maimonides was to achieve lasting literary fame, as many historians believe that he was the inspiration for the character of the physician El Hakim in Sir Walter Scott's tale of the crusades, *The Talisman* (1825).

Court Physicians Come of Age

As the Moslem Empire declined, the gilded days of Arabian medicine passed and a new era of medical practice evolved from the ashes of the western Roman Empire, to be dubbed 'monastic medicine'. That the secrets of the ancient medical practitioners should have passed into the grasp of the Church is not startling. The ancient works of the Greek masters of medicine had been retained, copied, illustrated and translated in every monastic *scriptorium* in Christendom. Further, it was a tenet of the *Opus Dei* for each monastery to take care of the sick in the convent's *infirmarium*, with a brother as *infirmarius* and another as *hortulus* (gardener) for the *herbarium*. Monastic physicians were encouraged to come to court and such men as the Dark Age ruler King Theodoric of the Ostrogoths (454–526) actively promoted monastic care for the poor. By the eleventh century, then, medicine had become largely the exclusive right of the Church in Britain, with Physic joining Latin Grammar and Classical Philosophy as one of the monastic Humanities.

The Pipe Rolls of the Exchequer, Patent Rolls and Close Rolls held at the Public Record Office give details of the holders of royal preferment as medical attendants to the English royal houses, whereas the chronicles, registers and cartularies of Britain's medieval monasteries tell of monkish royal physicians. One of the earliest mentioned is Baldwin (d. *c.* 1097), Abbot of the Abbey of St James, Bury St Edmunds, Suffolk. A native of Chartres, it is likely that he studied medicine at the famous cathedral medical school there and he is chronicled in the documents of Bury St Edmunds Abbey as court physician to Edward the Confessor (r. 1042–66), of the House of Cedric and Denmark.[18] When this line was replaced by the House of Normandy, Baldwin became physician to William the Conqueror (r. 1066–87), joining Brother Nigel, who was already in the conqueror's suite and was one of the first recipients of royal largesse for medical attendance.[19]

Another man made wealthy through royal medical service was Gilbert Maminot, Bishop of Lisieux (d. 1101). The first personal physician to William's queen, Matilda, he is known to have attended William after he was injured in 1086 at the sacking of the garrison of Mantes (during William's laying waste of the French Vexin).[20] The chroniclers William of Malmesbury (in his *Gesta Regnum Anglorum*) and Matthew Paris (*Chronica Maiora*) both concur in describing the activities of the royal physicians Baldwin, Nigel and Bishop Gilbert at William's deathbed. They record that at Mantes William's horse, 'in leaping a trench burst the bowels of the rider. Much disabled . . . his physicians, on being called, they declared after an examination of his urine that his death was inevitable.' William was further examined and treated at the Priory of St Gervais, Rouen, then known for its skilled medieval brethren, taught by men such as Guntard, Abbot of Jumièges. William is likely to have ruptured his urethra, for which no surgical repair was available; he died on Thursday, 9 September 1087 and his bloated corpse was buried at the Church of St Stephen, Caen.[21]

During the eventful reign of William II (r. 1087–1100), John de Villula (d. 1122), Bishop of Bath and Wells and founder of the monastery of St Peter and St Paul at Bath, became the official royal physician, this post being combined with the role of chaplain to the royal household. De Villula restored the Roman hot springs at Bath and is said by some – based on very little evidence – to have lived on long enough to give medical advice to Henry I. The unpopular William Rufus, by the by, met his death from a crossbow bolt while hunting in the New Forest. Most historians aver that he was murdered.

Of all the Anglo-Norman monarchs, Henry I, 'Beauclerk' (r. 1100–35), the youngest and only English-born son of William I and Matilda of Flanders, 'enjoyed the company of medical men, sought them far and wide, and rewarded their special services'.[22] The Pipe Rolls of Henry's reign show that he had eight prominent physicians severally at his court, although data on them is sparse. There was Ranulf, a monk of the Cluniac priory of Montacute, Monmouthshire, who also served as royal chaplain. He took the title *Ranulfus domini Henrici Regis medicus*. Clarembald, Canon of Exeter (and London; d. *c.* 1133) was another royal physician and chaplain, who made a study of the medical miracles said to have taken place at the Cathedral of St Peter, Exeter. He was also physician to the powerful prelates Bishop William Warelwast and Richard de Beaumaris, Bishop of London. Another chaplain to Henry I, Nigel of Calne, Wiltshire (*c.* 1107–1230), is also mentioned as a physician, along with the Spanish layman Pedro Alfonso (fl. 1062–1142), a Christian convert from Judaism who served at the court of King Alfonso of Aragon; he was at Henry's court around 1100–21. Another physician was Serlo of Arundel, a secular clerk at Waltham Abbey who had served as physician to Adeliza of Louvain, Henry I's second wife, from 1136 to 1160.[23]

Perhaps the most celebrated of Henry I's physicians were Faritius and Grimbald. Faritius, Abbot of Abingdon (d. 1117), was a native of Arezzo in Tuscany, and held the post of cellarer-infirmarer at Malmesbury Abbey. He was also principal physician at the court of Henry I's first wife Matilda, daughter of Malcolm III of Scotland.[24] Grimbald (d. *c.* 1138) also originated in northern Italy and served as Henry's travelling physician both in England and in Normandy from 1101. As with most of his colleagues,

Grimbald was proud to proclaim his royal prerogatives and was another of the king's *medici* who served as religious advisers and bureaucratic agents. Grimbald was thought to have been with Henry I in France and was present at the monarch's death.

Henry I was not the first sovereign to ignore his physician's advice. On 1 December 1135, at the prodigious age of 67, Henry was at Lyons-la-Forêt in Normandy. Returning from the hunting field he sat down to a favourite feast of lampreys (a type of eel), and almost immediately became ill with a fever and vomiting followed by a rapid death. Determined to exonerate themselves, the royal physicians present attested that they had warned the king not to gorge himself with lampreys. Today doctors believe that Henry did not contract a supposed fatal food poisoning but actually succumbed to peritonitis.

The court of King Stephen (r. 1135–54) produced no medics of note, yet physicians like the little-known Iwod and Ernulf are identified as witnesses to royal papers. Stephen also may have died from peritonitis, for Gervase, monk of the Priory of Christ Church, Canterbury, wrote: 'The King was suddenly seized with pain in the iliac region, along with an old discharge from haemorrhoids.'[25]

Henry II (r. 1154–89), the first of the House of Anjou, also has shadowy physicians like Johannes and Radulfus listed in the Pipe Rolls as *medicus*. Ralph de Bellomonto has a longer mention in the Court Rolls, as he was drowned off Normandy in 1171, when the royal fleet came to grief in a storm. Henry II was a very active man, and chroniclers do not identify him as a sickly individual, although he did share the Plantagenet manic-depressive curse. He is said to have died of a 'lingering fever'.

When Henry's successor Richard I, 'Coeur de Lion' (r. 1189–99), took part in the Third Crusade with Philip Augustus in 1191–2, he took with him Ranulphus Besace (d. *c.* 1243) as his personal physician, while another prominent royal physician, John de Bridport (*c.* 1178–1215), remained at court in London and Normandy. Richard I died from a wound received at the siege of Châlus in Poitou. Gervase of Canterbury recorded his end: 'The king was fatally wounded in the left shoulder by an arrow in such a way that the bolt, driven down from the shoulder, reached the neighbourhood of the lung or liver, nor could it be checked by any skill of the physician.' It appears that Richard died from septicaemia.

The Pipe Rolls of King John (r. 1199–1216) identify both Master Alan and Matthew Macy (practised *c.* 1200–18) as physicians to the king, but little is known of the former. The chronicler Matthew Paris avers that John died of gluttony after 'indulging too freely in peaches and copious draughts of new cider'. At his deathbed at the castle of Newark-on-Trent, on 19 October 1216, John was attended by the physician Abbot Adam of Croxton, Leicestershire. Abbot Adam subsequently dissected the king's cadaver, a procedure that had its technical roots in Ancient Egypt. John had long wanted to be entombed at Worcester Cathedral, between the shrines of St Oswald and St Wulstan, so Adam removed the king's internal organs and preserved them in salt. Thus, he believed, the body would be less corrupt for its journey to Worcester. John's heart and viscera were later buried at Croxton Abbey.[26]

During the reign of Henry III (r. 1216–72), we begin to glean from the Court Rolls more details about the rights, duties and status of royal physicians. Throughout medieval society, physicians were deemed to rank between canon lawyers (those learned in the laws of the Church) and civil lawyers. Surgeons were deemed low-life. Julius Leopold Pagel describes them thus: 'illiterates – barbers, sorcerers, landlords, tricksters, counterfeiters, alchemists, bawds, go-betweens, midwives, old women, converted Jews, Saracens – all those who have foolishly squandered what they have and proclaim themselves surgeons so that they can make a living, hiding their wretchedness, poverty and lies under the cloak of surgery'.[27] In what might be called the 'pre-professional age', and certainly within court circles at this period, the distinction between medicine and surgery was hardly observed. Yet physicians kept themselves aloof from 'the butchers' who performed surgery; and for those with a surgical background a court appointment was a rich, plum job. Henry III's Court Rolls show that trusted medics received annuities, ecclesiastical benefices, wood from royal forests and fish from crown fishponds.

The *Calendar of Patent Rolls* shows that Henry III built up a strong medical staff at his court, although he appears to have lived a reasonably healthy life for the time and he lacked the symptoms of 'Plantagenet manic-depression'. These records also show that a very early recipient of the title 'Surgeon to the King' was the cleric Master William, who flourished at court during the period 1233–54.[28] In 1233 he was presented with the living of Haukerinton, in the diocese of Lincoln, establishing the custom of Henry bestowing ecclesiastical properties on his *medicus regis* with generosity. In 1241 William's contemporary, Master David, was granted one hundred *escheats* of land in Ireland for his medical services to the king.[29] In 1243, the year of his death, David was also given land that had formerly belonged to one John of Kaerdiff (Cardiff).[30] Henry III made further provision for David's widow, Mistress Alice, whereby she was given three *obolus* in 1248 by way of an early example of a widow's pension.[31]

In 1251 Henry de Saxeby (*c.* 1250–71) appears as 'Serjeant-Surgeon', a new title for the royal appointment,[32] with an annual fee by 1253 of ten pounds sterling.[33] This surgeon also received ex-judiciary land in Ireland to the extent of ten *liberates*.[34] Henry III expected his medical staff to work hard to earn such largesse and we are told that Henry de Saxeby ministered to seven workmen who were injured when a wall fell down in Westminster Hall during renovations.[35] Nevertheless the *Close Rolls* in particular show that Henry de Saxeby was one of the best paid and most richly rewarded of all the royal appointees, who, together with surgeon Sir Thomas de Weseham (*c.* 1252–72), saved the king's life. De Weseham, by the by, was perhaps the earliest instance of a physician being knighted for medical service. The British Library preserves a rare prescription of the physician Roger de Lacoc (d. 1233), who seems to have treated Henry III for an eye infection. The prescription details treatment with an ointment of fennel, rue, musk and attic honey.[36]

In 1253 Henry III made his second expedition to Gascony, which had fallen to Aquitaine in 1052 and to the English Crown when Henry married Eleanor of Provence in 1252. Among his entourage were the royal clerk and physician Ralph Necton, Henry's saviour Sir Thomas de Weseham and the physician Patrick de Carliolo (Carlisle). Sir Thomas, by the by, was to rise to greater heights in gifts of royal property: in 1255 he was given possessions in Colchester that had been sequestered from the usurer Isaac the Jew; in 1256 he received a bailiwick of the Forest of Cannock; and by 1260 he had been granted the right to mint his own coins.[37] This allowed Sir Thomas to live in prosperous retirement until around 1281.

It may be noted that Henry III founded a separate medical staff for his queen consort; Eleanor's entourage included Peter de Alpibus, Raymond de Bariamondo and Nicholas of Farnham, professor of medicine at the University of Bologna, and later Bishop of Durham. In 1255 Queen Eleanor became anxious about the health of her 15-year-old daughter Margaret, wife of the 14-year-old Alexander III (r. 1249–86), King of Scotland, and her physician Reginald of Bath was dispatched to investigate. Matthew Paris recorded that Reginald observed Margaret's 'melancholy and pallor', which evidently derived from the repressive way in which she was treated by the Scots courtiers. Reginald berated the young couple's Scots guardians, who had even denied them a matrimonial bed. Alas, Reginald was soon seized with a severe illness and died; some said he was poisoned by the Scots for his outspokenness. Later that year Henry III visited Scotland 'to put things right'.

Education, Disease and Court Roles

By the end of the twelfth century more up-to-date knowledge was coming from the medical schools at Montpellier, Bologna and Salerno, while several of the court physicians were graduates of Paris. This meant a significant shift in who was being employed at court. In Norman and early Angevin times it is clear that most medical practice was carried out by monastic personnel, but as the houses of Normandy and Anjou declined, non-practising clergy and non-clergy appear in the lists of court medics. Slowly the quality of medieval knowledge was improving, but throughout the Middle Ages medicine was taught as a philosophy and little practical expertise was offered. Surgery was taught by apprenticeship in the houses of barber-surgeons, whose novice attendants were called *garciones*.

Most poor folk relied on herbal medicines and made pilgrimages to saints' shrines to cure their ills. Many suffered from malnutrition, which often led to deformed or crippled limbs, impaired sight and skin diseases. Poor hygiene also contributed to the nation's ill-health, as did exposure to the wet and cold climate, which exacerbated rheumatism and arthritic disease.

Physicians and surgeons at court were presented with patients who were better fed and housed, but by the reign of Edward I (r. 1272–1307) medics were able to isolate the possible causes of particular diseases, encouraged by a better quality of medical education on the curricula of Oxford and Cambridge colleges. Royal doctors of the period had to cope with eight diseases in particular: gastro-enteritis, endemic in the Middle Ages, largely because of the insanitary conditions; smallpox, another scourge of medieval times; measles, scarlet fever and diptheria, all fatal diseases at this time; tuberculosis, both of the bovine (through milk products) and human (by airborne droplet infection) forms; plague (typhus, typhoid and bubonic); and venereal diseases.

Although Edward I's court was always adequately staffed by prominent physicians like William of York and William of St Père, perhaps influenced by his father he encouraged certain royal physicians to take an interest in the medical needs of his war machine. Certainly Philip de Beauvais (*c.* 1279–*c.* 1320), son of the royal surgeon Simon de Beauvais (*c.* 1276–90), was present during Edward I's initial campaigns in Scotland in 1296, and is referred to as *cirurgicus regis*. De Beauvais tended the king's wounds – including fractured ribs – at the House of the Knight's Hospitallers at Torphichen, West Lothian, after the Battle of Falkirk, 22 July 1298, where he was joined by another royal physician, John de Kenley.

For his campaign in Galloway in July and August 1300, Edward I had with him de Kenley, de Beauvais and a physician identified as Peter of Newcastle. The *Liber Quotidianus Contrarotulatoris Garderobae*[38] tells us that both the surgeon and the physician received two shillings per day, equivalent to the fee of a knight, and Peter one shilling, the fee of an esquire. The *Liber* also speaks of clothes allowances and free sustenance while on campaign. Each senior medic was attended by two *valetti* (junior assistants) and two *socii* (associates). Taken ill at Carlisle, Edward I was attended by the royal physician Nicholas Tingewick (*c.* 1291–1339), described as 'the best doctor for the king's health'.[39] In his medical bags Tingewick carried turpentine, aromatic flowers, carminatives, electuaries and various ointments.

Both Edward I's mother Eleanor of Provence and his (second) wife Princess Margaret of France had their own identified personal physicians. William le Provençal came to Britain in Eleanor's entourage, while John de Fontaines treated Margaret for measles in 1305.[40]

After Edward's death at Burgh-by-Sands on 7 July 1307, his son Edward II (r. 1307–27) continued the Scottish campaigns, leading to his defeat at Bannockburn in June 1314, and the last Scots expedition of August–September 1322. This campaign reveals one snippet of interest in the study of doctors in royal military service: contemporary documents show that the king's surgeon Stephen de Paris had his own baggage-horse carrying panniers of drugs and instruments.[41]

The *Calendar of Patent Rolls* for Edward II's reign lists Adam of Southwick, Albert, John, Nicholas of Corwenne (in Scotland), and Robert de Sidesterne as royal doctors; the latter had been in the king's suite since his days as Prince of Wales. Yet in Edward II's reign it seems that, just as the Roman aristocracy had done, English monarchs used physicians from outside the court on an ad hoc basis, the reputation of these doctors being enhanced by peripatetic royal patronage. One who benefited was John of Gaddesden (*c.* 1280–1361), Professor of Merton College, Oxford. He had learned his skills almost entirely in England, although some scholars aver (on little evidence) that he was once a student at the medical school at Montpellier. In his great work *Rosa Anglica Medicinae*, Gaddesden describes how he treated the little son of Edward II, John, Earl of Cornwall, for smallpox by wrapping him in a red cloth, within a room hung with red curtains, in a bed with red counterpane. It is thought too, that Geoffrey Chaucer immortalised John of Gaddesden in *The Canterbury Tales* as the 'Doctor of Physick'. In 'The Prologue' to the *Tales* Chaucer mentions Gaddesden by name, lists well-known medics of the day and gives an overall description of what folk might think of contemporary doctors:

A Doctor too emerged as we proceeded;
No one alive could talk as well as he did
On points of medicine and of surgery,
For, being grounded in astronomy,
He watched his patient's favourable star
And, by his Natural Magic, knew what are
The lucky hours and planetary degrees
For making charms and magic effigies.
The cause of every malady you'd got
He knew, and whether dry, cold, moist or hot;[42]
He knew their seat, their humour and condition.
He was a perfect practising physician.
These causes being known for what they were,
He gave the man his medicine then and there.
All his apothecaries in a tribe
Were ready with the drugs he would prescribe,
And each made money from the other's guile;
They had been friendly for a goodish while.
He was well-versed in Aesculapius too
And what Hippocrates and Rufus knew
And Dioscorides, now dead and gone,
Galen and Rhazes, Hali, Serapion,
Averroes, Avicenna, Constantine,
Scotch Bernard, John of Gaddesden, Gilbertine.[43]
In his own diet he observed some measure;
There were no superfluities for pleasure,
Only digestives, nutritives and such.
He did not read the Bible very much.
In blood-red garments, slashed with bluish-grey
And lined with taffeta, he rode his way;
Yet he was rather close as to expenses
And kept gold he won in pestilences.
Gold stimulates the heart, so we're told.
He therefore had a special love of gold.

Edward II's horrific death is worthy of note as it was far beyond the skills of his royal doctors to avert, either in cause or in effect. In 1327 Edward II had been forced to resign the throne and was in the custody of Thomas de Berkeley and Sir John Maltravers at Berkeley Castle. There, said the historian Ranulph Higden in his *Polychronicon: Cum veru ignito inter celanda confossus ignominiose peremptus est.* (He was ignominiously slain with a red-hot spit thrust into the anus.)

Three royal doctors stand out in the service of Edward III (r. 1327–77). One of them, Jordan of Canterbury (d. 1361), served the royal house for some three decades and was present in August 1346 when the king and his son Edward, the Black Prince (1330–76), inflicted their terrible defeat on the French at Crécy. For this Jordan was awarded a war purse of 109 shillings.[44] His colleague, the surgeon Roger de Heyton (d. 1349), showed so much loyalty and devotion to the king that he was gifted land and property.[45] The third was Adam Rous (d. 1379), whose will is preserved, showing he was a prominent property-holder who left a number of buildings to the Augustinian Priory of St Bartholomew.[46] It is likely that Rous was an alumnus of the medical school within the priory, founded by the Frankish prebendary of St Paul's, Rahere (d. 1144), and which later developed into St Bartholomew's Hospital, West Smithfield, London. Jordan, de Heyton and Rous are mentioned most frequently in the *Calendar Rolls* because of their accumulation of property from royal service, but Edward III and his queen Philippa of Hainault had a staff of a dozen more medics, including the 'Doctor of Medicine and Master of Medicine' Godfrey Fromond (*c.* 1335–51). When on the continent the king was served by extra-surgeons like the Irishman William O'Hannon, who is known to have treated the monarch's young son Prince Lionel (d. 1368).

A search through the state papers of Edward III reveals that some of his doctors, like John Bray, went on to serve Richard II. One of the Black Prince's personal surgeons was his protégé John Arderne (fl. 1370), one of the most capable practitioners of his day; another was the surgeon Adam de la Poeltrie. The king's daughter Isabella, Countess of Bedford (d. 1382), had a 'personal physician for her lifetime' in William Holm, who received £10 per annum for his services.

Despite his rather arbitrary style of rule, Richard II (r. 1377–99) was magnanimous to his surgeon John Leche (d. *c.* 1410), to whom he gave land, a pension and clothes for his lifetime when his eyesight declined.[47] He was also generous to the 'king's servant' surgeon John de Bury in his old age. Richard died in 1400 while in custody, possibly poisoned on the orders of his rival Henry Bolingbroke.

For his royal doctors Henry IV (r. 1399–1413), the first of the House of Lancaster, chose two medics – Louis Recouchez and David de Nigarellis de Lucca (d. 1412) – who had been with him in exile on the continent when he was still Duke of Hereford. Recouchez added 'Keeper of the King's Mint' to his duties as physician and 'king's servitor'. They worked alongside the sergeant-of-arms cum military medic William Bradwardyne (d. 1445), inherited from Richard II's court. Henry's medical entourage also included the physicians John Malverne (d. 1422), Peter Albocasse (d. 1427) and Geoffrey Melton (d. *c.* 1411), who also served in the medical household of Queen Joan of Navarre, Henry IV's second wife. We know from the Patent Rolls that the surgeon Thomas Morstede had an annual salary at this time of £40.[48]

Both Bradwardyne and Morstede were to enter the court service of Henry V (r. 1413–22). Morstede became chief surgeon to the king's army which was successful against the French at Agincourt on 25 October 1415. For this he was paid 40 marks, with 20 marks for his assistants, and a purse with which to buy medical equipment and drugs, and their conveyance. Bradwardyne was among the surgeons who had their own personal assistants, as was Henry V's personal physician Nicholas Colnet (d. 1421), principal physician at Agincourt.[49]

On the death of Henry V the crown was inherited by the infant Henry VI (r. 1422–71). Because of their prominence, Bradwardyne and Morstede can be traced in the new reign as they continued at court. Morstede became Sheriff of the City of London and Master, in 1422, of the association known as the Enfranchised Art of Surgery. He died in 1450 and was buried in the Church of St Olave, Upwell Old Jewry, London; his surgical instruments were inherited by his apprentice Roger Brynard.[50] Bradwardyne eventually became Vice-Master of the Enfranchised Art of Surgery.

In his *Foedera, Conventiones et Cujuscunque Generis Acta Publica*, the historiographer royal, Thomas Rymer (1641–1713), cites an interesting recommendation to the King's Council (*Curia Regis*) regarding the royal surgical staff. The recommendation came about in preparation for Henry VI's second coronation; he was first crowned at Westminster in 1429, but now he was crowned again at Paris in 1430. The document reads:

> May it please your Sovereign Majesty, of your special grace, and on the advice of your wise Council, to ordain that four surgeons take residence in your most honourable household, and to be obedient and answerable to William Stalworth (later Steward of Cheillesmore, Warwickshire), and to have each of them sixpence a day. And, in addition, to make a grant of twenty pounds sterling for sundry medicines, instruments, *estuffes* (dressings), and other necessaries and pertaining to the office of Surgery for the use of you and the people of your household in this your present journey.[51]

In 1453 Henry VI temporarily lost his reason. Thereafter his health was monitored by three physicians, John Arundell (d. 1477), Bishop of Chichester, John Faceby and William Hatclyff, and two surgeons Robert Wareyn, sergeant-surgeon to the royal household, and John Marshall. Within the records of the *Curia Regis* the duties of these advisers were set out, along with allowances for baths; confections; clysters (a liquid introduced to the intestines; an enema); electuaries (a honey, or syrup-based medicine; a common one being electuary of senna made of senna, syrup and tamarind pulp); gargles (to remove catarrhal fluids); head shavings; laxatives; suppositories; and other sundries.[52] The Court Rolls of the period also list the physicians James of Milan and Walter Leinster, with surgeons Michael Belwell and William Marshall, while Henry VI's queen, Margaret of Anjou, was tended by William Forest and Francis Panizonus of Alexandria, who came to England in her retinue. Because of his supposed sanctity and martyrdom, much has been written about Henry VI's illness, and thus about his royal doctors. Medical historians believe that he inherited his proclivity to weakmindedness from his schizophrenic grandfather Charles VI of France. The stresses on his mind produced by such events as Jack Cade's rising (1450), the loss of his French possessions (1451–2) and his mounting debts drove him to a mental breakdown, featuring periods of manic elation and depression. All of this may have caused Wareyn and Marshall to make a head incision, to relieve what was then considered to be the seat of madness, the brain.

Whether or not his doctors' ministrations were effective is not known, but Henry VI did regain his reason for a while. In June 1455, however, Gilbert Kymer, Dean of Salisbury, a recognised and skilled physician who had treated the family of the king's uncle, Humphrey, Duke of Gloucester, was called in to attend Henry, once again in the depths of his depressive-mania.[53] Civil strife ultimately tore Henry's realm apart; his Lancastrian army was routed by the Yorkists in the Wars of the Roses and his son and heir, Prince Edward, was killed as he fled from the Battle of Tewkesbury on 4 May 1471. Henry himself met a violent death in the Wakefield Tower of the Tower of London on 24 May 1471. At first Henry was buried at the distant Benedictine Abbey of Chertsey, Surrey, and doctors and relatives began to take the insane there to pray for cures at his shrine. Over 170 miracles were said to have taken place at his tomb. In 1448 Richard III had Henry's cadaver removed to St George's Chapel, Windsor, which became a new site of pilgrimage.[54]

As the first representative of the House of York, Edward IV (r. 1461–83) made some interesting grants in the early months of his reign. The Patent Rolls show how international was the pool of royal doctors he employed. Dominic de Serego was granted some £66 for 'good service to the king and his consort and daughters'. Together with William Hatclyf and Roger Marshall, he examined alleged cases of leprosy on the monarch's behalf. The king gave a life-grant of £40 per annum to James Fryse, his personal physician, who hailed from Friesland, the northern province of the Netherlands.[55] The king's generosity encouraged Fryse to stay in his service for two decades. In 1462 Edward IV appointed William Hobbys his surgeon, to be advanced by 1470 to principal surgeon. Hobbys was already, in 1461, a prominent citizen of London as warden of the Company of Barber-Surgeons, and much later he went on to serve King Richard III as his personal physician. Both Fryse and Hobbys served during Edward IV's invasion of France in 1475, receiving a daily fee

A ROYAL DOCTOR COLLUDES AT MURDER

In 1483 the Italian cleric Domenico Mancini wrote an invaluable account of his stay in England under the title *Ad Angelum Catonem De Occupatione Regii Anglii per Riccardum Tercium*. In it he comments on the supposed fate of King Edward V and his brother Prince Richard, Duke of York, who were presumed murdered after imprisonment in the Tower of London, by the orders of King Richard III. In his account Mancini also cites the royal doctor John Argentine as a colluder with the murder of the princes.

Dr John Argentine had been called in to attend to Edward V's toothache, and Mancini suggests he was the last person to see the two princes alive. Dr Argentine (*c.* 1422–*c.* 1507), future physician to Prince Arthur, and Provost of King's College, Cambridge, sensed that Edward V knew that he was doomed. Mancini wrote:

> Edward V and his brother were withdrawn into the inner apartments of the Tower proper, and day by day, began to be seen more rarely behind the bars and windows, till at length they ceased to appear altogether. The physician Argentine, the last of his attendants whose services the King enjoyed, reported that the young King, like a victim prepared for sacrifice, sought remission for his sins by daily confession and penance, because he believed that death was facing him . . .

of two shillings and one shilling and sixpence respectively. Incidentally, the *Annals of the Barber Surgeons Company* show that several of its wardens served Edward IV, including Richard Brightmore, Simon Cole, Thomas Collard and Richard Cambre, all of whom were members of the 1475 French campaign.

During 1474 the duties of royal physicians and surgeons were reorganised through new ordinances.[56] The duties of the physicians included advising on the monarch's diet and the 'devysing' of his medicines. The physician must also be watchful 'to espie if any of the courte be infected with leperiz (leprosy) or pestylence (plague) and to warne the sovereignes of him (and) till he be purged clenely to keep him out of courte . . . The costes of all medycines belonge to the chamberlayne his audyte in the jewellhouse.' For the comfort of the monarch's eldest son (later Edward V, supposed murdered in 1483), a physician and surgeon was to be employed 'sufficiente and cunninge and that they enforce themselves to make him joyoux and merry towards his bedde'.[57]

Because of his short reign, records of the medical household of Richard III (r. 1483–5) are thin, save for a mention of Edmund Albon (d. 1485), who had been physician to Edward IV for a while. After Richard's death at the battle of Bosworth Field on 22 August 1485, Henry VII (r. 1485–1509) assumed the throne as the first monarch of the House of Tudor. Little is known about his royal doctors. Thomas Denman administered physic to Henry VII and his mother Lady Margaret Beaufort and there is a mention of payment of 40 marks life-grant per year to one William Altoftes of Atherston for services as surgeon.[58] Others like John Baptiste Boerio and John Chamber went on to serve Henry VIII.

By this time a greater sense of professionalism was growing among the doctors in royal employment and court medics were becoming more and more influenced by continental medical knowledge. From around the end of Henry VII's reign royal doctors really had come of age and went on to new and better defined medical court roles.

PART ONE:

ROYAL PROGRESS

CHAPTER ONE

LEARNING FROM THE GREATS: STEPS TOWARDS THE THRONE

Around the end of the fourteenth century a revival of the classical learning of Greece and Rome took place; it was a prelude to the great climax of the Renaissance in the fifteenth and sixteenth centuries. Untrammelled by the 'tyranny of dogmatic scholasticism' formerly imposed by the Roman Catholic Church, medicine made huge forward steps, with men such as the anatomist Andreas Vesalius and Bartolomeus Eustachius (1520–74) leading the field.

Andre Wesel, bynamed Andreas Vesalius, is worthy of a detailed note. Born in Brussels in 1514 within a medical family, Vesalius was educated at Louvain in classics and studied anatomy at Paris under Jacobus Sylvius and Johannes Guinterius. His dissection samples were boldly purloined from the cadavers of criminals executed at the judicial killing-grounds of Montfaçon, or from the graves of the *cimetière* of Saint Innocents. Vesalius returned to Louvain to teach in 1536, but despaired of the ambience of the priest-ridden campus; he yearned to follow the bright lights of the Renaissance at Venice and the University of Padua. In 1543 was published his great tome *De Humani Corporis Fabrica*, illustrated by Jan Stephan von Calcar. Attacked by jealous colleagues, incensed by his repudiation of the teachings of Galen, Vesalius resigned his teaching post and became court physician to the Holy Roman Emperor Charles V (1500–58) and later to Philip II of Spain (1527–98).

Vesalius's indiscreet use of bodies snatched from new graves, however, brought him to the attention of the Holy Inquisition and he was sentenced to death, although his sentence was commuted to a pilgrimage to Jerusalem. He died on the return journey at Zante in the Ionian Sea in 1564. Nevertheless his reputation as a giant among medical practitioners and court physicians was assured.[1]

The 'greatest surgeon of the Renaissance', Ambrose Paré also became one of the most famous court physicians of all time. Born in 1510 at Bourg Hersent (modern Laval) in the province of Maine, France, Paré was poorly educated. Apprenticed to a barber-surgeon in Paris he then became a 'companion surgeon' at the Hotel Dieu, a hospital near the Cathedral of Notre Dame. When he was 27, Paré became the personal surgeon (and barber) to one Montejon, who campaigned in the French wars. He also earned a few coins tending wounded soldiers. All the while he experimented with concoctions of his own devising to salve wounds. His extant writings show that, while he was of a realist, practical mind, Paré also retained a foot on the 'superstitious medicine' of France's culture. Here is an example of one of his salves:

> (Take) 2 new-born puppies, 1 pound earthworms, 2 pounds oil of lilies, 16 ounces Venice turpentine, 1 ounce aqua vitae.
> (Method) Boil the puppies (alive) in the oil. Add the worms, which have been drowned in white wine. Boil and strain. Add the other ingredients.[2]

After his service for Montejon, Paré returned to Paris and began to write about his campaign discoveries, overturning common practice by composing in colloquial French rather than in Latin. As he was not a trained academic his treatments of war wounds did not find favour with the intellectually snobbish *Faculté de Médecine*. Paré furthered his experience by joining more campaigns as a non-combatant, and when he returned to Paris succeeded in obtaining a licence by examination to practise as a barber-surgeon.

Paré now married and practised the barber-surgeon's trade in Paris, while working on a volume on gunshot wounds. His book, published in 1545, became a standard work on the subject; this was followed by a handbook on anatomy in 1549. Soon he was off to the wars again, with Henry II's expedition against the Holy Roman Emperor Charles V in 1552. His success in the field of war surgery won him a place as surgeon to Henry II, although only with the lowly station of barber-surgeon. In 1554 his low rank was put aside by the authorities at the medical school of the Collège de Saint Côme, and he passed their examinations to become a Master Surgeon.

During a hunting trip on 29 June 1559 Henry II was accidentally struck by Count Montgomery's lance, the point of which remained lodged in the monarch's skull. Alas, the wound was severe and, despite being assisted by the famous Vesalius, Paré was unable to save the king, who died eleven days after the accident.

Paré now became surgeon to Henry II's son, the frail Dauphin, who succeeded as François II; on 28 April 1558 he married Mary Stuart, Queen of Scots. François lived only eighteen months after his accession, dying from a form of meningitis. He was succeeded by his brutish brother as Charles V, and then by Henry III. All the while, as these reigns succeeded one another, Paré remained in royal service, his career buffeted by civil war and the politico-religious intrigues of the French court. In 1562 there appeared his famous *Cinq Livres de Chirurgie*, which was immediately condemned by the *Faculté de Médecine*. The practical usefulness of the work cut across the legal opposition mounted by the *Faculté*, whose public denouncements of Paré gave his work the oxygen of publicity. Ambroise Paré remained in royal service for the rest of his life; he died in 1590 and was buried at the Church of Saint André des Arts. As 'the Father of Modern Surgery' his work was recognised and admired by the medics at the English court, which had entered a new reign in 1509.

On his accession to the throne English King Henry VIII (r. 1509–47) appointed his own physicians and surgeons, the first being Marcellus de la More in 1510 at 40 marks per annum. Later he became medical officer to the king's household and by 1513 he was raised to the post of sergeant of the king's surgeons. Within the king's household, and under the direction of de la More, were three royal doctors who had served Henry VII: the Genoese physician and astrologer John Baptist Boerio (d. *c.* 1514), the physician John Cambre (d. 1549) and the surgeon William Altoftes (d. 1521). In due course Sir William Butts (d. 1545), principal of St Mary's Hostel, Cambridge, was added to the staff.

The reign of Henry VIII witnessed great advances in professional medicine and out of the new colleges of medical excellence were to come generations of court physicians and surgeons. In 1518 Henry VIII granted a charter for the founding of the Royal College of Physicians of London, following a petition to this end from John Chambre, Nicholas Haslwell, John Francis, Robert Yaxley and Ferdinand de Victoria (d. 1529), physician to Queen Catherine of Aragon. One of the first fellows admitted to the new Royal College was the royal physician Richard Barlatt (1470–1557).[3]

Instrumental in the founding of the college was Thomas Linacre (*c.* 1460–1524), its first president. Linacre had gained degrees from All Souls College, Oxford, and Padua University. In 1509 he was one of Henry VIII's court physicians, combining this with his other court duties, including being the Latin tutor to the Princess Mary Tudor; he had already been responsible for the health and education of Henry VIII's eldest brother, the deceased Prince Arthur. At first the Royal College of Physicians held its meetings at Linacre's house in Knightrider Street, near St Paul's Cathedral, and after his death it progressed to a series of other homes. Linacre sustained his position as court physician through three successive reigns, a precedent copied by John Caius (1510–73), another graduate from Padua. Caius was called to court from his practice at Shrewsbury, where he observed and wrote on the 'Sweating Sickness', and he remained as court physician to Edward VI and Mary I; he was, however, expelled from Elizabeth I's court for his fervent Roman Catholicism.

> 'Mirth is one of the chiefest things in physic.'
> **Andrew Boorde**
> *(d. 1549), Physician to Henry VIII*

Although the Royal College of Surgeons of England did not obtain its first royal charter until 1800, its origins lay deep in the Middle Ages when London had its own Guild of Surgeons. In 1540 the Surgeons united with the Barbers Company, which had been chartered as a City Livery Company in 1462. From early monastic times the barbers had assisted monks in surgical procedures, and when the monks were forbidden by Pope

Innocent III's 4th Lateran Council of November 1215 to shed blood – i.e., to practise surgery – the barbers took over. The first Master of the United Company of Barber-Surgeons was Thomas Vicary (1495–1561), who became surgeon to Henry VIII in 1528; from 1536 to 1561 he served as sergeant-surgeon to the king in succession to de la More. The surgeons left the barbers in 1745 to form their own company, which evolved as the Royal College in 1800.

Because he was a larger-than-life character whose reign encompassed learning, splendour, mayhem, murder and rapaciousness in equal measure, the health of Henry VIII has been closely examined by chroniclers. Even so, historians must treat contemporary accounts of his health with circumspection, as the irascible king considered any bulletins on his health that were other than most encouraging to be treasonable. Much has been made of the possibility of him having syphilis and of his obesity. In 1521 his medical records show he had a bout of quartan fever, and certainly malaria was prevalent in the Middle Ages. He also suffered a series of minor jousting and tournament wounds. By 1537 his gluttony and hard drinking had increased, although the court painters were cautious not to show any swelling or bandaging in their portraits of him. At length Henry died at Westminster on 27 January 1547 of his obesity with accompanying renal and hepatic failure.

Henry VIII was succeeded by his 10-year-old son as Edward VI (r. 1547–53). Following the birth of Prince Edward, and on the advice of his royal doctors, Henry had subjected the young prince to important protocols to keep him away from infection. Anyone in the young prince's suite who fell ill was removed from the dwelling where the prince might be, and no one on the prince's staff could visit foetid London without permission; should they make a visit on official or private business they had to go into quarantine before rejoining the prince's court. A regime of unprecedented cleaning was ordered for the prince's rooms. Nevertheless by Christmas 1541 the prince had fallen ill with what is now thought to be the tubercular condition that would eventually shorten his reign.

After the death of Edward VI, Lady Jane Grey, the 16-year-old niece of Henry VIII, was proclaimed queen, but she was deposed in

July 1553 and executed in February 1554 after a reign of just nine days. Mary Tudor (r. 1553–8), Henry VIII's eldest surviving child, was now proclaimed queen as Mary I. The medical attendants of Henry VIII were largely still in place, but by 1558 Mary had added one Adelmar Caesar (d. 1569) to be a medical adviser; he was to carry on his duties into the reign of Elizabeth I.

Mary seems to have been healthy enough when she married Philip II of Spain at Winchester on 25 July 1554. By November the queen thought she was pregnant; it turned out to be a 'phantom' pregnancy and the queen now suffered from a series of gastro-intestinal problems. A second false pregnancy was diagnosed and eventually she died on 17 November 1558 of an ovarian tumour.

Elizabeth I (r. 1558–1603) formed a new medical household which included Lancelot Browne (d. 1605), the president of the College of Physicians Roger Giffard (d. 1597), the physician Robert Jacob (d. 1588), the physician-in-ordinary Edward Lister (d. 1620), and Richard Master (d. 1588), another president of the College of Physicians (1561). Lister and Browne would serve into the next reign and others would be added to the royal medical household as time went by, but one of the most curious of all doctors who vacillated at the court of Elizabeth was Dr John Dee (1527–1608).

A mathematician, astrologer and dilettante physician, Dee was introduced to the queen by her Master of the Horse Robert Dudley and William, Earl of Pembroke. Dee's academic career as a Fellow of Trinity College, Cambridge, was marginalised by his penchant for magic, sorcery, crystallomancy and necromancy. He was arraigned by the Star Chamber accused of practising sorcery against the life of Mary I and was placed under the surveillance of Edmund Bonner, Bishop of London, as a suspected heretic. To folklorists, Dr Dee became 'Queen Elizabeth's Merlin'. Dee cast the queen's horoscope and showed her his 'magic looking-glass' through which he claimed to conjure up spirits. She consulted him on her lifelong martyrdom to toothache and other health matters, and marvelled at his own regimen for a healthy life of 'eight hours a day study, two hours eating, and four hours sleeping'.[4] In 1578 Dee was sent to the continent to consult with physicians on the queen's health.[5]

War and increasing colonial ambition led to the broadening of medical and surgical knowledge. Two more royal medical men at the court of Elizabeth I are examples of this development. John Woodall (*c.* 1556–1643) became a military surgeon in Lord Willoughby's regiment and was to be the first surgeon-general to the East India Company when it was formed into a joint-stock company in 1612. As a member of the Barber-Surgeons Company he became surgeon to Elizabeth and some historians give him credit for promoting citrus juice as a cure for scurvy.[6]

William Clowes (*c.* 1540–1604) began his career as an army surgeon in France, then served as a naval surgeon during the period 1563–9. He was to retain his interest in military medicine throughout his term as surgeon at St Bartholomew's Hospital and Christ's Hospital, London, and he became a trusted surgeon to Elizabeth.

Another of Queen Elizabeth's physicians who spiced up his court career with adventure was Roger Marbeck (1536–1605), Provost of Oriel College, Oxford, and Registrar to the Royal College of Physicians. Marbeck joined Lord High Admiral Charles Howard, 1st Earl of Nottingham, on an expedition against the Spanish at Cadiz in 1596 and wrote an account of the events.

Throughout her life Elizabeth I deliberately employed only a small personal staff, mostly through thrift and a fear of her own safety. Even so, she was not averse to adding a new member if his worth had been proved. One such was the Italian-born doctor Giulio Borgarucci (fl. 1563–79), who came to England as a Protestant refugee. Borgarucci had studied medicine at Padua and graduated MD at Cambridge in 1567. He won public notice by treating plague victims in London by the bleeding process, and Elizabeth I appointed him physician to her royal household for life. The appointment of another foreign national, though, could have cost the queen her life.

Roderigo López (d. 1594) was a Portuguese Jew who settled in England in 1559 and became a house physician to St Bartholomew's Hospital. In 1586 he was appointed chief physician to the queen. He became implicated in the plot to murder Antonio Pérez and the queen; at trial, he was found guilty and was executed at Tyburn. Scholars believe that he was the original of Shakespeare's Jewish usurer Shylock in *The Merchant of Venice* (printed 1600).

Queen Elizabeth is known to have suffered from smallpox in 1562, when the royal physicians warned the privy council that her life was in danger. She rallied, however, to complete a reign dogged by war, plots and assassination attempts. She died in 1603, suffering from several conditions, including cancer. In an ironic quirk of history she was succeeded by the son of her sworn enemy and cousin Mary, Queen of Scots. King James VI ruled Scotland as a separate kingdom from 1567 (when he was one year old) to his accession to the English throne on 24 March 1603.

Some historians have called the seventeenth century the 'Golden Age' of medicine,[7] as it witnessed a welter of new practices and many new diagnoses were made. Yet one foot was still placed firmly in the past. Physician Sir Thomas Browne (1605–82), for example, appearing as an expert witness at a trial of witches at Bury St Edmunds in 1662 before presiding judge Sir Matthew Hale, stated that he believed in the reality of the Black Arts.[8] It was hardly surprising that such trials took place when James VI & I himself played a role in the persecution of witches, particularly through his book *Daemonologie* (1597).

Yet out of this period came a physician who greatly influenced medical science and established the foundations of modern clinical practice. Born in 1578 at Folkestone in Kent, William Harvey studied at King's School, Canterbury, and at Caius College, Cambridge, and then followed the well-worn trail to study at the world-famous University of Padua in 1589. Here he was influenced by his tutor Hieronymous Fabricius (1537–1619), who introduced him to original research into valves in the veins. Thus Harvey's spark of interest in the human circulatory system was ignited. He graduated Doctor of Medicine at Padua in 1602. In 1604 he married Elizabeth, daughter of Lancelot Brown, whom James VI & I had inherited as a physician from Queen Elizabeth's reign, and thus Harvey was introduced into royal circles. By 1609 he was physician to St Bartholomew's Hospital and was named physician-extraordinary to King James in 1618. As Lumleian Lecturer in Anatomy and Surgery he did much practical research into the function of the hearts of animals and

SECRETS FROM A ROYAL PHYSICIAN'S JOURNAL

Sir Thomas Browne was born in London in 1605 and educated at Winchester and Pembroke College, Oxford, and around 1635 he produced his *Religio Medici*. Browne studied medicine at Montpellier and Padua, and received a doctorate in the subject at Leiden, and his volume, first published in 1642 (without his permission), was an assessment of his attitudes as a Christian and as a physician towards God and the Church. Its wit and style made Browne famous, but his other beliefs sat incongruously on his credibility as a royal physician.

Thomas Browne – knighted by Charles II in 1671 – was to be an expert witness in the trial of the Bury St Edmunds witches in 1662, an episode described by Lord Chancellor John, 1st Baron Campbell (1779–1861) in his *Lives of the Chief Justices* (1849) as 'a most lamentable exhibition of credulity and inhumanity'. The case concerned two old widows, Amy Duny and Rose Cullender, of Lowestoft, Suffolk, who were accused of various acts of *maleficia* (sorcery) against seven children, causing them bewitchment and death. In his testimony, couched in circumlocutary language, Browne assured the jury of his belief in diablerie:

> [My opinion is] that the Devil in such cases did work upon the bodies of men and women upon a natural foundation, that is, to stir up and excite such humours super-abounding in their bodies to a great excess; whereby he did in an extraordinary manner afflict them with such distempers as their bodies were not subject to, as particularly appeared in these children . . .

The two women were hanged four days after the trial.

sea creatures and in 1628 he publicly stated his theory of the circulation of the blood, which was published at Frankfurt, then the centre of the book trade, as *Exercitatio Anatomica de Motu Cordis et Sanguinis in Animalibus*. Like Sir Thomas Browne, and most other seventeenth-century medics, Harvey believed in witchcraft and at the Essex Lent Sessions in 1634 he examined women so accused for signs of the 'witch's-mark' – i.e., strange spots and blemishes.

Other physicians to James VI & I caught the public eye

through circumstances different from Harvey's, yet amid gossip about supernatural influences. Henry Frederick, Prince of Wales, was born in 1594 and was being groomed as the future king of the still new dual kingdom of England and Scotland, and for a French or Spanish marriage, when he was struck down with typhoid. He died on 6 November 1612. It was a national calamity, and there were those who believed that witches had attacked the monarch's family, just as they were purported to have attacked the king's person back in Scotland in 1590, when the 'North Berwick Witches' had cast spells on the waters as King James sailed to Norway to claim his bride Anne of Denmark. Physicians Henry Atkins (1558–1635), Theo Diodati (d. 1651) and the eccentric William Butler (1535–1618) were called in to treat the prince, and after his death physician John Hammond (d. 1617) was selected to conduct a post mortem. As Hammond worked the court waited to hear if the prince's cadaver exhibited any internal evidence of witch-inspired cankers. Hammond reported that the prince had died of typhoid after all, but some courtiers remained unconvinced.

When he left Scotland for his new throne in England, James VI brought with him physician John Craig (d. 1620) and surgeon John Nasmith (d. *c.* 1619) to establish a new royal medical household. To this staff were added four physicians of note. Sir Simon Baskerville (1574–1641) and Sir William Paddy (1554–1634) were skilled clinicians, while Sir Theobald de Mayerne (1573–1655) won distinction for his writings on typhoid. The rebel of the four was Helkiah Crooke (1576–1648), who earned a reputation at court of being an implacable intellectual enemy of fellow royal practitioner William Harvey and his theories on the circulation of the blood.

On 5 March 1625, during a hunting trip at Theobald's, his country house 12 miles from London, James VI & I went down with a tertian ague, an acute fever which induced convulsions. His eccentricities, impatience and tantrums increased, but when he was feeling somewhat better he pursued his lifelong custom of ignoring the advice of his royal physicians and went back to the habits that shocked and repelled many. His 'dirty ways did not inspire respect', one commentator remarked. His blatant homosexual flirtations and his alcoholism deterred many from attending court; they were further repulsed by his slobbering speech (his tongue was too big for his mouth) and his habit of grabbing courtiers with his filthy hands as he passed them to support himself – from birth his spindly legs had been unable to support his weight. What was worse he stank abominably; it was reported that, while at the hunt, James did not dismount to relieve himself but defecated in the saddle so that by the end of the day he was in a filthy state. His custom of having one bath a year made little difference.

After a few hours' remission at his country house, James's convulsions returned and he descended into a profound melancholy. The monarch's favourite and Master of the Horse George Villiers, Duke of Buckingham (1592–1628), secretly sent for certain herbal remedies from one John Remmington, who had previously treated the duke's own family. The powders were administered to the king without the knowledge of the royal physicians. As his condition worsened, his physicians, led by John Craig, accused Buckingham of poisoning James. They were dismissed for their boldness.[9] As the king's condition deteriorated further Buckingham became more nervous, for James himself had cried out that he had been poisoned. James's chief physician Sir William Paddy realised that there was nothing that he could do. James VI & I succumbed to a stroke and finally died of the complications of pulmonary tuberculosis on 27 March 1625. Even before the monarch's cadaver had cooled Buckingham 'desired the physicians who attended His Majesty to sign with their own hands, a writ of testimony that the powder that he gave him was a good safe medicine'. They refused.[10] In due course Sir William Paddy released the results of his autopsy on the body. He deemed the king's head 'very full of brains', yet his 'blood was wonderfully tainted with melancholy'.[11] Strange stories circulated that the nails on James's fingers and toes had become loose, and the skin of his head had stuck to the pillow of his deathbed. This led later royal doctors to aver that the monarch had been poisoned with arsenic. Whether or not this had been contained in the powder administered at Buckingham's instructions remains a mystery.

James VI & I, first of the Stuart dynasty of the United Kingdom, was succeeded by his son Prince Charles, who had been born at

Dunfermline Palace, Fife, Scotland, on 19 November 1600; as Charles I he reigned until his execution on 30 January 1649. He was always a frail child and his royal doctors were never far away. They included his physician in Scotland Sir John Wedderburn (1599–1679), William Denton (1605–91), Walter Charleton (1619–1707) and Sir Matthew Lister (*c.* 1570–1656), who had also been in the medical household of Charles's mother, Queen Anne of Denmark. Sir Thomas Cademan (*c.* 1590–1651), the prominent Roman Catholic recusant, joined Sir Theodore de Mayerne as physicians to Charles's wife Queen Henrietta Maria. Several of these doctors went on to serve Charles II, but one who stands out as an example of secure tenure was George Bate (1608–68) who served not only Charles I but also his mortal enemy Oliver Cromwell (Lord Protector 1653–8) and later Charles II.

Another tenacious survivor was William Harvey, whom Charles I appointed physician-in-ordinary to his court. Harvey accompanied the monarch's entourage to Scotland in 1633 to attend the coronation at the Abbey Church, Holyrood. Just as he had done on continental trips on the king's business, Harvey took the opportunity to study the flora and fauna around Edinburgh for his research notes on anatomy, which were to include observations on deer in the royal parklands.[12]

Prompted by Charles I, Harvey conducted a post mortem on one Thomas Parr, who was claimed to have been born in 1483. Thus at his death in 1635 he was deemed 152 years old. Twice married (at 88 and 120), Parr lived a countryman's life for many decades and came to London among the household of Henry Howard, 3rd Earl of Arundel. Harvey's post mortem showed that Parr died of pleuropneumonia brought on, it is thought, by London's polluted atmosphere.[13]

In the years 1642–8, when England was devastated by Civil War, Harvey confirmed his royalist loyalties. He was with the king at the battle of Edgehill on 23 October 1642, but had no real interest in war medicine. He withdrew with the king to Oxford, and Oxford University conferred the degree of Doctor of Physic on him in 1645. He retired to London when the parliamentarian siege of Oxford was lifted. In 1646 he lived at the house of his rich brother at Laurence Pountney Hill. Now an old man, Harvey was distressed at the execution of his royal employer, but he continued his researches and in 1657 was elected president of the Royal College of Physicians. He died in the year of his election, racked with gout but clear of mind, and was buried at a private chapel at Hampstead. He was a remarkable example of the 'Golden Age' medic.

Out of the seventeenth-century 'Golden Age' also came the Worshipful Society of Apothecaries of London. Constituted by royal charter of King James VI & I in 1617, it is worthy of some mention. Because they did not rank highly in the social scale, details about royal apothecaries are scanty before their specific appointments, noted in the *Curia Regis Rolls*, as 'spicers' to King John. Herein we have the first mention of a *speciarius regis* to King John in William, Mayor of Winchester (1249), who also supplied wine and ale to the king.[14]

Incidentally, little is known of the specific costume effected by royal medics, although a simple black gown was common, yet in the period 1236–7 we find Jasceus of London, purveyor of spices and electuaries, sporting 'a robe of green, tunic and supertunic, to be trimmed with squirrel fur'.[15]

By the fourteenth century the 'spicer-apothecaries', as they became known, had established their Guild of St Anthony. A goodly number of spicers were Lombards. As the rule of the House of Anjou came to an end with Richard II, the status of the spicer-apothecary had risen to 'serjeant' rank in the royal household, with some recorded as 'king's clerks'. When King Henry VI was taken ill in April 1454, the king's apothecary Richard Hakedy was much involved in the monarch's treatment, on the instructions of physicians Arundell, Faceby and Hatcliffe, and surgeons Warren and Marshall.[16] He was instructed to supply the following materials:

Electuaries, Potions, Syrups, Confections, Laxative Medicines, in whatever form they thought best, Clysters, Suppositories, Cataplasms, Gargles, Baths, complete or partial, Removal of the skin (epithemata), Fomentations, Embrocations, Shaving of the Head, Ointments, Plasters, Waxes, Scarification, with or without rubifacients, and to do whatever was necessary to relieve and bring back the King's health.[17]

A ROYAL APOTHECARY REMEMBERED

Sometimes the only remembrance of a royal medical man is his epitaph. Hugh Morgan, apothecary to Queen Elizabeth I, was one such. Appointed in July 1583, Morgan was an Essex man who became a Freeman of the City of London on 4 February 1543. His shop was sited near Coleman Street but prosperity brought by royal patronage earned him a substantial house and garden at Battersea, where he grew specimens of rare herbs for use at court. He died at his home and was buried at St Mary's Church, Battersea, on 13 September 1613. His epitaph runs:

> HUGH MORGAN
> Sleepeth here in peace
> Whom men did late admire for worthful parts
> To Queen Elizabeth
> He was Chief 'Pothecary, till her death
>
> And in his science as he did excel.
> In her high favour he did always dwell.
> To God religious, to all men kind,
> Frank to the poor, rich in content of mind:
> These were his virtues, in these dyed he,
> When he had liv'd an 100 years and 3.

The Worshipful Society of Apothecaries was reputedly founded by Gideon de Laune (*c.* 1565–1659), apothecary to Queen Anne of Denmark. In those days the apothecary was still a compounder and dispenser of medicines, and assisted physicians in their treatments. Thus they became regular attenders at court by the sixteenth century. In 1815 the Apothecaries' Act allowed the Society to grant licences to practise medicine. In the seventeenth and eighteenth centuries many members devoted their studies to botany and herbalism, establishing physic gardens to research vegetable medicines. In 1632 the Society purchased its own hall at Blackfriars, where it remains today.

A little forward in time from the reign of Charles I, but none the less relevant here, was one royal physician who had an interest in the apothecaries trade. The scientific polymath Sir

Hans Sloane (1660–1753), a student of Paris and Montpellier, was variously secretary then president of the Royal College of Physicians. Sloane was a physician to Queen Anne and 'first physician' to George II and to Christ's Hospital from 1694 to 1730. By 1712 he had purchased the manor of Chelsea, where he founded a botanical garden (1721). The Society of Apothecaries had established their famous Physic Garden in 1673 and through Sir Hans's generosity it became their property outright.

In a relatively long reign of thirty-six years, from 1649 to 1685 (encompassing the Commonwealth and the Lord Protectorates of Oliver and Richard Cromwell), Charles II had a long series of royal physicians:

John Archer (fl. 1660–84). Court physician, 1671. Published a self-advertising volume, *Every Man His Own Doctor*, the year of his appointment.

Sir John Baber (1625–1704). Personal physician, 1660.

Peter Barwick (1619–1705). Physician-in-ordinary, 1660.

John Betts (d. 1695). Physician.

John Browne (1642–d. *c.* 1700). Surgeon. Surgeon at St Thomas's Hospital.

Peter Chamberlen (1601–83). Physician.

Timothy Clarke (d. 1672). Physician.

Edmund Dickenson (1624–1707). Physician-in-ordinary.

Sir Alexander Fraizer (*c.* 1610–81). Physician and political agent.

Sir Edward Greaves (1608–80). Physician.

Walter Harris (1647–1732). Physician.

Sir John Hinton (*c.* 1603–82). Physician also to Queen Henrietta Maria, Charles's mother.

Sir Edmund King (1629–1709). Physician, 1676.

Fernando Mendes (d. 1724). Physician.

Sir John Micklethwaite (1612–82). Physician also to Queen Catherine of Braganza, Charles's wife.

Sir Thomas Millington (1628–1704). Court physician.

James Molines (1628–86). Surgeon-in-ordinary.

Sir Charles Scarburgh (1616–94). Physician, 1660.

Thomas Shirley (1638–78). Physician-in-ordinary.

Thomas Whitaker (d. 1666). Physician-in-ordinary to the royal household. His volume *The Tree of Humane Life* became popular through its advocacy of the use of wine as a universal remedy against disease.

Other physicians at Charles II's court won fame – or notoriety – for other reasons. Sir George Wakeman (fl. 1668–85), physician to Queen Catherine of Braganza, was accused in 1679 by the Roman Catholic perjurer Titus Oates (1648–1705) of plotting to kill Charles II with poison; he subsequently acquitted himself. As physician-in-ordinary, Sir Robert Sibbald of Kipps (1641–1722), President of the Scottish Royal College of Physicians, combined his medical role with that of geographer-royal for Scotland.

Another distinguished court medic to Charles II, Richard Wiseman (*c.* 1622–76) served in the royalist army, then as surgeon-in-ordinary for the Person in 1660, and finally as principal surgeon and sergeant-surgeon in 1672. Known as the 'Father of English Surgery', Wiseman wrote the volume *Severall Chirurgicall Treatises* (published 1676), wherein he discussed one of the most curious aspects of 'royal medicine', the 'king's evil', wherein the monarch was deemed to be able to cure scrofula by 'divine touch'.

The events surrounding Charles II's death reveal the curious practices royal doctors had developed for the mortally ill. On the night of Sunday, 1 February 1685, the king retired to bed with a sore foot. By the morning he was clearly quite ill. His physician Sir Edmund King attended to the foot but as the barber was preparing to shave the king Charles was struck with an apoplexy. Sir Edmund immediately drew 'Sixteen Ounces of Blood' – risking his own death for treason by not first obtaining the permission of the privy council for the bloodletting.[18]

As the historian Thomas Babington Macaulay was to recount, on his deathbed poor Charles was 'tortured like an Indian at the stake'.[19] By now a dozen physicians were around his bed, all anxious to draw off the 'toxic humours' assailing the monarch. He was bled and purged, his head shaved and cantharides plasters applied to his scalp to cause blistering, with plasters of spurge for the feet to induce more vesicles. When they did not work, red-hot irons were applied to the skin. All this was conducted in the

DR WHITAKER AND THE ROYAL CRAMP RINGS

Dr Tobias Whitaker, physician-in-ordinary to Charles II's royal household, was known for his less-than-contemporary attitude to medical practice. He was a keen designer and promoter, for instance, of 'cramp rings'.

From early times rings made of metal were favourite artefacts for magical medicine. Made from various metals, the rings were used as protection against muscular cramps and epilepsy, much as copper bangles are worn today against rheumatic pain.

These *annuli vertuosi*, first mentioned in English history in July 1323, in the reign of Edward II, were usually made from rendered down gold and silver coins that had been consecrated by royalty at the Adoration of the Cross ritual on Good Friday. A man of superstitious tendencies, Dr Whitaker averred that the most potent rings were those made from old coffin nails or from a public gibbet.

Dr Whitaker encouraged his royal patient Charles II to sanctify the cramp rings that he made for use both within and without the court. Whether he considered this a perk of his position is not known.

presence of some seventy-five people, all crowded around the monarch's bed as family members and state officers witnessed the last hours of their king.

For five days the royal physicians laboured on the monarch, applying enemas of rock salt and syrup of buckthorn, and 'orange infusion of metals in white wine'. The king was treated with a horrific cabinet of potions: white hellebore root; Peruvian bark; white vitriol in paeony water; distillation of cowslip flowers; sal ammoniac; julep of black cherry water (an antispasmodic); oriental bezoar stone from the stomach of a goat and boiled spirits from a human skull. Somehow retaining his sense of humour the king remarked to his physicians: 'I am sorry, gentlemen, for being such an unconscionable time a-dying.' To which he added, with much understatement: 'I have suffered much more than you can imagine.' By 6 February 1685 the exhausted king, his body raw and aching with the burns and inflammation caused by his treatment, was given heart tonics, but to no avail. He lapsed into a coma and died at noon on 7

February. Today historians cite Charles II's death as a case of iatrogenic regicide.

Charles was succeeded by his 52-year-old brother James, Duke of York and Albany, who had married the Roman Catholic Princess Mary Beatrice d'Este of Modena as his second wife in 1671. Royal physicians such as Sir John Micklethwaite and Edmund Dickinson continued in royal service, as did Charles's personal physician David Bruce (fl. 1660). The Roman Catholic religion was the new king's downfall. The Whigs had always opposed James II & VII, but now he alienated the Tory nobility and gentry, the Church, the universities and the non-conformists. These various Protestant groups feared that James would turn the United Kingdom into a Roman Catholic state, especially when Queen Mary of Modena gave birth to a son, Prince Francis Edward Stuart, on 10 June 1688. The Protestants now envisaged a Catholic dynasty ruling Britain in perpetuity. Thus the Protestant Prince William of Orange (nephew and son-in-law of James) was invited to 'invade' England, to seize the throne, restore national liberty and protect the Protestant religion. James fled on Christmas Day, 1688. In exile he appointed Francis Bernard (1627–98) his physician-in-ordinary (1698). In 1701 James suffered a cerebral thrombosis and died at St Germain.

Thus began the reign of William III and Mary II; William would rule until 1702 and Mary until 1694. They had their own medical households, with John Browne and Walter Harris still in harness from the reign of Charles II. William's medical appointments included William Blackadder (1647–1704), who had already conducted secret diplomatic missions for the new king; Sir Richard Blackmore (*c.* 1655–1729), who became physician-in-ordinary with William Briggs (1642–1704), the distinguished physician and oculist; and John Hutton (d. 1712). Hutton, who had attended Queen Mary in Holland, became William's first king's physician in Ireland. Queen Mary continued to employ Walter Harris and Sir Charles Scarburgh from her late uncle Charles II's medical household.

In mid-December 1694 Queen Mary fell ill and her doctors diagnosed smallpox. Among his copious medical works Walter Harris left a record of her last hours:

She took Venice treacle the first evening, and finding no sweat appearing as usual, she took the next morning a double quantity of it before she asked the advice of her physicians. The smallpox was of the very worst and most dangerous sort, being united with the measles as is such as is usually accompanied with the erysipelas in the face, pustules and spitting of blood. On the third day of the illness her eruption appeared, with very troublesome cough and they came out in such a manner that the physicians were very doubtful whether they would prove the smallpox or measles. On the fourth day the smallpox showed itself in the face and rest of the body under its proper and distinct form. On the sixth day in the morning the various pustules all over her breast were charged into the large red spots of the measles. And the erysipelas called 'rosa' swelled her whole face, the former pustules giving place to them. That evening many broad and round petechiae appeared in the forehead above the eyebrows and on the temples. About the middle of the night there began a great difficulty in breathing and a little afterwards a copious spitting of blood. On the seventh day the spitting of blood was succeeded by bloody urine. On the eighth day the broad spots of the measles continued on the breast, but in the lower limbs where there had been many pustules of the smallpox all the swelling of them immediately disappeared and they changed into round spots about the bigness of the pustules, of a deep red or full scarlet, their surface being smooth and not at all elevated like the penitential stigmata. There was one large round pustule filled with matter having a broad scarlet circle round it like a burning coal which I then observed above the region of the heart and under her body. Lasting about the middle of the night she breathed out her pious soul.[20]

Mary died at Kensington Palace on 29 December 1694. She was anxious that after her death her body would be autopsied and instructions were left for her doctors that she was not to be 'opened'. However, as she was embalmed, her cadaver had to be 'opened' before she was entombed.

After Mary's death William's health continued to deteriorate;

his asthma worsened and he suffered from a constant swelling of the legs. In February 1702 he sustained a broken collar-bone after falling from his horse, and died at Westminster on 8 March 1702.

Queen Anne, William III's successor and sister-in-law, had been introduced to royal doctors in France, when she was only four years old. At her grandmother Queen Henrietta Maria's palace at Colombes she was attended by a French oculist for 'deflusion' (constant watering) of the eyes. This condition, likely in modern times to be diagnosed as stenosis of the nasolacrimal ducts, was to trouble her all her life. Although she had a mild attack of smallpox, it was her obstetric history that caused her royal physicians the most anxiety. She had seventeen recorded pregnancies, but none of her children survived to inherit her throne.

At the age of seventeen, on 28 July 1683, Anne married the dull, gluttonous Prince George of Denmark (1653–1798). George was more remembered in royal circles for his asthma than for his intellect; John Mulgrove, 3rd Earl of Sheffield, remarked that George's heavy breathing was necessary to alert courtiers to the fact that he was still alive. After three miscarriages, one stillbirth and two infant daughters dead from smallpox, Anne at last gave birth in 1689 to a son. But William, Duke of Gloucester, seems to have suffered from hydrocephalus, known as 'dropsy of the brain'. He was attended by royal physicians John Radcliffe (1652–1714) and Sir Edward Hannes (d. 1710). The former's blunt speaking caused him to be dismissed; he averred publicly during one of her indispositions that the queen was not ill but suffering from 'nothing but the vapours'. Radcliffe was replaced by William Gibbons (1649–1728) and the physician and satirist John Arbuthnot (1667–1735).

Following the firework party staged for his eleventh birthday, the young Prince William fell ill with a fever and nausea, with an accompanying sore throat. Gibbons and Arbuthnot ordered that the child be bled, but his condition worsened. Anne stifled her antipathy and summoned Dr Radcliffe back to court. He immediately fell out with Gibbons and Arbuthnot concerning the treatment, commenting: 'Then you have destroyed him and you may finish him for I will not prescribe.'[21] Four days later the young prince died.

His professional attitude towards the prince resulted in Arbuthnot's appointment as physician-in-ordinary to Queen Anne, whose medical household now included Sir Richard Blackmore from William III's court, serjeant-surgeon Charles Bernard (1650–1711), physician-extraordinary Sir John Shadwick (1671–1747) and Sir Hans Sloane.

Poor Queen Anne now gave birth to a son and then a daughter, neither of whom survived more than twenty-four hours, and a further series of eight pregnancies failed to produce a living heir. When Anne succeeded to the throne in 1702 she had no legitimate heir. Her own health now began a slow deterioration. She suffered so acutely from degenerative arthritis that she had to be carried to her coronation in a sedan chair. This, combined with her obesity, gave her difficulty in walking for the rest of her life.

> The queen:
> 'What time is it,
> Dr Arbuthnot?'
> Arbuthnot:
> 'Whatever it may
> please Your Majesty.'
> **John Arbuthnot**
> *(1667–1735), while
> attending Queen Anne*

One physician closely associated with Queen Anne in her declining years was Sir David Hamilton (1663–1721). He was to be attacked by fellow doctors for not spotting, or ignoring, the queen's supposed condition of dropsy. After her death at Kensington Palace on 1 August 1714 Hamilton became publicly irate with his attackers at the autopsy, especially at the accusation that he had hastened her death.[22]

In truth, Queen Anne's royal doctors were seemingly reluctant to record a detailed description of her health. She was undoubtedly a woman of many ills. There are suggestions of convulsions and a *petit mal* attack in her final days. But did she really die of septicaemia from an 'impostulation' (abscess) of her leg? Hamilton was vague, and her other doctors added nothing on record to solve the mystery.[23] It has been left to modern doctors to suggest that Queen Anne died of, *inter alia*, kidney failure.

ROYAL DOCTORS' QUALIFICATIONS

By the early years of the nineteenth century physicians were distinguished from 'surgeons and quacks' by the possession of university degrees. MDs – Doctor of Medicine degrees – were mostly acquired on the continent for cash, or, for very little study, for around £20 from universities such as St Andrews. These 'parchments' allowed the purchaser – and no other – to be dubbed 'doctor'. As in medieval times surgeons remained as 'Mr' and had few formal qualifications, except for those who were members of the Company of Surgeons. After 1800, the year of the foundation of the Royal College of Surgeons, applicants could take the examination for membership and advertise themselves, if successful, as MRCS. Following the pioneering work of men such as John Hunter (1728–93), surgeons were on a par with physicians in terms of professional status. Thus for a surgeon to be called 'Mr' was no insult.

All this was taken a step further with the advance of the surgeon-apothecary, the forerunner of today's general practitioner. Many of the latter were MRCSs and holders of the degree (after the Apothecaries' Act of 1815) of LSA – the Licence of the Society of Apothecaries. The mark of the 'pure surgeon' was recognised in the degree of FRCS in 1843. In 1884 the degree of LRCP (Licence of the Royal College of Physicians) was conjoined to the MRCS. To complicate matters for the general public, obstetricians up to the end of Victoria's reign called themselves 'physician-*accoucheurs*' and were addressed as 'Dr'. All of these features are extant on the succeeding roll calls of royal doctors.

CHAPTER TWO

'A THRONG OF THE KILLING PROFESSION': ROYAL DOCTORS UNDER SCRUTINY

After the death of Queen Anne, the House of Stuart could supply no legitimate heirs, as defined by the Act of Settlement of 1701, and a quantum leap across the next forty-two genealogical successors was effected, and fate selected Anne's second cousin, the 54-year-old German-speaking George Lewis, Duke of Brunswick-Lüneberg, Elector of Hanover, and grandson of King James VI & I, to rule as King George I from 1714 to 1727. On the succession of the House of Hanover, royal doctors began to have a higher public profile – with all the attendant gossip, innuendo and falsehoods that such a profile entails.

Because of his inherent shyness and hatred of ceremony George I's court in Britain was to be very different from any other in the history of the realm and reflected in part the appalling dullness of his former court at Herrenhausen, a country house outside Hanover. His limited interests – horses and women – also added to his narrowness of mind, which took in little outside the needs of the Hanoverian cause. His interests in Britain were thus minimal; he never learned English and was hardly the stuff of great monarchy.

At Zelle, on 21 November 1682, George married his first cousin Sophia Dorothea, daughter of the Duke and Duchess of Brunswick-Lüneberg and Zelle. From 1694 George and Sophia Dorothea were separated and she was confined in the castle at Ahlden on account of her indiscreet flaunting of her relationship with Count Philip von Königsmark; although they were never formally divorced, Sophia Dorothea was never to be acknowledged Queen of Great Britain. Their son George Augustus, Duke and Marquess of Cambridge, later became

George II, while their daughter, Sophia Dorothea, named for her mother, married Frederick William II, King of Prussia.

George I enjoyed a complicated network of mistresses, although only Sophia von Kielmansegge (whom he created Countess of Darlington) and his official *maîtresse en titre* Ehremgard Melusine von der Schulenberg (later Duchess of Kendal) came to England with him. After the death of Queen Anne's son and heir, William, Duke of Gloucester, in 1700 – which made George's mother heir to the British throne – George played a waiting game for fourteen years, indulging only in hunting and his mistresses, but he watched over Hanoverian interests in Britain through his ambassador to the Court of St James's, Baron Johan Caspar von Bothmar. At last Queen Anne died and on 18 September 1714 George set foot on English soil as the lawful sovereign; he was crowned at Westminster Abbey on 20 October.

In the thirteen years of his reign George I built up only a small medical household of prominent doctors to add to a few he inherited from his predecessor as consultants when needed. Richard Mead (1673–1754), was a physician from a Stepney practice who had been educated at Utrecht and Leiden, graduating MD at Padua in 1695. He survived the family shame of the supposed involvement of his father, the Revd Matthew Mead, in the Rye House Plot, by which extreme Liberals planned to murder Charles II as he returned from Newmarket. Despite the scandal, Mead became physician at St Thomas's Hospital during the period 1703–15. He was an expert in toxicology and wrote a treatise on snake poisons, but like so many of his medical contemporaries he also studied the more esoteric afflictions that might affect patients. His 1704 treatise on the influences of the Sun and Moon on the human body was one example. While treating George I, Mead also included the scientist Sir Isaac Newton and Sir Robert Walpole, the Whig prime minister, among his patients.

The physician and naturalist Sir Tancred Robinson (d. 1748) was appointed physician-in-ordinary to George I, but was better known for his philosophical writings than for his royal connections. Sir John Shadwell (1671–1747) continued as physician-in-ordinary to the monarch, as he had done at Queen

Anne's court. The eighteenth-century upsurge in the interest in anatomy prompted George I to add an anatomist to his medical household. This was Nathaneal St André (1680–1776), a surgeon at Westminster Hospital. St André's beliefs and activities brought him some scrutiny and no little ridicule at court. First there was his involvement in the 'Mary Toft case'. On 26 December 1726 one Mr Howard, a surgeon from Guildford, announced to the public that he had safely delivered Mary Toft, a woman from Godalming, of a litter of rabbits. The woman claimed that conception had taken place when she was startled by a rabbit while she was weeding in her garden. Later she told the credulous that she had dreamt about rabbits in her lap. Her case was studied by Sir Richard Manningham (1690–1759), the leading male midwife of the day, who wrote up his findings in his *Exact Diary of the Case* (1726); Dr St André added his credence to the occurrence and recommended that Mary Toft be given a civil pension. The case caused so much public interest that it was examined by the authorities – and eventually Mary Toft admitted the fraud. Howard, St André and Manningham were all lampooned in Hogarth's cartoon depicting the birthing scene and St André's credibility was shattered. If this were not bad enough, St André's marriage came under severe court scrutiny. In 1728 St André had married Lady Elizabeth Capel, daughter of the Earl of Essex and widow of the astronomer and MP Samuel Molyneux (1689–1728), former secretary to George Augustus, Prince of Wales. At court, St André was now accused (probably erroneously) of having hastened Molyneux's death.

None of George I's English court doctors was with him at his death. On 3 June 1727 George set out for Hanover in the company of his mistress the Duchess of Kendal, his Turkish servant Mustapha, and a small suite. Before departing, the king had suffered 'a few minor fits' but he insisted on travelling to his 'real home' at Herrenhausen. The crossing of the North Sea from Greenwich was uneventful, and by 9 June the small royal party was at Delden in the Netherlands. There they stayed overnight and the king over-indulged in oranges, strawberries and melons, 'an act of imprudence to which was subsequently ascribed (by his doctors) the disorder that caused his death'.[1]

After breakfast on 10 June the royal party left, without

the Duchess of Kendal, who remained in Delden, and made their way towards Osnabrück. The king was beginning to feel faint as they left the environs of the town, but where George I actually died remains a mystery. Some sources aver that he had a stroke and died in his carriage while being attended by his *Kammerherr* (gentleman attendant) Fabrice and physician Dr Steigerdahl. Others say that when he was taken ill in the coach, it was stopped so that the king could be lifted on to the grass verge by the road where he was bled by Steigerdahl, who had rushed from King Frederick Wilhelm II's court at Lingen. Comments on his treatment say that plasters were applied to his hand (now somewhat immobile) and his (distorted) neck, while he was dosed with 'strong spirits'. Still others say that the king was taken to Osnabrück, where he lapsed into unconsciousness and died during the night hours of 10–11 June.

News of the king's death was sent to London by fast courier and on 14 June a report by the court doctors was published in the broadsheets. The doctors noted the received circumstances of the monarch's demise, describing him in the bulletin as 'a Prince endowed with all the royal virtues'. The court doctors ascribed the king's death to a 'a fit of an apoplexy'. George I was buried in Hanover at the Leineschloss Church.[2]

King George I was succeeded by his only son, Prince George Augustus. Born at Hanover on 30 October 1683, George II had become a naturalised British citizen in 1705 and was Prince of Wales from his father's accession. On 22 August 1705, at Hanover, Prince George Augustus married Wilhelmina Charlotte Caroline (1683–1737), third and youngest daughter of the Margrave of Brandenburg-Anspatch and his wife Eleanor of Saxe-Eisenach. As Queen Caroline she was crowned with her husband at Westminster Abbey on 11 October 1727.

The dysfunctional existence of the House of Windsor in the late twentieth century is reflected in the family tree of the House of Hanover. George II had formed an antipathy for his father because of the incarceration of his mother Sophia Dorothea at Ahlden. A soldier who had distinguished himself at the battle of Oudenaarde (11 July 1708), one of the Duke of Marlborough's major victories over the French in the War of the Spanish Succession, George II was limited in intellectual achievements but he did speak English, albeit with a heavy German accent. Yet he formed a hatred for his eldest son, Prince Frederick Louis (1707–51), whom he described as a *Wechselbalg* (changeling).

The situation became so bad that Prince Frederick set up his own court and lived a life of scandal and inconsideration. He was refused both access to his mother (even on her deathbed) and audience with his father. Prince Frederick died suddenly on 20 March 1751, the doctors citing a burst abscess. George I's cruel but memorable comment on his son's death was: 'I have lost my eldest son, but I am glad of it.'[3] The Jacobites, the Hanoverians' political enemies, promoted an epitaph-jingle on Prince Frederick, the authorship of which remains a mystery. At the battle of Culloden in 1746, five years before the prince's death, there was a young army surgeon called James Grainger (d. 1766), who served in Pultney's Regiment in the army of Prince Frederick's brother, Prince William Augustus, Duke of Cumberland (1721–65). Grainger was a poet and Latin versifier, and after his death the following lines on his Hanoverian masters were found among his papers. Was he their author, or did he obtain them from a medic in royal service? We shall never know – but it remains one of the most famous of all royal doggerel epitaphs gleefully disseminated by the Jacobites:

> Here lies Fred
> Who was alive and is dead:
> Had it been his father,
> I had much rather.
> Had it been his brother,
> Still better than another.
> Had it been his sister,
> No one would have missed her.
> Had it been the whole generation,
> So much the better for the nation.
> But since 'tis only Fred
> Who was alive and is dead,
> There's no more to be said.[4]

Richard Mead and Sir John Shadwell continued to serve in George II's medical household but the new king was to add four prominent medics to his household. Benjamin Hoadly (1700–57), a distinguished medical orator, also dabbled in playwriting; his comedy *The Suspicious Husband* (1747) was performed at Covent Garden and the distinguished actor David Garrick took a role. Charles Peters (1695–1746) came to court as physician-extraordinary to the king in 1733 and became physician-general to the army six years later. Robert Taylor (1710–62) joined the medical household as physician, as an adjunct to his large and flourishing London practice.

Perhaps the most flamboyant and best-known court surgeon of his age was the idiosyncratic Sir Caesar Hawkins (1711–86), surgeon to St George's Hospital. He was sergeant-surgeon to George II from 1735 to 1760, and continued in the post for fourteen years into the next reign. Hawkins won professional renown as the inventor of the cutting gorget (an instrument used to guide a surgical knife in performing a lithotomy). He was reputed to earn the huge amount of £2,000 per year with his lancet alone, as well as garnering fees from those apprentices who 'walked the wards' in his wake. Supported by his particular apprentice John Gunning (d. 1798), bearing his books and papers, Hawkins' booming voice told all in the vicinity that the panacea for all ailments known to humanity was 'heroic cupping' and 'vigorous blooding'. (The former was the art of raising blisters on one part of the body to draw off deep-seated pain or poisons, while the latter was the puncturing of veins to draw off blood in varying amounts.)

A hearty, blustering, larger-than-life character, Hawkins became the quintessential eccentric court physician, who paced the royal corridors rapping on doors (and the heads of anyone who got in his way) with his gold-headed ivory physician's cane – shaped like a femur. The cane was packed with herbs to sniff in the presence of more noxious patients – and he is said to have sniffed it particularly deeply when encountering the king's sergeant-surgeon John Ranby (1703–73). Hawkins was reported to be incandescent with rage when Henry Fielding gave Ranby a mention in his novel *The History of Tom Jones* (1749). Hawkins's usual greeting to George II, while rising from a deep bow, was: 'How are Your Majesty's piles today?' Yet it was not the monarch's haemorrhoids that caused the distressing events of 1737.

Queen Caroline of Ansbach had formed her own medical household. It included James Douglas (1675–1742), the physician and bibliographer of anatomy, and John Freind (1675–1728), MP for Launceston, who was involved in some political skirmishing. During the period 1705–7, Freind had acted as physician in Admiral Charles Mordaunt's expeditionary force to Spain. Mordaunt (1658–1735) was involved in a number of financial irregularities and was subject to an official enquiry; Freind wrote pamphlets in his defence. In 1720 Francis Atterbury (1662–1732), Bishop of Rochester, was involved in several attempts to restore the Stuarts to the throne. As leader of the 'Atterbury Plot', the bishop was tried before the House of Lords; he was found guilty of Jacobite complicity and banished. John Freind, also implicated in the plot, was arrested and it is said that court physician Richard Mead arranged his release from the Tower. Surgeon John Shipton (1680–1748), however, lived a more sedate life but as one of a group of royal doctors he was brought into the limelight in the events of 1737.

Queen Caroline of Ansbach brought intelligence to the House of Hanover, and was so trusted by her husband and his ministers that she acted as regent during his absences from London. Following several pregnancies, her health declined and after her sixth confinement in 1723 she developed an umbilical hernia, a condition she hid from those around her. Obesity added to her troubles.[5]

During a court reception on 9 November 1737 she was taken ill with acute abdominal pain and vomiting. She became so indisposed that the assembled company was dispersed. On hand was physician to the household staff Dr George Tesier, who called in Dr Noel Broxholme (d. 1748) of St George's Hospital and surgeon John Ranby. The queen was bled, purged and administered with a clyster, to no avail. Then they tried the various 'panaceas' of the day – snake root and brandy, Daffy's Elixir and Sir Walter Raleigh's cordial,[6] but once more there was no relief for the patient. At length, and contrary to protocol, the queen agreed to a physical examination by Ranby.[7] On 10 November she was bled again and attended, at the king's request, by Sir Hans Sloane and Dr (later Sir) Edward Hulse

(1682–1759), the leading Whig physician, who advised further aperients and blistering.

On 11 November the king made public the fact that for years the queen had suffered from an umbilical hernia and this had now strangulated, causing her the severe symptoms. The medical team now caring for the queen was augmented by John Shipton and the distinguished surgeon and Huguenot-exile Paul Buissière (d. 1739), who recommended that the abdomen be opened to reduce the hernia. The procedure was opposed by John Ranby, who averred 'all the guts . . . would come out . . . on to the bed'. Ranby instead lanced the swelling, and incisions were made daily, without ease to the patient. The queen submitted to the unanaesthetised cutting with great fortitude and sense of humour. At one point Buissière bent low over the work in progress, holding a lighted candle which set fire to his wig; the queen begged that the lancing be stopped for a while to enable her to laugh.

By 18 November the queen was worse; the physicians' log of the day recorded 'the Queen's vomiting returned with as much violence as ever and in the afternoon one of the guts burst in such a manner that her excrement came out of the wound in her belly . . . the running of the wound was in such immense quantities that it went through all the quilts of the bed and flowed all over the floor . . .'.[8]

The queen realised she was dying and called upon her friend, Sir Robert Walpole to look after 'the King, my children and the Kingdom'. Her strangulated bowel became gangrenous and Queen Caroline died at St James's Palace on 20 November 1737 and was buried at Westminster Abbey.[9]

During her suffering one of her court ladies had said: '(Queen Caroline was) among a throng of the killing profession trying their utmost to prolongue her life in adding more torment to it.' Her words were to be mirrored to a greater extent by royal doctors during the treatment of King George III.

George II lived for twenty-three years after the death of his wife, his reign troubled by war with Spain and the Jacobite rebellion of 1745. The writer Horace Walpole said this of the monarch's end:

[*The King*] rose as usual at six, and drank his chocolate. A quarter after seven he went into the little closet (i.e., his privy). His German valet de chambre in waiting heard a noise and running in found the king lying dead on the floor. In falling he had cut his face on the corner of the bureau. He was lain on the bed and blooded, but not a drop followed; the ventricle of his heart had burst.[10]

Thus George II died on 25 October 1760 at Kensington Palace and was buried at Westminster Abbey.

CHAPTER THREE

'TOADS WITH THEIR POISON, DOCTORS WITH THEIR DRUG': PHYSICIANS AT SCOTLAND'S COURTS, 1568–1853

In his epistolary poem of the later 1780s to Robert Graham (1749–1815), 12th Laird of Fintry in the County of Angus, the Scots poet Robert Burns made the unconscious link between poisonous toads – once the stock-in-trade of the wandering Scots medieval medic – and the 'bloody dissectors'. The latter with their scalpels and potions were still more famous in his day outside Scotland than in their native land.[1]

Development of medical knowledge came to Scotland in the wake of the incursion of Norman civilisation. It was only with the accession of David I, on the death of his brother Alexander I (r. 1107–24), that Normans settled the Scottish Lowlands by royal invitation, though some cultural and religious ties had been fostered by Malcolm III's second wife Margaret (1046–93), queen and saint.

David I is known in Scottish history as a great patron of the Church and a builder of abbeys from Kinloss in Moray, to Melrose on the Scottish borders. These religious houses, mostly manned by the Augustinian Canons and the Cistercians, both powerful eleventh-century orders, were the keepers of contemporary medical knowledge. Up to his death the medical needs of David I's Anglo-Norman court were usually tended to by the Augustinians. David I is also credited with founding, in around 1153, the only house of the Knights Hospitalers in Scotland. The Knights belonged to the religious military Order of the Hospital of St John of Jerusalem, and they were the sworn protectors of the pilgrims to the Holy Land from around 1070. Their headquarters were at Torphichen, West Lothian, and the

Knights survived as a land-wealthy group into the 1560s. One of the most distinguished royal patients treated at Torphichen was Edward I, who was kicked by a horse before the battle of Falkirk (July 1298). He was tended by the chief practitioner at the time, Alexander de Welles, who was himself killed in the subsequent battle.

From the days of David I, Scotland developed a whole range of medieval hospitals like Torphichen for travellers and pilgrims, whose administrators (both male and female) attended to the court's medical needs on an *ad hoc* basis wherever the royal family and court happened to be.

Although almost nothing is known of individual practitioners of medicine in the early medieval royal courts of Scotland, one name does stand out. Some 35 miles south of Naples lies the town of Salerno, where 'the seat of the first organised medical school in Europe was established'.[2] Several of its graduates and tutors were to practise at European royal courts, and one of the most mysterious was Michael Scot (*c.* 1160–*c.* 1235). Today he lives on in Scottish folklore as 'The Wizard', largely because Sir Walter Scott alluded to his magic powers in *The Lay of the Last Minstrel* (1805):

> In these far climes it was my lot
> To meet the wondrous Michael Scot;
> A wizard of such dreaded fame . . .[3]

A man of myth and many mysteries Michael Scot is claimed by the Diocese of Durham for his birth, by the Castle of Balwearie, Fife, for his home, and by the Abbey of Melrose for his burial, but no one knows much about his personal background. Yet it is recorded that Michael Scot studied at Oxford and Paris, and then at the 'school of magic' at Padua, and the English chronicler Raphael Holinshed (d. *c.* 1580) describes him as 'Michael Medicus'.

He was in medical practice at Salerno in 1220 and was (probably) entourage physician to Pope Honorius III, who recommended his skills to Stephen Langton, Archbishop of Canterbury. On slight evidence, some writers place Scot at the court of Frederick II, King of Sicily and afterwards Emperor of

Germany. Some suggest that it was for Frederick II that Scot composed his *Liber Physionniae*, a guide, *inter alia*, to character, personality and disease. Indications are, though, that Scot spent the latter years of his life variously as physician and occult dabbler in the court of the Scots king Alexander II (r. 1214–49). In these latter years too, Michael Scot defined his treatments of leprosy, gout and dropsy, and his cure for headaches within his *Pilulae Magistri Michaelis Scoti*; this headache cure was also purported to be an elixir for happiness and a retarder of baldness.

Medical historians are on stronger ground a few years later with records of Adam of Kirkcudbright. On 3 July 1282 Prince Alexander Stewart, second child of Alexander III (r. 1249–86) and Margaret Plantagenet, daughter of Henry III of England, wrote to his uncle Edward I of England, begging him to arrange that Adam be given leave from his duties to attend him at the Scottish court. Prince Alexander had always been sickly and his letter notes that he had no confidence in the (unnamed) doctors who were then administering his physic. It was a lot to ask, even for a prince. Adam of Kirkcudbright was an important man.

Adam was papal chaplain to Pope Urban IV and held many benefices in England and Scotland as priest, rector and landowner. But Edward I allowed Adam to journey north. Prince Alexander was seriously ill and Adam tarried long at the Scottish court, and was rebuked for it by the bishops of the diocese in which he held the benefices. So the prince further petitioned his uncle to ask the bishops to withdraw their objections.[4] The letter also emphasises that Adam was physician to Alexander III and Robert Bruce, Lord of Annandale and grandfather of the future King Robert I, the Bruce. Alas, though Adam 'brought the Prince back from the very gates of death', the prince later died in 1282, aged 20.

During the reign of Alexander III there was a move to ban clergy from studying medicine. The *Corpus Juris Canonici* details a decree on the subject by Alexander III:

> The Devil, after his accustomed fashion, transfiguring himself into an Angel of Light, under colour of caring for the bodies of sick brethren and of administering ecclesiastical business

for the faithful, entices certain monks from their cloisters in order to study law and to weigh out medical prescriptions. Therefore, lest men of spiritual profession should again involve themselves in worldly actions by occasion of learning, we decree that no man whatsoever, after he has taken the vows and made his profession in any place of religion, may be permitted to go out for the the study of physic . . .[5]

The penalty was excommunication, for the practice of medicine by clergy encouraged them to sidestep their 'true vocation' in pursuit of enrichment from fees from patients. In Scotland, as elsewhere in Christendom, the practice of surgery by clergy was forbidden by canon law specified by Pope Innocent III.

The best known of all Scotland's medieval kings was Robert I (r. 1306–29), who achieved hero status by defeating Edward II's English army at Bannockburn on 24 June 1314, and played a crucial role in Scotland's struggle for independence. Consequently his health and final illness have long been the subject of interest – and controversy. Historical records show that Robert I was seriously ill in the autumn of 1307 as he campaigned against the English garrisons at Elgin and Banff before the battle of Inverurie on 23 May 1308. He was so ill that he could not mount his horse unaided and had to be supported in the saddle by two soldiers riding on each side of him. The doctors in his entourage feared for his life, as Archdeacon John Barbour records in his epic poem:

> The King his way to Inverurie made;
> And fell into a grave sickness,
> That put him to such great distress,
> That soon he neither drank nor ate,
> No medicine could his company get,
> For his distress, that might prevail
> And all his strength began to fail,
> On horse or foot he could not go.[6]

On the opinion of the medics of the day, Barbour attributed Robert I's illness to the hardships and setbacks the king had suffered and the poor diet and inadequate shelter endured on his many military ventures. But his health does not appear to have caused the royal doctors too much anxiety until his last days, although what he suffered before the battle of Inverurie seems to have recurred from time to time. Here's Barbour again, recording that after the Treaty of Edinburgh, made on 17 March 1328 and ratified at Northampton on 4 May, the illness so worsened that the king was unable to attend the marriage of his five-year-old son Prince David to the five-year-old Joanna Plantagenet, daughter of Edward II, on 12 July:

> For such an illness did he bear,
> That he himself could not be there,
> A numbing sickness struck him down,
> From lying cold upon the ground,
> When in his troubled days of yore,
> Misfortunes hard upon him bore.[7]

Whatever ailed Robert I, his debilitation was slow but relentless in its effect; the king himself, says Barbour, thought that it was the punishment of Heaven for such wicked deeds as the murder of John Comyn of Badenoch on holy ground:

> For through my strife I bear the guilt
> Of blood that has been freely spilt
> And harmless men that have been slain,
> Therefore this illness and this pain
> My recompense I take to be.[8]

Robert I died at his *manerium* of Cardross, Dumbartonshire, on 7 June 1329 and was buried at the Abbey of Dunfermline, near the shrine of his predecessor, Queen Margaret. During 1818–21 the eastern part of the ruined Dunfermline Abbey was renovated to serve as a parish church, and a tomb was discovered that was identified as 'the last tomb of Robert the Bruce'. The clincher for the identification was the interred skeleton's split breastbone. At his own request, as he approached death, Robert I had asked that his heart be removed at death and transported to the Holy Land in Holy Crusade.[9] Before the skeleton was reinterred a plaster cast of the preserved skull of Robert I was made by W. Scoular. This skull has been the source of vigorous medical speculation.

For five hundred years the death of Robert I was attributed to leprosy but contemporary records do not speak of Robert I having this disease. Barbour for one makes no mention of what the royal doctors thought about the monarch's ailments. It has been suggested that there would be 'a natural reluctance on their part to attribute to a hero-king a disease regarded with superstitious dread and loathing'.[10] At the time of disinterment the extant bones were examined by Robert Liston (1794–1847), teacher of anatomy and operating surgeon at the Royal Infirmary, Edinburgh. He pronounced that Robert I stood 5ft 6in tall and was of slight stature. He also described other aspects he deemed 'interesting' – that the skull showed large orbits and a huge mandible with complex nasal bones. Missing teeth indicated the possibility of the leprosy supposition being correct.

Certainly leprosy had become prevalent in Scotland in the fourteenth century and the numerous monastic-run leper houses would suggest that Robert I's royal doctors at the last were clerics. Finally, the Exchequer Rolls of the period identify one Janvin as the king's apothecary and mention is made of John the Apothecary who supplied spices to the royal family. The latter may refer to the embalming unguents for the king's cadaver.[11]

David II (r. 1329–71), son of Robert I and Elizabeth de Burgh, lacked the essential qualities of leadership enjoyed by his father, and he lost all his father had gained. His chroniclers identify one royal physician called Hector, who in a single year drew in excess of £27 from the Scottish Exchequer.[12] A player in the French invasion of England in 1346, David II was defeated and captured at the battle of Neville's Cross and spent eleven years in English captivity. While in the Tower of London he was prescribed medicines and *electuario condayle* by John Adam of Lucca, the royal apothecary.[13]

On 4 September 1379 Prince Alexander Stewart, Earl of Buchan and Ross, bynamed the 'Wolf of Badenoch', son of Robert II (r. 1371–90), rewarded his royal physician Farquhar Leiche with land endowments, which were topped up with more royal beneficence by Robert II in 1386.[14] Robert II's royal physician Maurice of Perth did less well, although in 1329 he was assigned houses and rents in Perth.

During the reign of Robert II we learn that the profession of physician was becoming hereditary in the ancient lands of the Northern Picts. Professor John Edgar of St Andrews has made a special study of these families and in his *History of Education in Scotland* (p. 282) he avers:

> The physicians were hereditary like the bards, father handing on to son whatever of his own science and skill he could impart. The MacLeans of Skye, and the Bethunes of Mull were specially distinguished in this important profession. One member of the latter family, Fergus Bethune, cured Robert II of a painful disease when the court physicians had failed. A charter still exists by which the King, to mark his gratitude, conveyed to this successful doctor a number of small islands on the West of Scotland. Though the office was hereditary, there was apparently a real scientific interest in their profession shown by these men, and the manuscripts (*in Gaelic belonging to the families*) are said to prove that they tried to extend their native knowledge by diligent perusal of the literature of early medicine.[15]

Farquhar Leiche, *Medicus Regis*, is recorded as one of these 'hereditary doctors'.[16]

Records of the reign of the murdered James I (r. 1406–37) reveal the name of James Alamanus (fl. *c.* 1431–53) as a physician who received cash gifts for his services along with ostrich plumes for his wife, furs and purple velvet.[17] Papers from the time of James II (r. 1437–60) identify three royal doctors. Nicknamed 'James of the Fiery Face' because of an unfortunate birthmark, the monarch employed Venetian (fl. *c.* 1445), Serapion (fl. *c.* 1455–62) and David Crannoch (fl. *c.* 1447–57); of the latter pair a little more is said in the state papers than was usual before.

David Crannoch was an arts graduate of St Andrews and Paris, who became procurator (administrator) of the German Nation from 1453 to 1454. Shortly before taking up this post he had graduated in medicine, probably at Paris, and returned to Scotland to serve as physician to James II.[18] Serapion is described as 'court physician', with a stipend of £20 per annum and gifts of a horse, saddle and bridle. He also prescribed for James II's wife Mary of Guelders.[19]

The court of James III (r. 1460–88) included royal doctors Andrew Alaman of Denmark (fl. *c.* 1480), who also served as royal astrologer. The king was somewhat mentally unstable, with delusions of grandeur and a keen interest in the occult, which might have attracted him to Dr Alaman. Certainly the king seems to have had great faith in his soothsaying, for Alaman's foretelling of the manner of the king's death led to the monarch's ultimate rash political behaviour. Alaman reported to the king that he had seen a vision of a lion strangled by its whelps. Was this to be James's mode of death, at the hands of his own family? Maybe he believed it, for James III fell foul of an army led by his son Prince James, and was said to have been murdered on the field of battle.[20]

Another royal doctor to James III was Michael Ker, student of medicine at Louvain, who is listed as a court physician during the period 1460–80. The Exchequer Rolls indicate that the king subsidised his studies. Little is known of him, but one of his medical compatriots from Louvain was to become a giant of Scottish ecclesiastical history.

Born of a well-to-do Aberdeenshire family around 1440, William Scheves studied astrology and medicine at Louvain under the astrologer Spiricus. He became master of the Maison Dieu (hospital) of the Poor of St Mary the Virgin of Brechin, in the county of Angus. His skills as an astrologer and medic brought him royal favour as court physician. Scheves also exploited his skills of ingratiation and by 1459 he was made Archdeacon of St Andrews Diocese. Thereafter he appears in the *Rotuli Scaccarii Regum Scotorum* as being in receipt of regular money and goods from the royal treasury. Soon he was combining his duties as physician with those of a further court prerogative, Officer of the Royal Wardrobe.

In 1478 Scheves received the pall (a lamb's wool vestment) of his new ecclesiastical appointment as Archbishop of St Andrews, at the church of Holyrood Abbey in the presence of the king and nobility. Scheves was frequently employed on political missions, but joined the conspiracy of nobles against James III. He nevertheless retained his powerful influence under the new king, James IV.

Scheves died at his palace-castle at St Andrews on 28 January 1496 and was buried before the high altar of the cathedral.[21] Making an assessment of Scheves's life for the *Dictionary of National Biography*, A.H. Millar commented: '(Scheves was) a scheming time-serving prelate, who obtained ascendancy over James III by astrological quackery.'

A leading historical character in Scotland's transition from the Middle Ages to the Renaissance was King James IV (r. 1498–1513), in whose reign there was a rebirth in the promotion of, and interest in, medicine. Impetus for the study of medicine came from the monarch himself, who regularly paid subjects to allow him to act as surgeon at their operations, and to draw teeth with his own set of 'equipment' purchased in 1503. James IV eagerly read the medical compendia of Mandino of Bologna and Henri de Mondeville of Paris and Montpellier, and was keen for medicine as a subject to be promoted in the colleges the foundation of which he was supporting.

A chair of medicine was established at Aberdeen University to lecture after the fashion of the school at Paris, and medics were encouraged to attend court to inform the king about recent developments in the science. James IV supplied cash from the royal treasury to buy medicines, books on alchemy and surgical instruments to be used by those who needed them, and he subsidised 'the Abbot of Tungland's researches' in particular.[22]

The Abbot of Tungland was one John Damien, who persuaded the king that he could make 'fine golde' from baser metals. This was long an occupation of medieval alchemists, who believed they could do this if they discovered the right touchstone, known as the 'Philosopher's Stone'. Damian managed to persuade James IV to equip a laboratory for his use at Stirling Castle. There he and James would potter happily testing various alchemical theories. In the manifest of goods the Scottish Exchequer bought for Damien were many stocks-in-trade of the contemporary Scots medic, from alum, cinnabar and aqua vitae to orpiment, sal ammoniac and vinegar. The inclusion of whisky and wine were seemingly not challenged by the Scots royal treasurers. Damien's useless experiments never lost the king's support nor was the alchemist's reputation ever dented – not even when Damien strapped on a pair of home-made wings and launched himself from the battlements of Stirling Castle and tried to fly. As the royal doctors treated him for impact injuries and a broken leg, Damien solemnly told the king that 'some of the feathers used in the wings were those of barn-door fowls little accustomed to flight'.[23]

James IV was also a leading light in the foundation of the Guild of Surgeons and Barbers at Edinburgh, which was incorporated under a Seal of Cause from the town council of 1505 and ratified by the king on 13 October 1506. An entrance fee to study at the Guild's school of medicine was fixed at Five Scots Pounds plus a dinner for the master of the craft on admission. Included in the privileges was one cadaver a year, for anatomical study and dissection, supplied by the public hangman.[24]

Hardly anything is known of the personal physicians at James IV's court, apart from the ubiquitous William Scheves. Yet it may be noted that in James IV's reign royal doctors were given areas of Scotland in which to promote health care. For instance, at the direct command of James IV and Queen Margaret, one Henry Railston was given a portion of the rents of Kere Lawmond and Little and Meikle Lupes, Bute, to care for the patients in the area.[25] This system formed a prototype national health service.

James IV was forty years old when he died – run through by an English 'brown bill' (an 8ft long halberd) at the battle of Flodden on 9 September 1513.

James V (r. 1513–42), who inherited the throne at the age of one, was no intellectual equal to his father; largely uneducated, he developed into a sensual and avaricious despot. Records on his royal doctors are somewhat thin but the Scottish poet and Lyon King of Arms, Sir David Lyndsay of the Mount (1490–1555), wrote a lampoon on three of them. He describes a joust between these doctors, which he said took place at St Andrews on Whit Monday in an unspecified year:

James was one man of great intelligence (*Dr James Watson*)
Ane medicinar ful of experience;

And John Barbour, he was one nobile leche (*leche=leech: a
pun on the name of Dr Thomas Leche*)
Cruikit carlings, he would gar them get speche.
(*i.e., Barbour would try to make fish speak*)[26]

Lyndsay reduces the joust to farce, with each royal doctor made
to fight the others with boxing gloves.

James V died on 14 December 1542, at his palace of Falkland,
amid an atmosphere of despair. Two infant sons, Prince Robert
and Prince James, had predeceased him in 1541; his army had
been defeated at the battle of Solway Moss on 20 November
1542; and the heir to his throne was a girl, just a few days old.
The chroniclers wrote that the king died 'of a broken heart'.
Court records show that some time in 1542 the soldier-surgeon
Antoine Brisset rendered some medical treatment to James V's
queen (and second wife) Marie de Guise-Lorraine. This is the first
mention in any Scottish source of a specific military surgeon.
Born into conflict, her Scottish realm riven in two by pro-English
and pro-French factions, at the age of six Mary, Queen of Scots,
was whisked away to safety in France by her widowed mother.
There she remained for twelve happy years, while her mother
ruled Scotland as regent from 1554 to 1559.

Marie de Guise-Lorraine's Scottish household was almost
entirely French, as were her physicians. In October 1559 her
regency was suspended by the Scottish Lords of the Congregation
and Scotland was now ruled by a Council of Regency. From this
time there exists an undated memorandum entitled *Advice of
the Queen's Doctor*, in which it is suggested that she should
avoid the pressures of state affairs.[27] This rare memorandum
records her symptoms: 'severe palpitations, resulting in
insomnia, a heaviness of the body, languor, a livid complexion
and a general feeling of melancholy'. A French court physician
pronounced the condition serious and difficult to cure because
of 'an abundance of humours spread through the body'.[28] In
modern terms Marie de Guise-Lorraine was probably suffering
from chronic heart disease. She died around 12.30 a.m. on 11
June 1560. From the papers of the French ambassador to her
court, Jacques de la Brosse, there comes a rare comment on the
work of royal doctors of the period. De la Brosse describes what

the doctors found when they were embalming the body of the recently dead queen:

> The liver and the heart were found to be without a single drop of blood: the gall very large and swollen, as yellow as saffron, inside and out: the heart rather small and covered with fat; the brain full of fluid.[29]

During the reign of Marie de Guise-Lorraine the Scottish court was visited from time to time by continental physicians who were called in to treat prominent court members. One such was Jerome Cardan, bynamed Hieronymous (or Girolamus) Cardanus (1501–78). A native of Milan, Cardan became professor of medicine at Padua and Pavia. In 1552 he journeyed to Scotland to treat John Hamilton (1512–71), Archbishop of St Andrews. His consultations while at the Scottish court throw light on the strange medico-magic practice of the time.

The bastard son of James, 1st Earl of Arran, John Hamilton was the half-brother of James, 2nd Earl of Arran and Governor of Scotland. He became severely ill in the early part of 1552. Asthma was diagnosed and Cardan began a regimen of therapeutic treatment. On one occasion he applied to the archbishop's shaved head 'an ointment composed of Greek pitch, ship's tar, white mustard, euphorbium, and honey of anthardus'. The English ambassador to the Scottish Court, Thomas Randolph (1523–90), reported to his royal mistress Elizabeth I that Cardan had hung the archbishop 'certaine houres a day by the heels' to allow better breathing. Cardan also laid down advice on diet (he fed the archbishop 'younge whelpes') and exercise, and added for good measure an astrological chart which, to the archbishop's discomfort, revealed that he would suffer 'a passion of the heart' in 1560 and succumb to a violent death. For all of this Cardan received gifts of gold, a horse and 1,800 gold crowns. About Hamilton's death Cardan had been accurate. As a leading supporter of Mary, Queen of Scots, he was captured by her enemies and hanged at Stirling Castle on 7 April 1571.

On 28 April 1558 Mary Stuart – she spelled her name in the French style – married Francis II of France. He died in December 1560. So at the age of eighteen, and already a widow, Mary

Stuart returned to her troubled Scottish kingdom to rule until she was deposed in favour of her infant son James in 1567.

Mary Stuart confirmed the Seal of Cause of the Guild of Surgeons and exempted all surgeons and physicians from having to bear arms in raids and wars by the dispensation of 11 May 1567. This was her only incursion into medical politics. As with the records of her mother's reign, Mary Stuart's royal doctors are shadowy characters, but from scattered sources a few names do stand out.

The life and reign of Mary Stuart are well documented. She enjoyed a robust childhood and developed a commanding figure, at just under 6ft tall. She suffered from the measles as a child and was treated for *petite vérole* (smallpox) by her French physician Jean Fernel. She had a virtual nervous breakdown at the news of her mother's death. Throughout her life Mary Stuart suffered gastric trouble, tertian fevers and bouts of depression brought on by the terrible traumas of her life. Her worst bouts followed the murder of her secretary David Rizzio (1566), in her presence at Holyrood, and the assassination by gunpowder explosion at Kird o'Field of her second husband Henry Stuart, Lord Darnley (1567). Her health was certainly affected by her periods of captivity, although the royal doctors were incarcerated with her.

In 1563 she suffered the curiously dubbed 'fashionable new disease' (influenza), and was desperately ill while at Jedburgh (1566), where she was attended by her French physician Dr Arnault. During her twenty-odd years in exile in England, as the captive of Elizabeth I – on whose mercy she had thrown herself for succour and asylum after her defeat at the battle of Langside in 1568 – Mary Stuart's health was closely monitored. Her early death would have been a weight off Elizabeth I's mind, as Mary Stuart was an obvious claimant to the English throne and a focus for Roman Catholic terrorist groups. While she was a prisoner at Tutbury, her jailer, George Talbot, 5th Earl of Shrewsbury, reported to Elizabeth I that his physician Dr Francis said that Mary Stuart was suffering from *obstructio splenis cum flatu hypochondriaco*, which Shrewsbury translated as 'grief of the spleen'.[30] Thus, after 1569 Mary Stuart's health was 'a chronic problem' to herself and to her captors.

From this point historians have begun to study Mary Stuart's health in some detail, noting that she suffered from gastric ulcers, rheumatism and hysteria. From her teenage years she had complained of terrible pains, vomiting, lameness and periods of mental instability. Medical historians have concluded that she suffered from porphyria, inherited from James V. Certainly her son King James VI & I shared similar symptoms.[31]

On 21 September 1586 Mary Stuart was transferred to her final prison at Fotheringay Castle, Northamptonshire, and there she was executed on Wednesday, 8 February 1587. Following her death an inventory of Mary Stuart's worldly goods was collated, with some indication of who in her household should get what. The inventory, dated 20 February 1587, identifies her physician, apothecary and surgeon, none of whom is named, but all received artefacts, apparel and money legacies. From other sources the three men can be identified as Dr Castel (physician), Jacques Gervais (surgeon) and Pierre Garin (apothecary), all of whom were in her employ at her death.[32]

Back in 1567, when Mary Stuart had been forced to abdicate, her one-year-old son James ascended the throne of Scotland as James VI. During his reign much more detail was to be recorded concerning doctors who served at the royal Scottish court.

By 1567 the Guild of Surgeons and Barbers had extended their influences beyond their clinical activities to play a part in various aspects of local government. It would be a role they would hold for another one hundred years. Their constant rivals were the apothecaries and pharmacists, who were only partially subdued by legal proscribement against interference in what was considered the Guild's 'business'.

Even at this date physicians in Scotland, whether home-grown or not, were few and far between, and those with any formal degrees had trained abroad. The Scottish royal court therefore still depended on foreign, or foreign-trained, medics until the 1670s. Although the royal court was subject to some extent to practitioners of medico-magic, the blatant quackery that passed for medicine among the poor folk was hardly present.

From 1568 Scotland's royal mediciners (physicians and surgeons) began to emerge as official court appointments, with practitioners selected by commission under the privy seal.[33]

SCOTS 'ORDINARY PHYSICIANS' AT COURT, 1568–1853

Alexander Preston. Appointed 13 July 1568. Re-appointed 20 March 1576.

Gilbert Moncrieff of Myreside. Appointed 21 September 1575. Re-appointed 8 January 1598. Died 24 February 1598.

Gilbert Skeyne. Born Bandole, Skene, Aberdeenshire, *c.* 1522. Appointed 16 June 1581. Known salary 200 Scots pounds. Retired 1593. Died June 1599.

Martin Schoner. Appointed 27 October 1581. Appointed physician to Queen Anne of Denmark, 22 July 1597.

David Kinloch. Born Dundee *ante* 1559. Appointed 21 March 1597. Died 10 September 1617.

John McCulloch. In place 24 April 1622. Died January 1623.

James McCulloch. Details not known. Died 1623.

Alexander Ramsay. In place 9 March 1631. Last mention 9 April 1650.

James Chalmers. In place 9 March 1635. Died September 1644.

John Craig. Appointed *c.* 4 April 1635. Died January 1655.

Sir John Wedderburn. Born Dundee 1599. Attended Prince of Wales (later Charles II) in Holland. Known pension 2,000 Scots pounds. Died July 1679.

Sir Robert Cunningham of Auchenharvie. In place 25 July 1660 to 1674.

Sir Alexander Martin of Strathendry. In place *c.* 1670.

Sir Thomas Burnet. Born 1638. Appointed 30 May 1672. Principal physician to Charles II at both courts, 1689. Died 1704.

Sir David Hay. Appointed 30 May 1672. Died June 1699.

Sir Archibald Stevenson. Appointed 24 September 1675. Principal physician to Charles II, November 1681.

Sir Andrew Balfour. Born Balfour Castle, Fife, 18 January 1630. Appointed 11 November 1681. Died 10 January 1694.

Sir Robert Sibbald. Born 15 April 1641. Appointed 30 September 1682. Died 1672.

Thomas Dalrymple. Appointed 15 December 1691. Principal court physician, March 1704.

Sir Edward Eizat. Appointed 31 March 1704. Resigned August 1717.

George Mackenzie. Appointed 22 March 1714. Third physician to Queen Anne. Appointment not renewed by George I.

William Douglas. Appointed 10 August 1717.

Alexander Dundas. Appointed 31 March 1719. Died 1 April 1732.

James Lidderdale. Appointed 18 April 1732. Resigned April 1761.

Francis Home. Born 1719. Appointed 13 April 1761. Died 15 February 1813.

James Home. Born 1760. Appointed 10 June 1806. Died 5 December 1844.

Andrew Combe. Born 27 October 1797. Appointed 20 December 1844. Died 9 August 1847.

John Scott. Appointed 31 December 1847. Died 3 May 1853.

'PRINCIPAL MEDICINER/PHYSICIANS' TO THE SCOTTISH COURT, 1603–1844

John Craig. Appointed 3 January 1603.

(Title changed from 'Principal Mediciner' to 'Principal or First Physician' in 1645.)

Sir Alexander Fraizer of Dores. Appointed 1645. Died 1681.

Archibald Stevenson. Appointed 12 November 1681.

Christopher Irvine. Appointed 20 September 1686.

Sir Thomas Burnet. Appointed 7 December 1689.

Joseph Black. Born Bordeaux 1728. Appointed 8 March 1790. Died 6 December 1799.

James Gregory. Born Aberdeen 1753. Appointed 18 December 1799. Died 2 April 1821.

Andrew Duncan. Born 10 August 1744. Appointed 1 April 1821. Died 1828.

John Abercrombie. Appointed 22 July 1828. Died 1844.

The office of First Physician in Scotland lapsed after the death of John Abercrombie.

The salary attached to the position was 50 pound Scots (a Scots pound was worth one-twelfth of an English pound).

A number of 'ordinary physicians' at the Scots court are worthy of particular mention. James VI's doctor Professor Gilbert Skeyne wrote the earliest medical treatise published in Scotland: *Ane Bereve Description of the Pest* (i.e., Plague) *quhair in the cavsis, signes, and sum speciall preseruation and cure thairof ar contenit*. In it Skeyne asserted that the plague was exacerbated by poor public health and sanitation, and that stray animals should be destroyed. He advised a treatment of bleeding and purging as a cure, and the regimen of herbal therapy.[34]

Another physician at James VI's court, David Kinloch, was greatly influenced by what he studied in the medical schools at Montpellier and Rennes. While travelling in Spain he fell foul of the Holy Office, and his execution for heresy was delayed because of the illness of the Inquisitor-General. Kinloch is said to have attended his accuser, who recovered – and the Scots doctor was spared the flames.[35]

David Kinloch was the first Scottish physician to write a detailed treatise on obstetrics, *De Hominis Procreatione*, in 1596. An anonymous hand detailed his appointment as *Medicus Regis* in this rare comment on an individual doctor of the period:

> . . . a most honourable man, of famous learning, and in his life adorned with many singular virtues; a most skilful physician to the King of Great Britain and France, by whose patents and seals the antiquity of his pedigree and Extract is clearly witnessed and proven . . .

Sir Robert Sibbald, appointed to Charles II's entourage in 1682, was a physician, naturalist and antiquary, as well as an early general practitioner. Along with fellow-medic Andrew Balfour, he established in 1667 a small botanical garden at Edinburgh, which in time grew into the capital's Royal Botanical Garden. Around 1678 Sibbald became physician to the Jacobite Roman Catholic James Drummond (d. 1716), 4th Earl of Perth and Chancellor of Scotland. Through Perth's influence Sibbald achieved his royal preferment and the additional post of geographer royal for Scotland. At the king's command he undertook the writing of the natural history and geography of Scotland, funded from his own pocket. Again mainly through the assistance of his friend Andrew Balfour and their contemporary William Stevenson, Sibbald helped to found the Royal College of Physicians of Edinburgh.[36] He is thought to have died in 1772, in which year his library was sold.[37]

Queen Victoria's Scots doctor Andrew Combe studied surgery and medicine at Edinburgh and Paris and won fame both as a physician and as a phrenologist. While in Paris he had come across the contemporary research in phrenology which had been propounded as a doctrine by Johan Christof Spurzheim and Franz Joseph Gall in Germany around 1800. Their doctrine held that portions of the human brain had separate functions and that if these were fully developed the brain and the area of the skull over that part was correspondingly enlarged. Thus, said the phrenologists, these 'lumps' could be 'read' to deduce character and intellectual capability. It led to an upsurge of quackery and repudiation by academics.

Undaunted by academic opposition, Combe established the *Phrenological Journal* in 1823. By 1836 he had won such a reputation that he became physician to the future Queen Victoria's uncle, Leopold, King of the Belgians, and physician-extraordinary to the queen in 1838.

Another title for medical practitioners at the Scottish court was Principal Mediciner, a post established by James VI at a salary of 100 pounds Scots.[38] The first man to receive the new commission was John Craig, who accompanied the king to the English court when he became James I of England. After an apparent gap in appointments for Scotland, the title of Principal Mediciner was changed to Principal (or First) Physician and the role was reconstituted by Charles II. Sir Alexander Frazier of Dores was an early recipient.

Frazier was a faithful royalist who attended and supported Charles II during his exile on the continent; after the Restoration of 1660, Frazier became a prominent courtier. Shortly before Christmas 1660 Princess Mary of Orange (b. 1631), the princess royal and sister of Charles II, was taken ill with smallpox. Frazier attended her until her death on Christmas Eve. Frazier also won a special mention in royal medical records for successfully trepanning the skull of Prince Rupert of the Rhine (1619–82), Charles II's cousin.

Flourishing from around 1638, the year that he was thrown out of the college at Edinburgh for refusing to support the National Covenant, Dr Christopher Irvine won fame as a physician, philologist and antiquary. As a royalist and Episcopalian he was a thorn in the side of the Presbyterian clergy in Scotland and somehow became embroiled in the troubles in Ireland, to such an extent that he was deprived of his estate and 'reduced' to school teaching. He resumed his medical studies in 1650–1 and joined Charles II's army. After the battle of Worcester in 1651, wherein Cromwell defeated the royal forces, Irvine's glibness of tongue enabled him to join the other side and he served as surgeon to General Monck's Army (1652–3), and thereafter to the Horse Guards.[39]

Dr Andrew Duncan was one of the most well-travelled doctors of his age, having studied medical practice at such places as Gottingen, Vienna, Pisa and Naples. A Fellow of the Royal College of Physicians of Edinburgh, Duncan was founder-physician to the Royal Public Dispensary at Edinburgh and to the Fever Hospital. Duncan was one of the most published doctors of his age.

The office of first physician in Scotland lapsed at the death of its last holder, Dr John Abercrombie, in 1844.

CHAPTER FOUR

TO SERVE THE 'KINGS OVER THE WATER': ROYAL DOCTORS OF JACOBITE SYMPATHY

When Queen Anne died at Kensington Palace on 1 August 1714, Britain was plunged once more into dynastic turmoil. After the Roman Catholic King James VII & II had been pushed off the throne in 1688, to be replaced by the Protestant William III and Mary II, most people in the northern kingdom backed the Scottish Parliament in accepting them as rulers. Others took a different view. They believed the rightful ruler was the Roman Catholic Prince James Francis Edward Stuart (1688–1766), Duke of Cornwall and Rothesay, and styled (but never created) Prince of Wales, the eldest son of James VII & II by his second wife Mary Beatrice, daughter of the Duke of Modena. In 1714 Jacobites jockeyed once more for their prince's proclamation as James VIII of Scotland and III of England. In the event, George of Hanover was crowned King George I, according to the Act of Settlement (1701), which secured the Protestant succession.

Historians note that a prominent royal apothecary was a player in the controversy surrounding the birth of Prince James Francis Edward Stuart. His name was James St Amand (fl. 1679–88, d. 1728) of St Pauls, Covent Garden, London. St Amand came into James VII & II's entourage when the king was still the Duke of York. On James's accession St Amand became first apothecary.[1]

Prince James Francis Edward, known as the 'Old Pretender' by future generations, was born at St James's Palace on 10 June 1688. Rumour had it that he was a supposititious child, but this was clearly nonsense – thirty people had crowded into Queen Mary of Modena's chamber to witness the birth. Yet the fact that the midwives and lady-in-waiting, the Countess of Sunderland, had taken the newborn infant into an antechamber, without first holding it up to the assembled courtiers, sparked the rumour that the legitimate child had been born dead and had been replaced by 'a healthy, male changeling',[2] smuggled into the chamber in a bed-warming pan. Foolishly, King James ordered an entirely unnecessary enquiry into the birth. For those who opposed the king, his enquiry altered nothing and they continued to believe in the 'Warming Pan' theory.

When Queen Anne came to the throne in 1702 St Amand was petitioned to give testimony as to the legitimacy of Prince James Francis Edward's counter-claim to the throne. St Amand was questioned closely by Dr George Hickes (deprived Dean of Worcester) and by Dr George Harbin (former chaplain to Viscount Weymouth), and on 2 April 1703 St Amand gave details of Queen Mary of Modena's pregnancy. He attested that the pregnancy was 'well assured' and that he had prescribed medicines to prevent miscarriage. He further averred that substitution was impossible; he had observed the midwives and had examined the afterbirth.[3] He also confirmed that he had attended the child for infant illnesses until it was quite well. St Amand had been paid £200 for his services.[4] His testimony was duly accepted as the truth by Hickes and Harbin and it entered the state papers as such under their signatures.

Jacobites had been active and rebellious in Scotland from 1688; in 1689, 1708 and 1718 there were unsuccessful attempts to restore the Roman Catholic Stuarts, but the best remembered Scots uprisings were those of 1715 and 1745. These two rebellions brought to light Jacobite doctors dubbed 'royal Stuart doctors', either because they were self-appointed volunteers of Prince James Francis Edward, or special appointees of his sons Prince Charles Edward (1720–88) and Prince Henry Benedict (1725–1807).

For historians, records on doctors involved in the Jacobite risings are sparse. This is not surprising, since to openly declare allegiance and active support for the exiled Stuarts could lead to custodial sentences, if not to execution. One of the most celebrated Jacobite physicians of his time, Archibald Pitcairne, born at Edinburgh on 25 December 1652, was an erstwhile theologian and lawyer turned medic. A Fellow of the Royal College of Physicians of Edinburgh, Pitcairne studied medicine at Paris and became Professor of Physic at Leyden by 1692.

He returned to Edinburgh the following year to pursue medical practice, authorship and his lampooning of the Presbyterian Church from his Episcopalian standpoint. In 1693 he married the daughter of royal physician Dr Archibald Stevenson.[5] Pitcairne died at Edinburgh on 20 October 1703. At the end he dedicated his life's work 'To God and his Prince (James Francis Edward) . . .'. In his will he left a jeroboam of claret to be opened at 'the Restoration of the House of Stewart (*sic*)'.[6] Pitcairne was an outspoken Jacobite who argued the case of the Roman Catholic Stuarts and propagandised on their behalf. He was one in a long line of Scots Episcopalians who supported the Stuarts against the 'upstart' Hanoverians. When Pitcairne's son fell into the hands of the Hanoverians and was imprisoned in the Tower of London, a former pupil of Archibald Pitcairne's at Leyden came to the rescue. Richard Mead, royal physician to George II, negotiated with Prime Minister Robert Walpole to have the young Pitcairne released.[7]

Perhaps the best known of the Jacobite royal doctors was Sir Stuart Threipland of Fingask Castle in the parish of Kilspindie, Perthshire. Threipland was born in 1716, while his father was in hiding from the Hanoverian troops occupying the family home – an incident resulting from the 1715 Jacobite rebellion. In 1742 Threipland graduated MD at Edinburgh University and was admitted Fellow of the Royal College of Physicians in 1744.

When Prince Charles Edward Stuart, known severally as 'Bonnie Prince Charlie' and the 'Young Pretender', landed at Eriskay in July 1745, in an attempt to win back his father's throne, Threipland joined him when he raised the Jacobite standard at Glenfinnan. Here, on 19 August, the prince heard his father proclaimed king of the united kingdoms of England and Scotland. Thereafter Threipland accompanied the prince on his ill-fated march from Edinburgh to the events of 6 December – 'Black Friday' in Jacobite parlance – when the Jacobite Army retreated. Threipland was also with the prince at the rout of the Jacobite army at Culloden on 16 April 1746, and fled with the prince in the 'fugitive wanderings' that followed the battle.

Threipland parted company with the prince when he and fellow Jacobite royal doctor Dr Archibald Campbell went into hiding in the lands of Badenoch. There, in a cave, Threipland

tended the wounds of Donald Cameron of Lochiel (*c.* 1695–
1748), who had received severe wounds to both ankles at the
battle of Falkirk (17 January 1745). Threipland then made his
way to Edinburgh disguised as a Presbyterian probationer.[8] In
various other disguises he escaped to France, where he rejoined
Prince Charles.

In 1747 an amnesty was effected for Jacobites in the form
of the Act of Indemnity and Threipland was able to return
to Edinburgh, where he established a flourishing medical
practice. In 1766 he became president of the Royal College
of Physicians of Edinburgh. A fervent Jacobite until his death
in 1805, he died at his family estate, which he acquired from
forfeiture. His medicine chest, which was with him at Culloden,
remains in the museum of the Royal College of Physicians
of Edinburgh. Of French origin, this chest is dubbed 'Prince
Charles's Medicine Chest' and was given by Threipland to
surgeon Alexander Wood (1725–1807). Known as 'Lang Sandy
Wood' because of his tall, lanky figure, Dr Wood treated Robert
Burns when he hurt his leg falling from a coach, and has gone
down in Edinburgh medical history as the first Scots medic
to own an umbrella. Wood bequeathed the chest to his son
Dr George Wood, who in turn gave it to Dr John Smith, who
donated it to the College. Dinner, by the by, at the table of Dr
(then Sir) Stuart Threipland was an event of 'Jacobite delight'
– as the Loyal Toast was drunk, Threipland carefully drew his
glass to his mouth over a strategically placed bowl of water.
Thus he drank 'To the King . . . over the water'.

With Dr Threipland on the 'fugitive wanderings' was another
Jacobite royal doctor, Archibald Cameron (1707–53), the
younger son of Sir Ewan Cameron of Lochiel (1629–1719), who
sent his clan to the 1715 Jacobite rebellion. Archibald Cameron
studied medicine at Edinburgh and Paris, returning to Lochaber
to act as physician to the Jacobite insurgents of the '45; he it was
who effected the escape of Prince Charles from Culloden.[9] In
time Dr Cameron became physician to a regiment in France, but
was arrested in Scotland in 1753 while collecting money thought
to be for Jacobite insurgency. Cameron was hanged, drawn and
quartered at Tyburn, the last Jacobite to be so executed.

Two other Jacobite royal doctors are worthy of mention. James

Grainger (*c.* 1721–66) was a physician and poet who graduated MD at Edinburgh in 1753 after three years as an army surgeon (1745–8). He saw action at the battles of Falkirk and Culloden, and escaped to the continent. Grainger died in the West Indies after attempting to combine commerce with medicine.[10] Then there was William Balfour of Aberdour who was with Prince Charles on the march to Derby.[11] Little is known about his personal life except that he appears as a character in Robert Louis Stevenson's *Kidnapped* (1886) and also in *Catriona* (1893).

The bloody aftermath of the Jacobite rebellion of 1745 brings to the fore another half-dozen Jacobite royal doctors. After Culloden there was much work for them. As the Hanoverian troops sought out rebels in the vicinity of the Highland capital of Inverness, records show that the prisons there held twenty-five surgeons who had either served in the Jacobite army, or declared sympathy with the cause.

The courthouse and jail, Inverness Tolbooth, were crowded with prisoners. After the provost marshal had dealt with the numerous deserters from the Hanoverian army – with trees serving as gibbets – his attention came to bear on the Jacobites. There was such a huge number of prisoners that they spilled out into cellars, requisitioned houses and graveyards. One strange medic attending them was Captain John Farquharson, of the Farquharson Regiment. He was a farmer and 'blooder', an unqualified doctor who served the sick in the prince's name by letting blood. He left this account of a scene that was witnessed scores of times by the Jacobite royal doctors:

But, Oh Heavens! what a scene opens to my eyes and nose all at once; the wounded feltered (i.e. matted) in their gore and blood, some dead bodies covered quite over with pish and dirt, the living standing to the middle in it, their groans wou'd have pirsed a heart of stone, but our corrupt hearts was not in the least touched, but on the contrary we began to upbraid them the moment we entered their prisons. Dr Lauder's case of instruments was taken from him for fear he should end any of the wounded, and, (my) lancet was taken out of (my) pocket for fear (I) should begin to blood them . . . to save some few of the wound(ed) to have fallen in fevers.[12]

The 'Dr Lauder' referred to was George Lauder, a surgeon who had volunteered to join Prince Charles. With another surgeon, John Rattray, he was physically restrained from tending the sick and wounded.

Captain Farquharson also testified to cruelty at sea. In order to 'de-louse' the prisoners, they were dropped into the sea from the yard-arms of Hanoverian vessels such as the *Alexander and James*. Farquharson testified thus:

> They wou'd take us from the hold in a rope and hoisted us up to the yard-arm, and let us fall into the sea in order for a ducking of us; and tying up to the mast and whipping us if we did anything, however innocent, that offended them; this was done to us when we was not able to stand.[13]

Among the other doctors who had rallied to the prince were the 'Highland blooder' and farmer Donald MacIntyre of Argyll, and Alexander Abernethie, another surgeon-farmer from Tipperty in Banff. Abernethie died in prison in London. Dr Colin Maclachlan was a Highland medic who had returned from the West Indies to assist the Stuarts. He made a point of pursuing a Hanoverian neighbour to his Scottish family home to avenge the violation of a female member of the family during the emergency.[14]

Tending the Jacobite wounded during and after the 1745 rebellion was deemed a treasonable act. Dr James Stratton was tried for tending the Jacobite garrison at Carlisle, and Chief Justice Wills made the ruling plain: 'It is objected that it don't appear [Dr Stratton] had arms. All are participants in aiding or assisting; and are parties in levying war, and surgeons are necessary, so are drummers.'[15]

During the ill-fated campaign Prince Charles suffered a series of illnesses en route and was treated, *inter alia*, for influenza at Bannockburn (5–16 January 1746), pneumonia and scarlet fever (February–March 1746) by the royal doctors in the entourage. Again the doctors are not identified in the official Stuart Papers. In exile, Charles's debauched and alcoholic life was brought to an end by the stroke that killed him on 30 January 1788. At first his cadaver was buried in the vaults of Frascati Cathedral, before being taken to St Peter's, Rome. His brother, dubbed

HRH and HE Henry Benedict, Cardinal Duke of York, succeeded him as King Henry IX in Jacobite parlance. He received a pension from George III and was tended by the Pope's physician Dr Laurenti, among others. Henry died at Frascati on 13 July 1801 and was buried with his family in the Stuart vault at St Peter's. The Stuart line of the exiled monarchs was passed on through Charles Emanuel IV of Sardinia (d. 1819), and thence to the descendants of Duke Albrecht of Bavaria (d. 1996). But the Stuarts in exile had no more use for royal doctors who risked a charge of treason for their collaboration.

CHAPTER FIVE

THE PRISONER AT WINDSOR: GEORGE III AND HIS ROYAL DOCTORS

It was during the long reign of King George III – 'Farmer George' to his subjects – that royal physicians began to enjoy greater political prominence in the public eye than ever before. The reason was the apparent declining mental state of the monarch and its consequences to state and people. Contemporary journals and diaries show in detail for the first time the difficulties royal doctors faced in dealing with royal patients, and illustrate with painful clarity the sufferings of royal patients at the hands of their chosen practitioners.

George III's court included physicians and surgeons of the highest achievement of their day. Doctors like Sir John Pringle (1707–82) had attained a position of great influence in scientific circles. Before he was appointed physician to George III, Pringle had been Joint-Professor of Pneumatics (Metaphysics) and Moral Philosophy at Edinburgh University and physician-general to George's forces in Flanders. He was present at the battle of Culloden as senior medical officer and physician-in-ordinary in the suite of Prince William Augustus, Duke of Cumberland. From 1749 he began to attend various members of the royal family. By 1761 Pringle was physician to the household of Queen Charlotte before progressing to physician-extraordinary and then physician-in-ordinary, and in 1768 he included among his patients the king's mother, Princess Augusta, Dowager Princess of Wales, with a salary of £100 per annum.

Then there was William Heberden the Younger (1767–1845), a prominent medical author who became physician-in-ordinary to Queen Charlotte in 1806 and to the king in 1809. Another man of European reputation was John Hunter (1728–93), the distinguished surgeon and anatomist who became surgeon-extraordinary to George III in 1776, while his brother William (1718–83) held the position of physician-extraordinary to Queen Charlotte.

Yet all of them laboured with great difficulty. Apart from a dearth of clinical apparatus and effective medicines, court etiquette and protocol hindered them from making a detailed clinical evaluation of the monarch, either physically or verbally. The king, for instance, could be neither touched nor questioned. The doctors further worked in a medical tradition that had not changed for decades and still gave credence to the body being affected by any of four 'humours', which were held to determine temperament and health. An example of this is found in the writings of the statesman George Grenville, 1st Marquis of Buckingham (1753–1813). On 20 November 1788 he wrote about a diagnosis the royal doctors had made concerning George III's first really noticeable phase of mental disturbance:

> The cause to which they all agree to ascribe it, is the force of a humour which was beginning to show itself in the legs, when the King's imprudence drove it from thence into the bowels; and the medicines which they were then obliged to use for the preservation of his life have repelled it upon the brain . . . The physicians are now endeavouring . . . to bring it down again into the legs, which nature had originally pointed out as the best mode of discharge.[1]

King George III was born Prince George William Frederick on 4 June 1738, at Norfolk House, St James's Square, London, the eldest son and second of the nine offspring of Frederick Lewis, Prince of Wales, and his wife Augusta, Princess of Saxe-Gotha-Altenburg (1719–72). He was two months premature and his survival was put down to the good feeding and attention given to him by his wet-nurse Mary Smith. Prince George's life was transformed in 1751 when his father died unexpectedly. The young prince now became Duke of Edinburgh and Prince of Wales, and heir to the throne of his grandfather George II. By now he had grown into a lad described by courtier Lady Louisa Stuart as 'silent, modest and easily abashed', but he was robust enough in health.

Just before Prince George came of age (at eighteen) in 1756, King George II proposed that his grandson have his own household at the residence of Savile House, Leicester Square. When necessary, however, he would be tended by doctors of George II's court. On 25 October 1760 news came of the death of his grandfather; Prince George was now King George III and his household was elevated to royal status.

A series of rapid and direct enquiries were undertaken in Germany to find a suitable bride for the young king. Skeletons were shaken out of dynastic cupboards within the aristocratic houses from Brunswick to Anhalf-Dessau. At length Princess Sophie Charlotte of Mecklenberg-Strelitz (1744–1820) was chosen, but with little enthusiasm by George III. They were married on 8 September 1761 and crowned at Westminster Abbey by Thomas Secker, Archbishop of Canterbury, on 22 September.

In the middle of February 1762, the eighteen-year-old Queen Charlotte was at chapel one Sunday, when events caused her to make a rapid exit. Sergeant-surgeon Sir Caesar Hawkins was called. He treated her 'giddiness' with his favourite of all remedies, namely 'blooding'. Three months later the 'giddiness' returned and the queen, who objected to the treatment, was bled again. The surgeon-*accoucheur* of the Middlesex Hospital, William Hunter, was called to attend the clearly pregnant queen, and he immediately terminated the bleeding regimes. The queen's labour began on 12 August and Prince George Augustus Frederick was born five days later at St James's Palace. He was the first of a long line: the family was to grow to fifteen children – eight princes and seven princesses – in the space of twenty-one years. Only the last three died at an early age; the remaining men survived long in spite of gluttony and gross lechery and the women despite the mind-numbing boredom of life at court.

Despite the fact that his reign had more than its fair share of wars, riots, political crises and domestic problems, from the Seven Years' War with France (1756–63) to the disastrous War of American Independence (1775–81), and from the Gordon Riots following the Catholic Relief Bill of 1780 to the desperate search for a trustworthy and capable prime minister, King George III was publicly remarkably well and level-headed. A study of the early

A BIZARRE ROYAL PATIENT

Eccentricity in Hanoverian royal patients was encountered daily by royal doctors and especially by James Lind, an Edinburgh medical graduate, former naval surgeon at Haslar Naval Hospital, and Fellow of the Edinburgh College of Physicians (1750).

As physician to the royal household (at Windsor), Dr Lind tended the daughter of King Frederick William II of Prussia, Princess Frederica Charlotte Ulrica Catherine (1767–1820), who was married to George III's second son Prince Frederick (1763–1827), Duke of York and Albany – the 'Grand Old Duke of York' of nursery rhyme. She was estranged from her husband and usually avoided her in-laws. But she loved animals – to the point of lunacy. At her home at Oatlands, near Weybridge, Surrey, she had some one hundred dogs; 'a yapping, baying horde', some of which were brought to Windsor. So Dr Lind had to remove a variety of Dutch pugs, French poodles and English miniatures from her bed whenever he attended her. Luckily he was spared the kangaroos, ostriches and monkeys which inhabited Oatlands.

Dr Lind knew her well enough to observe her surprisingly small feet. He recorded their length at 5.5 inches. Copies of her small, elaborate shoes were sold in all the best fashion houses and women risked deformity by trying to squeeze their feet into them. Dr Lind, it seems, visited her once at Oatlands, which he described as a 'household resembling a kennel'.

years of his life does not produce any instances of George III suffering from any very serious bodily or psychological debility. Yet in 1758, when he was Prince George of Wales, his governor, John, 2nd Lord Waldegrave (1715–63), commented:

> [*The Prince of Wales has*] a kind of unhappiness in his temper . . . When he is displeased . . . he becomes sullen and silent, and retires to his closet not to compose his mind by study or contemplation, but mainly to indulge the melancholic enjoyment of his ill humour. Even when the fit is ended, unfavourable symptoms may frequently return.[2]

By the time he was in his twenties some courtiers were noticing temperamental traits they would remember and pore over when

George III's deteriorating mental behaviour began to promote concern.

George III's health began to show signs of severe trouble during his wife's first pregnancy. From January to March 1762, and twice more in May and July, he complained of fever, coughing and insomnia, and royal physicians noted a rapid pulse and weight loss. They diagnosed consumption, and prescribed bleeding and blistering, and dosed him with asses' milk. In 1765 the king suffered a recurrence of the symptoms. Despite the application of the useless remedies of the day the king recovered – and remained free from the symptoms for over twenty years.

On 2 August 1786 royal doctors rushed to King George's side. As he alighted from his coach to attend a levée at St James's Palace, a woman approached him bearing a sheet of paper. Thinking she had a petition for his attention he reached for the paper, whereupon she produced a knife and lunged at his chest. The blade (of what was later discovered to be a fruit knife) was thin and the blow was awkward. So the king was unharmed save for a tear in the linen of his waistcoat. The woman, one Margaret Nicholson, was grabbed roughly by the sentries, at which the king intervened: 'The poor creature is mad. Do not hurt her. She has not hurt me.' The queen and her daughters were greatly upset when hearing of the attack and were dosed by the royal doctors with sal volatile.

In mid-October 1788 the king was assailed by a grave and puzzling illness. Although he had access to the best medical minds of the age, they were completely baffled by George III's ills. In the long term, the illness was to trigger several political crises and actions by royal doctors that were unprecedented in the history of the monarchy.

The king began to act out of character. Stomach pains led to loss of concentration. The resultant frustration preceded abrupt outbursts of bad temper. At 7.25 a.m. on the morning of 17 October 1788 the king sent for his physician Sir George Baker (1722–1809). A graduate of Cambridge, Baker was a prolific medical writer and important diarist. He wrote:

> I found His Majesty sitting up in his bed, his body being bent forward. He complained of a very acute pain in the pit

of the stomach shooting to the back and sides, and making respiration difficult and uneasy. This pain continued all day, though in a less degree of acuteness towards the evening; but it did not cease entirely until the bowels had been emptied. It was observable that, during the extreme severity of the pain the pulse was only at sixty strokes in a minute, and that the pulse became quicker in proportion as the pain abated. At night it was at ninety.[3]

Unperturbed, Sir George cautioned his royal patient to be sure to change his stockings when returning from walks on wet grass. The previous day the king had walked to St James's and gorged on pears at supper. Sir George prescribed castor oil and senna to purge his system, and laudanum to placate it again.

Sir George further records his consultation with the king on the afternoon of 22 October 1788:

I was received by His Majesty in a very unusual manner, of which I had not the least expectation. The look of his eyes, the tone of his voice, every gesture and his whole deportment represented a person in the most furious passion of anger.[4]

At first Baker diagnosed the stomach pain as a dose of biliousness and consulted with the other royal physicians, including Benjamin Hoadley – erstwhile physician to George II – and Thomas Gisborne (d. 1806), and they concluded that the bile in the king's stomach was not going the right way through his system, and pronounced him to be suffering from gout. By this time the king had formed a derogatory opinion of his physicians and refused to take their prescribed medicines, as well as ignoring their advice to stop riding. He did agree, however, to go to Cheltenham to take the waters. The king now pronounced himself well enough to tour the Gloucestershire countryside and his curious, eccentric caravan was witnessed by crowds of bemused onlookers. Worse was to come.

Courtiers began to note the king's long periods without sleep and his strange garrulousness. Baron John Baker Holroyd, later 1st Earl of Sheffield (1735–1821), noted at an audience how the king 'talked incessantly for sixteen hours, to divert him from

GEORGE III'S MEDICAL HOUSEHOLD

ote: This list is *not* comprehensive. Right up to the nineteenth century official royal household lists were not all-embracing and even the Court Rolls compiled by Clippingdale, Munk and Plarr should be treated with caution. Dates of appointment are unclear in many sources. The medical and surgical practitioners herein listed were 'official appointments', not just doctors who 'attended' the court from time to time.

George III: Born 4 June 1738. Reigned 1760–1820. Died 29 January 1820.
Matthew Baillie (1761–1823). Physician-in-extraordinary.
Sir George Baker (1722–1809). Physician, 1776.
John Dollond (1706–61). Optician.
Sir James Earle (1745–1817). Surgeon-extraordinary.
Thomas Gisborne (d. 1806). Physician-in-ordinary.
Sir Henry Halford (1766–1844). Sergeant-surgeon, 1809.
Sir Caesar Hawkins (1711–86). Sergeant-surgeon.
William Heberden the Younger (1767–1845). Physician-in-ordinary.
John Hunter (1728–93). Surgeon-extraordinary.
James Lind (1736–1812). Physician to the royal household.
Sir Francis Milman (1746–1821). Physician, 1806.
Sir Lucas Pepys (1742–1830). Physician-extraordinary 1777; advanced to Physician-in-ordinary, 1792.
Sir John Pringle (1707–82). Physician, 1774.
Henry Revell Reynolds (1745–1811). Physician-in-ordinary, 1806.
Peter Shaw (1694–1763). Physician-in-ordinary, 1760.
Sir Noah Thomas (1720–92). Physician-in-ordinary, 1775.
Sir Jonathan Wathen Waller (1769–1853) also known as Dr Phipps.
Robert Whytt (1714–66). First Physician to George III in Scotland – a country the king never visited.

A number of doctors who attended the king during his periods of mental distress were not official appointees. They included: Samuel Foart Simmons (1750–1813) in 1803 and 1811; Francis Willis (1718–1807) in 1788; and William Heberden the Elder (1710–1801).

which (courtiers) endeavoured to turn to writing, at length he began to compose notes on Don Quixote'.[5]

The royal doctors informed the enquiring government ministers of William Pitt's administration that the monarch was suffering from 'delirium', while Sir George Baker described the condition as 'an intire alienation of mind'; Baker agreed that the king was becoming less capable of carrying out his duties as monarch.

The situation deteriorated. George III began to suffer hallucinations. He believed London was drowning, he aimed blows at his servants as they tried to dress him, and wrote a flurry of memos to fellow monarchs abroad on a variety of farcical subjects. To the embarrassment of the court ladies his language became obscene and he fancied himself in love with, and married to, the straitlaced lady-in-waiting, Elizabeth, wife of Henry Herbert, 10th Earl of Pembroke (1734–94). Lapsing into fluent German, which itself was out of character, he told the queen that he had always disliked her and that she was completely mad. The next minute, in a sideswipe at his doctors, he was saying: 'The queen is my physician.' Yet he had some insight into his own condition. Out of the blue one day he sank his head on the shoulder of his son Frederick, Duke of York (1763–1827), and cried: 'I wish to God I may die, for I am going to be mad.'

Baffled by the royal malady, the court physicians went into a huddle. Was the monarch's obvious mental condition of organic or psychological origin? None knew for sure and none was able to advise on the best form of treatment. Sir George Baker was approaching the end of his tether. When the king was assailed by his worst outbursts it was exhausting following him from room to room as he went on the rampage, shouting: 'What? What?' or, 'Hey, Hey,' at all he met, or who tried to converse with him. He alternately lashed out at servants or bestowed state honours on them when he encountered them in corridors. In a state of near nervous collapse Baker consulted colleague after colleague.

Groom of the bedchamber, the Hon. William Harcourt noted that a whole 'medical tribe' parlayed with Baker in the corridors and ante-chambers of wherever the king happened to be. First Dr Heberden the Elder (1710–1801) was brought out of retirement at Windsor to consult, then Dr Richard Warren (1731–97), physician to the Prince of Wales, was called in, with the prominent private practitioner and medical lecturer Henry Revell Reynolds (1745–1811), to compare notes with physician Sir Lucas Pepys (1742–1830).

The presence of Dr Warren caused the king to fly into a paroxysm of rage. One of the Prince of Wales's set, Warren was a Whig. The queen considered Warren to be a Whig spy at the Tory court, and the king ordered the doctor from his presence, endeavouring to assist the medic's exit with blows. Courtiers believed that in revenge for this Warren prescribed a cruel regime for the king's illness, including a blistering of his shaven scalp to coax out 'the poisonous matter from his brain'. The king now suffered a whole welter of appalling treatments: plaster of cantharides and mustard were set to draw the 'humours' from his legs, and leeches were applied to his forehead. Purges, emetics, sedatives followed one after another. Warren went about scandalously telling all who would listen that the king was a lunatic; he told Lady Spencer, the Duchess of Devonshire's mother, '*Rex noster insanit*', couching his words in Latin for dramatic effect.

For the first time the opinions of the royal doctors were solicited on a large scale for public consumption. The Whigs, in particular, were eager to have news of the king's condition. As the opposition to Pitt's Tory administration, they were eager for proof that the king was so incapable of ruling that a regency might be needed – bringing their willing tool the Prince of Wales to prominence. Newspapers like the *Morning Post* and *The Times* jockeyed for news and rumour took the place of reality. The political, literary and social salons of London were the breeding grounds of ridiculous tales. One such tale, which was to end up in print, recounted how the king, when out walking in Windsor Great Park, had approached an oak tree. After shaking one of its lower branches in greeting

> Here well-dressed Reynolds lies.
> As great a beau as ever;
> We may perhaps see one as wise,
> But sure a smarter never.
>   *On Henry Revell Reynolds*
>   *(1745–1811), medical attendant*
>   *to George III*

he entered into conversation with its bole, apparently believing it to be his kinsman and fellow-monarch Frederick William II, King of Prussia.

The novelty of royal doctors issuing public reports on the king's health became commonplace as the capital thirsted for news. The royal doctors were circumspect, but lack of news often led to individual doctors being threatened. Sir George Baker's carriage was stopped by a mob who jostled for news, and Sir Lucas Pepys and others were sent intimidating letters by the king's lowly supporters, who were fearful that their monarch was being murdered. Sir Lucas complained to the Prince of Wales that he feared for his life.

A curious physician now entered the royal milieu. Dr Francis Willis (1718–1807), former Vice-President of Brasenose College, Oxford, and erstwhile physician at Lincoln General Hospital, had entered holy orders before embarking on a medical career. It is clear that he first practised medicine without a licence, but the University of Oxford granted him medical degrees. Willis had an easy expertise in the treatment of mental cases and in 1776 opened an asylum at Gretford, near Stamford, Lincolnshire. There he implemented his own idiosyncratic way of dealing with patients. He dressed males and females in the garb of the senior servant class and set them to labouring and domestic tasks around the hospital estate. Willis came to court on the recommendation of Elizabeth, Countess of Harcourt (d. 1833), whose demented mother had been successfully treated by Willis.

Since he was not a member of the Royal College of Surgeons, Willis was deemed a 'mountebank' by the royal doctors at court. His opinions were sniggered at behind his back. Loud guffaws met the retelling of the fact that Willis forswore China tea for his patients as it stimulated 'nervous disorders'. Few who met him for the first time at Dr Warren's house in London could stand Willis's 'basilisk' stare for more than a few seconds. The stare was his stock-in-trade to 'master' patients to his will and the king himself was soon to be subject to its hypnotic power.

Nor was Willis welcomed with open arms by the king. Colonel the Hon. Robert Fulke Greville recorded their first encounter on 5 December 1788:

The King: 'Sir, your dress and appearance bespeaks of the Church. Do you belong to it?'

Dr Willis: 'I did formerly, but latterly I have attended chiefly to Physick.'

The King: 'I am sorry for it. You have quitted a profession I have always loved, and you have embraced one I most heartily detest.'

Dr Willis: 'Sir, our Saviour Himself went about healing the sick.'

The King: 'Yes, yes, but had not £700 (a year) for it.'[6]

In agreeing to treat the king, Willis insisted on three stipulations. He was to address the king directly with comments and questions without the protocol of 'leave to do so'; he was to have complete authority over the patient in matters of treatment; and he was to have access to the royal patient at all times. With some reservations, his terms were agreed by the king's ministers.

From the first Willis subjected the king to a strict regime, and the trio of 'keepers' he had brought with him from his Lincolnshire asylum forced the king into a straitjacket when he became difficult. Willis also had him confined to a custom-built chair for restraint, which the king dubbed his 'coronation chair'.

Assisting Dr Willis was his son Dr John Willis, who kept a journal of the king's condition. An example of his entries shows how the king's progress was monitored: 'Ungovernable through the night . . . Constrained at 5. Tongue whiteish. Pulse 108. Under constraint most of the day. High spirits, jocose and pertinent.'[7] It was through John Willis that the other royal doctors enquired of the king's condition, although none of them considered him to be a 'proper physician' because he was also not a member of the Royal College. Still they suffered him, for it kept them away from the king's verbal abuse and physical blows.

Willis continued to use the more traditional medicines of the day, with a strict regime of calomel and camphor, quinine and digitalis, but had his own firm methods of controlling the king. Although he despised all doctors, the king seems to have grown to respect Dr Willis Sr and cooperated with him more than with any other; one key to this was that at no time was Willis in awe of his patient's position, and he boldly 'fixed' the king with his eye.

Slowly the king began to be more controlled in Willis's presence. Previously he had loudly raged in the presence of royal doctors, yet he seems to have calmed himself more when Willis was in attendance. This was rewarded by Willis, who allowed the king to shave himself, under supervision, and organised meetings for the king with close members of the royal family, which previously had caused him much anxiety. Of one such visit Willis recorded:

> I led Princess Amelia [*the unmarried, youngest surviving royal child*] myself. His Majesty showed the greatest mark of parental affection I ever saw. The other physicians protested, but I told them I was sent to make use of my own discretion, and they could not think themselves proper judges of it. That or the next evening he had a quarter-hour interview with the Queen . . . Such occurrences can scarce be too frequent, as it comforts the patient to think that he is with his family and they are affectionate to him.[8]

Although still largely hostile to him, George III did respond to the treatment Dr Willis prescribed. On the appropriate occasions Willis would express the opinion that the king might make a full recovery. The other royal doctors shook their heads in disagreement. It was they and not Willis who prepared the bulletins on the king's health for public consumption, and Richard Warren continued to emphasise that the monarch was permanently in 'a decided state of insanity'. Queen Charlotte pressed to see the bulletins before they were issued and asked that they be toned down if she felt that his insanity was given too much emphasis, or that his periods of remission were overlooked.

Certainly the king's indisposition prompted a political crisis and his eldest son, the Prince of Wales, had to deputise for him on state and administrative occasions. Of all the royal doctors, Richard Warren was the most politically orientated and he encouraged the Prince of Wales and his brother the Duke of York to promote the Whig interest. On 12 February 1789 the Regency Bill was passed in the House of Common; as the Whigs were already riven with factions, William Pitt and the Tories deployed various tactics to limit Whig influence over and through the Prince of Wales.

As these political developments took place the king's health improved, and he was able to endure the three-hour Thanksgiving Service in his honour at St Paul's Cathedral on St George's Day, 23 April 1789. Despite the international repercussions of the storming of the Bastille in Paris during July 1789, George III's health continued stable and remained so for the next twelve years. Many rejoiced at the king's recovery but his royal doctors had better reason than most to celebrate. Handsome monetary rewards were now disbursed. For every visit a royal doctor made he was paid 30 guineas when at Windsor and £10 at Kew. Records show that Sir George Baker received £1,380, Dr Francis Willis £1,000 per annum for twenty years, and Dr John Willis £500 per annum for life.[9]

During February 1801 the king's symptoms returned. Historians have opined that his mind was disturbed by the Roman Catholic Emancipation legislation (which he had opposed) and the situation was exacerbated by the change of prime minister, Henry Addington (1757–1844) replacing William Pitt. Whatever the cause, the royal doctors now recorded the reappearance of dark-coloured urine, stomach pains, a fast pulse, muscular weakness and the frightening delirium. It was clear to the royal doctors that the events of 1788 were to be repeated, and to the king's dismay the Drs Willis were summoned to attend. As before, they were optimistic of a complete recovery, and the monarch was soon well enough to receive ex-Prime Minister Peel and to chair a meeting of the Privy Council.

> When patients come to I,
> I physics, bleeds, and sweats 'em;
> Then – if they choose to die –
> What's that to I –
> I LET'S 'EM.
> *Pun on the name of John Coakley Lettsom (1744–1815), who once attended George III*

Despite this improvement, his family remained worried about George's progress and Princess Elizabeth (1770–1840), his third surviving daughter, persuaded the Willises to stay, although both George III himself and the other royal doctors fumed at their continued presence. This time, though, the king rebelled against the Willises' treatment regime and they threatened to detain him by force. When their 'keepers' arrived to do just that, the king said to Francis Willis: 'Sir, I will never forgive you whilst I live.'

From March until May the Willises kept their royal patient confined at the White House, Kew, despite the accusation of 'kidnap' by the other doctors. By June the king was well enough for sea-bathing at Weymouth and a period of remission ensued.

Some of the royal doctors always averred that the King's mental problems were aggravated when he caught a chill. So they nodded in self-satisfaction when a sniffling king had another of his 'attacks' following a chill caught from wearing wet clothes in February 1804. The new Prime Minister Henry Addington was keen to send for the Willises but the king's sons, the dukes of Kent and Cumberland, were adamant against it, threatening that the Willises would be refused access to the royal grounds.

Instead Samuel Foart Simmons (1750–1813), Physician to St Luke's Hospital for the Insane, London, was called. Simmons's treatment was similar to that of the Willises, and the king liked him no better – that 'horrid doctor', he called him. Fortunately this attack was short-lived and the king was on the mend by March.

Although in a state of irritability, the king was able to undertake his royal duties and went once more to Weymouth to recuperate. This time physician Sir Francis Milman (1746–1821) advised against sea bathing. All the time pressures were building on the king; he was worried that his kingdom was suffering politically and economically from the long war with France; his sight was starting to fail and his capacity to concentrate had shortened. Then, on 2 November 1810, Princess Amelia died at Augusta Lodge, Windsor, from pulmonary tuberculosis. Very soon, the king was gripped again by his malady.

Each of the monarch's physicians did a tour of duty and a succession of doctors came and went at Windsor: Matthew Baillie, Henry Reynolds, Robert Battiscombe, William Heberden and the Willises were assisted when required by Windsor apothecary David Dundas, surgeon-apothecary John Meadows and one Mr Briand, keeper of the mad-house at Kensington. Yet it fell to Sir Henry Halford to advise that Dr Simmons be recalled to Windsor. This was agreed and Simmons arrived with an entourage of assistants demanding 'sole management of the King'.

THE MEDICAL HOUSEHOLD OF QUEEN SOPHIA CHARLOTTE

(19 May 1744–17 November 1818. Married George III, 8 September 1761)

Mark Akenside (1721–70), 1761.
Sir George Baker. Physician, 1776.
William Bromfield (1712–92). Surgeon.
William Heberden the Younger. Physician-in-ordinary.
William Hunter (1718–83). Physician-extraordinary.
Joseph Letherland (1699–1764). Physician.
William George Maton (1774–1835). Physician-extraordinary, 1816.
William Wright (1777–1860). Surgeon aurist-in-ordinary.

THE MEDICAL HOUSEHOLDS OF GEORGE III'S CHILDREN

Prince George Augustus Frederick, Prince of Wales (later Prince Regent and George IV)

Anthony Addington (1713–90). Physician, 1788.
John Birch (*c.* 1745–1815). Surgeon-extraordinary (as Prince Regent).
Sir Gilbert Blane (1749–1834). Physician-in-ordinary, 1785.
Thomas Christie (1773–1829). Physician-extraordinary (as Prince Regent).
Sir Walter Farquhar (1738–1819). Physician-in-ordinary, 1796.
John Latham (1761–1843). Physician-in-ordinary, 1795.
Sir William Rawson (1783–1827). Surgeon and oculist-extraordinary (as Prince Regent).
William Saunders (1743–1817), Physician (as Prince Regent).
Richard Warren (1731–97). Physician, 1787.

Princess Caroline Amelia Elizabeth (1768–1821), Princess of Wales.

John Mayo (1761–1818). Physician.

Prince William Henry, Duke of Clarence and St Andrews (later William IV).

Sir Andrew Halliday (1781–1839). Domestic Physician, *c.* 1822.
William Beattie (1793–1875). Physician.

Prince Edward, Duke of Kent and Strathearn (1767–1820).

Augustin Sayer (1790–1861). Physician.
Sir Joseph de Courcey Laffan (1786–1848). Physician-in-ordinary.

Princess Victoria Mary Louisa (1786–1861), Duchess of Kent. (Daughter-in-law of George III.)
David Daniel David (1777–1841). Obstetric physician: attended the duchess at the birth of the future Queen Victoria, 1819.
William George Maton.
John Merriman (1714–1839). General medical attendant.

Prince Ernest Augustus, Duke of Cumberland (1771–1851).
Thomas Jones. Physician, 1803.
Sir Jonathan Wathen Waller (or Phipps). Physician and surgeon.

Prince Augustus Frederick, Duke of Sussex (1773–1843).
Charles Badham (1780–1845). Physician.
Edward James Seymour (1796–1866). Physician.

Prince Frederick Augustus, Duke of York and Albany (1763–1827).
James Atkinson (1759–1839). Surgeon.

Reluctantly this was agreed to. George III became so violent that he once more had to be placed in a straitjacket. Again he sank back into his old eccentric ways, including his infatuation with Lady Pembroke, who was now seventy-three years of age. His behaviour became more 'indecent and obscene', with constant blasphemings and ramblings. As the queen refused to 'pleasure him', he threatened to take a mistress, identifying court ladies such as the Duchess of Rutland and Lady Georgina Buckley as candidates.

For some time responsibility for the care of the king had fallen to the Cabinet, as most of the royal family had signed a declaration to this effect. By now it was clear that the king had moved into a phase where he was incapable of ruling and a regency was again necessary. George, Prince of Wales, was sworn in as Prince Regent on 6 February 1811 and on the advice of Sir Henry Halford – who opined that a change would adversely affect the king's health – he desisted from replacing the administration of Prime Minister Spencer Percival (1762–1812).

George III, under strict restraint and kept apart from his family, slipped further into dementia at Windsor, which became the backcloth for his own fantasy world. Following a short visit to his apartments in June 1812, Queen Charlotte was never to see her husband again. Demoralised by years of anguish over his condition, the queen herself became progressively bad-tempered, quarrelled with her children and lived a solitary existence at Frogmore, where she sought solace in the gardens she created there.

Blind and deaf, George III was unable to register the death of Queen Charlotte at Kew Palace on 17 November 1818, although they had been estranged for years. Charlotte died a lonely and sick old woman, muttering to the end that the royal doctors had made her a pauper. The king's medical bills had drained her funds so much that the contents of Frogmore House were sold at Christie's in 1819 to provide income for her remaining daughters. Amusing himself by playing the flute and harpsichord, singing, and talking for hours to people long dead about his insane imaginings, the king grew weaker but more docile. Occasionally he would be well enough to take a walk with one of his sons. Waterloo veteran Colonel Rees Howell Gronow (1784–1865) recorded in his *Reminiscences*:

I once saw George III walking with his favourite son, the Duke of York, with whom he talked incessantly, repeating his 'Yes, yes, yes, Frederick' in his usual loud voice. His beard was of unusual length, and he stooped very much. He wore the Windsor uniform with a large cocked hat, something like that in which Frederick the Great is usually represented. The doctors walked behind the King, which seemed greatly to annoy him, and he was constantly looking round.[10]

By Christmas 1819 George's paroxysms had returned. Charlotte Georgina, Lady Jerningham, recorded a little of the king's last hours in her letters:

A few minutes before (he died) he extended his Arms, and bade his Attendants raise him up. The doctors signified to his Attendants not to do so, in the Supposition that the Effort would extinguish life but upon his repeating the request, they obeyed and he thanked them. His Lips were parched and

Occasionally wetted with a Sponge. He, with perfect presence of mind, said: – 'Do not wet my Lips but when I open My Mouth.' And when done he added, 'I thank you, it does me good.' This was told by the Duke of York, who was present, to the Duchess of Clarence [his sister-in-law]. She said that it gave her pleasure to see how much he was affected in speaking of his Father.[11]

The royal doctors recorded the king's death at 8.32 p.m. on 29 January 1820.

During his reign – and long after – the royal doctors puzzled over the king's condition. They never knew what they were trying to treat. Speculation remained rife even among the most scientific minds within the royal medical household. What had caused the king to go mad? Royal doctors did not demur when the word mad was used in connection with the king, and for decades the supposed royal insanity was accepted. George III's granddaughter, Queen Victoria, feared that she would go mad just like him.

Gossips created a whole range of reasons for the king's madness, and the *London Chronicle* even suggested: 'The King's late disorder was owing solely to his drinking the water of Cheltenham.'[12] Long after his death royal doctors tried to plumb the king's character for clues. Just after the Crimean War, and in consultation with his kinsman Sir William Fergusson (1808–77), surgeon-extraordinary to Queen Victoria, Dr John Fergusson sifted through the extant papers of George III's royal doctors and courtiers to see if he could find any hints to identify the king's malady. He drew up this chart of character traits, and starred certain of the characteristics that he deemed of relevance:

	collected		good humoured
	considerate	X	resentful
	courageous		hatred of flattery
	courteous	X	impatient
X	critical		kindly
	curious		meticulous
X	disconcerted	X	nervous
X	easily upset		niggardly

X	eccentric	X	obsessive
	expectant	X	obstinate
	faithful		pious
	fortitudinous		priggish
	friendly		self-congratulatory
	generous	X	shy
	genial		tactless
	gentle	X	worried and anxious

Fergusson also plotted a chart of the king's illnesses from the age of fifty to his death at seventy-five, and marvelled at the fact that the king was only 'deranged' for a 'a few months in total'. Again, the king's blindness and deafness, his isolation at Windsor and his ultimate senile dementia added to the untrue perception of the monarch's perpetual madness.

Dr Fergusson strongly believed that there was an impalpable and undivorceable link between bodily and mental health, and that George III's condition was caused by pressure on his mind from his royal duties. He wanted to pursue the matter further. Would Queen Victoria be willing to cooperate? Fergusson consulted his royal doctor kinsman on how to approach the queen, to seek permission to study any royal papers in the collection at Windsor Castle that might be relevant. Sir William Fergusson wrote back to his cousin: 'Her Majesty is very sentient on the state of her royal grandfather's mind and says that any examination of his health would be "TOO HORRID".' Fergusson dropped his researches.[13]

In the 1920s doctors speculated that George III was suffering from either depressive mania or schizophrenia, but no firm conclusions were reached. Then, in 1967, two medical researchers set out a new assessment of George III's ills. Dr Ida Macalpine, erstwhile psychiatrist at St Bartholomew's Hospital, London, and her son Dr Richard Hunter, physician in psychological medicine at the National Hospital for Nervous Diseases, London, averred that George III had suffered from *variegata porphyria*. The disease porphyria is fundamentally 'a group of largely inherited disorders which interfere with the ability of the body to make the red pigment of blood'. Dubbed the 'royal malady', variegata porphyria is the form that affects the skin, causes abdominal pains, temporary mental disorder, discoloured urine and a variety of other ailments – all of which were exhibited by George III.

Drs Macalpine and Hunter based their researches on the diaries and papers of royal doctors such as Sir George Baker and Sir Henry Halford, on the official letters of royal appointees Drs Warren, Pepys, Addington and Reynolds, and on the observations of royal physicians Drs Matthew Baillie and the Willises, as well as those who proffered 'systems' for dealing with the insane, like doctors Thomas Arnold, William Battie and John Brown. Their now well-publicised porphyria theory is widely accepted, but George III's malady still stirs up interest, with its ramifications for the descendants of Queen Victoria in Britain and Europe.

A recent theory is that George III suffered from lead-poisoning – and so the theorising goes on. But whatever caused the king to be ill, the whole episode certainly baffled his royal doctors.[14]

CHAPTER SIX

ASSASSINATION ATTEMPT AT ST JAMES'S: ROYAL DOCTORS AND THE DUKE OF CUMBERLAND

Three royal doctors were involved in one of the most curious assassination attempts ever to be perpetrated at the British court. Sir Henry Halford, erstwhile physician to the Middlesex Hospital, was already a frequent visitor to the royal court, having been appointed physician-extraordinary to George III in 1793. Sir Everard Home (1756–1832), surgeon to St George's Hospital since 1793 and sergeant-surgeon to the King, 1808, was a prominent member of the Royal College of Surgeons and well known too as a consultant to the aristocracy. Surgeon Dr J. Wathen Phipps (1769–1853) was a regular attender to the health of the Duke of Cumberland.[1]

Prince Ernest Augustus, Duke of Cumberland and Teviotdale, was born at Queen's House, St James's Park, on Wednesday, 5 June 1771, the fifth son and eighth child of George III and Queen Charlotte. His birth was supervised by the distinguished surgeon-*accoucheur* William Hunter, who had been physician-extraordinary to Queen Charlotte since 1764. Prince Ernest Augustus grew up in the 'spartan simplicity and stern morality' of his father's court. At the age of fifteen he was sent with his brother, Prince Adolphus Frederick, Duke of Cambridge (1774–1850), to Hanover, of which state his father was Elector, to study at the University of Göttingen, which had been founded by his great-grandfather George II.

To enhance their station the princes were promoted Knights of the Garter before leaving England. From Göttingen the princes went on to undertake training with the Prussian army. On 20 April 1792 France declared war against Leopold of Austria, a conflict which the Prussians joined in July, and the princes now served in the subsequent Flanders campaign. Prince Ernest

Augustus continued his military career, leading his own regiment as Lieutenant-Colonel of the 9th Hanoverian Hussars. He was wounded at Tournai and returned for a while to convalesce at the court at Windsor. In due course and now a major-general he rejoined his regiment and completed his military duties in February 1796.

For some time Prince Ernest Augustus had been suffering with inflammation of the eye, about which he consulted the oculist Dr Wathen Phipps. He now settled down to a life of privilege and a little real work, although he was promoted privy councillor in 1799, the year his father created him a royal duke. The title Duke of Cumberland had been held before him by Charles I's nephew Prince Rupert, Count Palatine of the Rhine, but by this time the title was associated with later and lesser holders, like Prince Henry Frederick, brother of George III and the infamous Prince William Augustus, dubbed 'Butcher Cumberland' by the Jacobites after the battle of Culloden.

As the war clouds continually loomed on the continent, the new Duke of Cumberland became involved in home defence. In 1805 he became Chancellor of Trinity College, Dublin. Today, justifiably or not, the Duke of Cumberland is remembered as a hate figure in royal history. The scar on his face and his 'dead eye' make him 'the pantomime ogre of Queen Victoria's childhood'.[2] The lifelong series of slanders, libels and calumnies against him were to begin with the events described here, but it is important to understand the contemporary public view of the duke in order to fully comprehend his persistently bad press. In 1829 it was asserted that one Captain Garth 'was the incestuous son of the Duke of Cumberland and his sister, Princess Sophia'.[3] His name was also linked in sexual liaison with court ladies, including Lady Graves, which led to her husband's suicide.[4]

The duke was particularly despised by one man, Sir John Conroy, comptroller of the household of the Duchess of Kent, Cumberland's sister-in-law. Conroy feared the duke's influence – and the demise of his own – over the duchess's daughter, the Princess Victoria, and sought to blacken the duke's name whenever he could. After all, the duke was next in line to the throne after Princess Victoria. Conroy terrified the Duchess of Kent with subliminal suggestions that the duke might poison

Princess Victoria, so that he could take the throne himself. This maternal disquiet alarmed Princess Victoria, turning her mind against her uncle Cumberland, whose radical views against the Catholic penal laws and the Regency Bill only exacerbated her enduring dislike of him when she became queen. All this lay in the future but the seeds of dissension were sown on 31 May 1810.

On that fateful Wednesday the duke dined with the administrators of the Royal Naval Hospital at Greenwich, of which he was a governor. He then returned to his apartments at York House, St James's Palace, to change for a charity concert of ancient music at Hanover Square Rooms. The duke came home about midnight and was attended by his valet, Cornelius Neale. The duke's bedchamber overlooked Cleveland Place and was set next to a dressing-room and lavatory in which were two large walk-in cupboards. The duke's bed was set in a recess. The room could be entered by two other doors, one leading into a sitting-room, known as the West Yellow Room, and the other into a narrow passage to the duty valet's room. Having seen the duke, sporting his thick-padded nightcap, safely to bed in his four-poster, Neale locked the door to the state apartment and returned to the valet's waiting-room.

Around 2.30 a.m. on 1 April, the duke was awakened abruptly, he later told physician Sir Henry Halford, by a swishing sound, which he thought was a bat fluttering about his bed canopy. Almost immediately he sustained a couple of heavy blows. Although he was short-sighted, he saw the flash of a blade descending. One blow sliced into his thick nightcap, and would certainly have gone deeper had it not been deflected by the bed curtains. The duke automatically fumbled for the bell cord to raise the alarm, all the while fending off the blows, one of which almost severed his fingers. Blood pouring from his wounds splattered the portrait of the French royalist soldier Charles Pichegru, some 8ft up the wall.

The duke managed to jump out of the bed and made for the door into the nearby passage, sustaining a wound in his thigh from another lunge by his assassin. The blow was then deflected, gouging a large splinter from the door, as the duke screamed: 'Neale, Neale, I am murdered.' Within seconds Neale was at his master's side. The duke indicated that his attacker was still in the room. Neale grabbed a poker from the fireplace and rushed into the duke's bedroom, noting that the door of the West Yellow Room, which he had previously locked, was standing open. On the floor of the room lay the duke's bloodstained regimental sabre. The perpetrator of the savage attack had vanished.[5]

Guiding his master to a chair, Neale set about raising the alarm. He stumbled downstairs to the porter's office and roused the duty porter Benjamin Smith with the words 'His Royal highness is murdered'. By this time the blood-drenched duke, sabre in hand, was making his way down the staircase shouting orders to the guards to fasten all doors. The group around the duke was now joined by his housekeeper, Mrs Anne Neale and his German servant Matthew Graslin.

Mrs Neale sent for Sir Henry Halford and the surgeon Sir Everard Home. The duke was almost fainting with loss of blood when he was examined by the doctors. The tendons and sinews of the duke's right hand were badly cut, as was the joint of his left wrist. There were deep wounds on his neck, head and arms. As Sir Everard dressed the wounds and Sir Henry prepared draughts, the duke enquired of his other valet, the Corsican Joseph Sellis, why he had not come when the duke shouted? On receiving no answer, the duke motioned to Mrs Neale, Graslin and Smith to go and look for Sellis. Obeying, they found the servant's door locked. Smith banged on it with the hilt of his sword. Again, there was no answer and they returned to the duke's chamber.

From his bed the duke, now swathed in bandages, instructed Neale to search the room for clues to his assassins. Inside one of the large walk-in closets was found a scabbard, a pair of slippers (marked in Indian ink with the name 'J. Sellis'), a water bottle and a shaded lantern. Moreover the presence of the crumpled linen and bed-cushions stored there indicated that it had been the assassin's hiding place.

Meanwhile the duke was still puzzled by the absence of his loyal Sellis and dispatched Mrs Neale and Smith to go again to the servant's room. Within minutes they were back in a state of agitation, reporting gruesome sounds coming from Sellis's room. Joined by Sergeants Creighton and Davenhall, and a group of Coldstream Guard sentries, the servants found Sellis's room door now ajar. Stealthily the door was pushed open and the porter was the first to react to the scene of carnage they witnessed: 'Good God,' he said. 'Mr Sellis has cut his throat.'

The group of servants and soldiers gathered in the doorway. Sellis's inert body lay on the bed. His throat was severed from ear to ear and the head lay unnaturally loosely. Blood was running from the gaping wound to soak the bedding, drench the cadaver and seep on to the floor. A cut-throat razor with a white handle lay on the chest of drawers, some 2ft away from the bed, alongside a basin of water tinted with gore.[6]

Sir Everard Home was just finishing his dressing of the duke's wounds when he was called to Sellis's room. Somewhat unnecessarily he pronounced the servant dead and examined the neck lacerations. Sir Everard did not demur from the opinion that Sellis had killed himself and was not murdered. Yet anyone with only a smattering of anatomical knowledge and common sense would have seen that Sellis could not have killed himself in such a manner. Later Sir Everard remarked to Sir Henry Halford that he thought Sellis's throat had been cut by a right-handed person (Sellis was left-handed). Sir Everard and Sir Henry also knew that their royal patient was short-tempered. Had he killed Sellis? Sir Everard dutifully composed this official report:

> I went to [*Sellis's*] apartment, found the body lying on his side on the bed, without his coat and neck-cloth, the throat cut so effectively that he could not have survived above a minute or two. The length and direction of the wound were such as left no doubt of its being by his own hand. Any struggle would have made it irregular. He had not even changed his position; his hands lay as they do in a person who has fainted; they had no marks of violence upon them . . .[7]

Back in the duke's room the Prince of Wales had arrived from Carlton House, and the Duke of Sussex from Brooke's club, to see their brother. While they commiserated with him, Neale searched Sellis's room and his clothes on the duke's instructions. He found a necktie which had been partially cut

CORONERS OF THE ROYAL HOUSEHOLD

The Sellis case brought to the public eye the role of the royal coroner, who had, significantly, chosen his jury from the City of London and not from St James's Palace.

The position of coroner to the royal household today is within the royal medical household. In medieval times the position was known as coroner of the verge. The holder had jurisdiction within the area where the monarch might be, or where the court was residing, and for twelve miles around. In those days the court had no fixed abode. Partly under the influence of the statesman Cardinal Archbishop of York, Thomas Wolsey (*c.* 1475–1530), who built Hampton Court Palace, King Henry VIII started to have his court at fixed palaces. Thus under the Act of Henry VIII 1541–2 a coroner was appointed to prevent bloodshed within the palaces.

As a crown appointment, the coroner of the verge was a member of the Lord Steward's department. Following the Coroners Act of 1887, the title of coroner of the verge was abolished. Today when a body has suffered death by violence or inexplicable causes, the case must be reported to the coroner of the queen's household if the event took place within stated areas at Buckingham Palace, St James's Palace, Windsor Castle, Royal Lodge (if the queen is resident), Kensington Palace, Hampton Court Palace and Sandringham House, or any house where the queen is resident at the time the body was lying there. (The jurisdiction does not apply to royal palaces in Scotland.)

Since 1835 holders of the office of coroner to the royal household have been as follows:

1835–88.	Frederick J. Manning.
1888–1934.	Arthur Walter Mills.
1934–55.	Lt-Col. W.H. Leslie McCarthy.
1955–9.	Sir William Bentley Purchase.
1959–83.	Dr A. Gordon Davis.
1983–6.	Dr Lt-Col. George McEwan.
1986–	Dr John D.K. Burton CBE.

through, and a key to the duke's apartments in a pocket. By 8.00 a.m. the royal family had been informed of the events and Sir Everard issued a medical bulletin: 'His Royal Highness's wounds are not immediately dangerous . . . he is as well as can be expected . . .'[8]

The events of 31 March–1 April caused a huge sensation in London and the fashionable crowds flocked to St James's to see the scene of the purported crime. Sellis had been a supporter of the Tory cause so the liberal Whigs naturally cried murder and named the Duke of Cumberland as the culprit. Meantime the duke was being treated by Dr Wathen Phipps. Diagnosing shock, Phipps suggested the duke be moved, so Cumberland was conveyed to Carlton House by the Prince of Wales, while the coroner and principal magistrate at Bow Street, John Read, began his legal investigation. He took his main depositions from the royal doctors and the servants, beginning work at 10.00 a.m. on 1 April. The depositions and facts were set before the coroner's jury which subsequently sat at the duke's apartments in St James's.

Apart from the Whigs, most people believed that Sellis had attacked his master. Assessing the case in 1867, Admiralty clerk turned historian John Heneage Jesse summarised contemporary opinion:

> after having attacked his master, [*Sellis*] had rushed back to his own apartment with the intention of washing the Duke's blood from his hands . . . but that the approach of the persons sent in search of him, told him that detection was inevitable and induced him to commit suicide in order to avoid the consequences of the crime.[9]

Popular though this opinion was, it was full of flaws – as the royal doctors' notes would show.

The official enquiry was conducted by the coroner to the king's household, solicitor Samuel Thomas Adams, who selected seventeen jurymen from independent local merchants in the Charing Cross area.[10] Francis Place, a tailor, was appointed foreman.[11] Coroner Adams also assembled two assistants, both coroners for the County of Middlesex, Gill and Hodgson, and solicitor to the Admiralty Thomas Bricknall, who also acted for the Duke of Cumberland. To supplement the royal doctors' testimony two further medics, Drs Thomas Jones and John Jackson, were summoned and the press was represented by journalists from four newspapers including *The Times* and the Tory *Morning Post*. The enquiry lasted six hours.

With Sir Henry and Sir Everard in tow, the jurymen, observers and advisers examined Sellis's corpse. Although most folk were happy to accept the death as suicide, there were clear signs of a struggle. The gory water in the basin and the cut necktie were noted, as well as Sellis's blood-stained jacket hanging over a nearby chair. Despite the comments of the royal doctors to the contrary, the jurymen formed the opinion that:

> the position of the body showed that Sellis had cut his own throat as he sat upon his bed, and had fallen backwards, while the razor had simply dropped from his hand to the floor where it had been found.[12]

Testimony was taken from housemaid Sarah Varley and under-butler Thomas Strickland as to Sellis's movements on 31 March. Nothing seemed to be unusual, although Strickland noted that when he took in the duke's late-night drink Sellis gave him 'such an extraordinary smile' that he found it a precursor of evil work.[13] The Duke of Cumberland was not called to give evidence but his statement was read to the jurymen. Without retiring, and with only one dissention, foreman of the jury Francis Place announced the verdict as *felo de se* (suicide).

The verdict caused great public disappointment. The Whigs were incandescent with rage that the 'murderous duke', who had not actually been legally accused of any misdemeanour, had 'got off lightly'. If he had not killed Sellis himself, he had hired someone to do it, said the Whigs in their fastness at Stowe, the seat of the liberal Earl Temple (later Duke of Buckingham and Chandos). It was in Whig society, too, that the rumour was hatched that the Duke of Cumberland had been having a homosexual liaison with valet Neale; this had been discovered by Sellis, who had been silenced by death (faked as suicide). Others unhappy with the verdict included Sir Francis Burdett

(1770–1844), the socilist MP for Westminster, who was among those who felt the suicide verdict had been 'fixed'.[14]

Dr Wathen Phipps was now permanently attending the Duke of Cumberland, who was in continual pain. It was reported:

> The slightest sound caused him excruciating agony. The Prince of Wales had to take off his shoes for slippers before approaching his brother's bed, and [*Dr Phipps*] said that if he accidentally touched the bedclothes [*the duke*] cried out with agony and could not bear the scratching of his pen, so he had to write in another room.[15]

Dr Phipps slept in the adjacent room to the duke for some two months, dispensing constant attention. On 2 June 1810 he issued this bulletin: 'His Royal Highness the Duke of Cumberland's wound in his head has been dressed for the first time. Though deep and large, it puts on as favourable an appearance as could be expected.'[16] *The Times* ran reports on the duke's condition, noting that 'he was operated upon and one of the wounds in his head was opened and a piece of fractured skull, one inch by a quarter, removed'.[17]

After 17 July Dr Phipps had no need to issue any further bulletins. On a visit by King George III to see his son, then at Queen's House, the duke was described thus: 'He was clad in a great-coat, with both arms in slings, and he had not the use of either hand; his head was bound with black silk and he also wore a black silk cap. He was pale . . .'[18] The duke had suffered extreme pain, for the treatment and surgery had all been done without anaesthetic, and he was to suffer for many months to come.

Still today historians mull over the inconsistencies of the Sellis death, particularly the records left by the royal doctors. For example, there is the attestation by Sir Everard Home that Sellis's throat was cut by a right-handed man, when Sellis was left-handed. Again there is the fact that Sellis's head was almost severed. It is impossible for a suicide to almost sever his own head. A suicide tends to lean the head back to cut the throat, making it difficult to sever. Again, suicides do not tend to have deep lacerations, only shallow cuts. Then there is the evidence of the cut necktie. Surely a suicide would have removed the necktie before trying to cut the throat it covered. And what about the bloody water in the basin? Sellis would hardly have washed his hands after the suicide. The whole looks like a carefully concealed murder. But by whom? The Duke of Cumberland? Valet Neale? Or a person, or persons, unknown? We are unlikely ever to know. And the royal doctors' part in the case is the most puzzling of all. Were they part of a cover-up? Academically, they knew it was no suicide; did they keep silent to protect their own royal positions?

CHAPTER SEVEN

PRINNY'S PHYSICIANS EXTRAORDINARY: COURT ROLES FOR DISTINGUISHED AND SHADY MEDICS

Those who knew him well called him 'Prinny', which was among the politest of the nicknames conferred on princes of the House of Hanover. For many folk the sentiments expressed by Percy Bysshe Shelley (1792–1822) summed up the general feelings about George III and his sons:

> An old, mad, despised and dying King,
> Princes, the dregs of their dull race, who flow
> Through public scorn – mud from a muddy spring –
> Rulers who neither see nor feel nor know
> But leech-like to their fainting country cling.[1]

Nevertheless, to the nation 'Prinny' was HRH George Augustus Frederick, Prince of Wales. At his birth at St James's Palace on 12 August 1762, the eldest son of George III and Queen Charlotte, he had succeeded to the dukedoms of Cornwall and Rothesay, with a myriad other titles; five days later the king created him Prince of Wales and Earl of Chester. From birth he was attended by physicians and surgeons of his mother's and father's households, but as Prince of Wales his own medical household was established by the mid-1780s.

To his physicians the Prince of Wales, who became George IV on the death of his father, remained an enigma. Although heir to the throne, he was educated for nothing; although destined for the monarchy, he was pushed into the arms of the political opponents of his father at best, and his outright enemies at worst, during George III's long sixty-year reign. Prinny's dalliances with Lady Melbourne and the wife of the (later) Prussian Foreign Minister Karl von Hardenberg led on to an illegal marriage. The Act of Settlement of 1701 decreed that no prince of Great Britain could marry a 'Papist' and succeed to the throne, and the Royal Marriage Act stated that no member of the royal family (under twenty-five) could contract a marriage without the monarch's consent. So Prinny's marriage to the 28-year-old Roman Catholic widow Maria Fitzherbert on 15 December 1785 was a constitutional and dynastic nonsense.

Ten years later, on 8 April 1795, at the Chapel Royal, St James's Palace, he married – legally – his first cousin Princess Caroline Amelia Elizabeth of Brunswick-Wolfenbüttel (1768–1821). The marriage was both a public embarrassment and a private nightmare, and it began in pure farce with a drunken wedding night. It led to a separation and a political pantomime when Caroline was forcibly excluded from her husband's coronation on 29 July 1821. The curse of the House of Hanover was further inflicted on the Prince of Wales with two cruel blows: the death at Claremont House on 6 November 1817 of his beloved heir Princess Charlotte Augusta, a day after the stillbirth of his grandchild.

George IV's amorous entanglements as Prince of Wales, regent and king, coupled with a love of the good life, threatened his health and added to his girth. It was not unusual for his French chef, Carème, to produce a *Menu de 36 entrées* – as he did at the prince's oriental building extravaganza, Brighton Pavilion, on 15 July 1817 – for the Prince Regent's soirées. *The Times* solemnly wrote about his weight and the despair of his doctors, and described the difficulty the Prince Regent had in mounting his horse:

An inclined plane was constructed, rising to about the height of two feet and a half, at the upper end of which was a platform. His Royal Highness was placed in a chair on rollers, and so moved by the ascent, and placed on the platform, which was then raised by screws high enough to pass the horse under: and finally, his Royal Highness was let gently down into the saddle. By these means the Regent was undoubtedly able to enjoy in some degree the benefit of air and exercise . . .[2]

By 1818 he was so large that Lord Folkestone wrote to the Whig MP Thomas Creevy: 'Prinny has let loose his belly which now reaches his knees . . .'[3]

During the period 1787–96, while he was still Prince of Wales, George's medical household included Sir Gilbert Blane, Richard Warren and the London physician Anthony Addington (1713–90). They were joined by his two physicians-in-ordinary Sir Walter Farquhar (1738–1819) and John Latham (1761–1843), a specialist in rheumatism and gout.

While tackling the effects of the prince's exogenous obesity and articular gout, these doctors were the first to record the prince's other 'weaknesses'. Apart from his craving for women and food, both the prince and his entourage suffered from his character traits of vanity, extravagance, self-indulgence and undependability, which led the diarist Charles Greville to declare him a 'contemptible, cowardly, unfeeling, selfish dog'.[4]

On becoming Prince Regent in 1811, Prince George added to his establishment John Birth (*c.* 1745–1815) as his surgeon-extraordinary, Sir William Rawson (1783–1827) as his surgeon oculist-extraordinary and William Saunders (1743–1817) as physician. A year later a baronetcy was arranged for Dr Gilbert Blane, who was to come to know the prince best of all.

Gilbert Blane was a remarkable physician. He was born on 29 August 1749 at Blanefield, Ayrshire. At first he was destined for a vocation in the Church of Scotland and took up religious studies at the University of Edinburgh. His observations of current medical practice in the capital, culled from roisterings with students from the university medical school, caused him to change career. His proficiency in the subject brought him to the notice of William Cullen (1710–90), Professor of Medicine at Edinburgh, who recommended him as pupil to the royal physician William Hunter. After graduating MD on 28 August 1778, Blane became private physician to the diplomat the Earl of Holderness, and then in 1779 to Admiral George Brydges Rodney (1719–92), then bound for the Leeward Islands station in the West Indies.

Ever since the days when he roamed the docks at Leith as a student, Blane had felt an affinity with the sea and during the years 1779–83 he was physician to the fleet. He saw action in the West Indies and observed at first hand the terrible medical service available to sailors. He did much to improve sanitary conditions in the Navy and in 1783 published his *Observations on the Diseases of Seamen*. By this time Blane had become physician to St Thomas's Hospital, and his contributions to naval medicine had brought him to the attention of Prince William Henry, Duke of Clarence, himself a naval lieutenant in the West Indies campaign. On the duke's recommendation, Blane became physician-extraordinary to his brother, the Prince of Wales, in 1785. In the same year Blane married Elizabeth Gardner. He combined royal service with the pursuit of his career as Commissioner for Sick and Wounded Seamen from 1795 to 1820. In 1820 he was appointed physician-in-ordinary to the nascent household of George IV.

While acting as Prinny's physician-extraordinary, Blane had often been called in for minor ailments. For instance, in 1811 George slipped and sprained his ankle while showing his daughter Princess Charlotte Augusta how to dance the Highland Fling. He was in bed for two weeks. Blane's advice to his royal patient – to curb his eating and keep more regular hours – was ignored, but Blane kept faith with his royal employer to the last. Blane died at his home in Sackville Street on 26 June 1864.

> 'If you are too fond of new remedies, first, you will not cure your patients; secondly, you will have no patients to cure'.
>
> **Sir Astley Cooper** *(1768–1841), Physician to George IV*

Another prominent physician of his generation was Sir Astley Paston Cooper (1768–1841), whom fate also brought within the royal milieu. Cooper had studied medicine at London, Edinburgh and Paris, becoming successively anatomy demonstrator and lecturer at St Thomas's Hospital (1789–1825).[5] A consulting surgeon with a lucrative practice, Cooper won a name for himself as an expert in arterial surgery, and he left this record of how he came to have a royal patient:

The King sent to Sir Everard Home, myself and (Benjamin) Brodie to go to Windsor to see a tumour on the summit of his head, which annoyed him from its appearance and was growing larger. When we saw it, it was tender, painful and somewhat inflamed; and we thought it best to delay the operation. The King was much disappointed, but yielded to our advice.[6]

The next year Cooper received a summons via the king's keeper of the privy purse (and acting secretary) Lt-Gen. Sir Benjamin Bloomfield (1768–1840) to attend the monarch at Brighton. The king was keen to have his 'tumour' (really a sebacious cyst) removed and came to the surgeon's room at one o'clock in the morning demanding an immediate operation. Cooper mollified the king thus:

> Sire, not for the world now, your life is too important to have so serious a thing done in a corner. Lady S. died of erysipelas after such an operation and what would the world say if this were to be fatal? No, too much depends upon Your Majesty to suffer me at 1 o'clock in the morning in a retired part of the Pavilion, to perform an operation, which, however trifling in general, might by possibility be followed by fatal consequences.[7]

Cooper was not keen to perform the operation at all. His wish was that the procedure be carried out by Sergeant-surgeon Sir Everard Home. Nevertheless, assisted by his old tutor Henry Cline (1750–1827), Cooper operated as the king sat in a chair by a window. Cooper remembered:

> I made an incision into the tumour and emptied it of its contents. Then I found it adhered strongly to the scalp . . . I with difficulty detached it from the skin without cutting the skin itself. On that side on which Cline stood I begged him to detach it which he did but it took up a great deal of time on the whole. The edges of the wound were brought together and lint and plaster applied. The King bore the operation well, requested there might be no hurry and when it was finished said, 'What do you call the tumour?' I said, 'A steatoma, Sire' (giving it its now archaic Latin name). 'Then', said he, 'I hope it will stay at home and not annoy me anymore.'[8]

A few days after the operation, the king complained of severe head pains; an anxious Cooper feared the onset of erysipelas. A day or two later the king suffered an attack of gout and the head pains cleared. Thereafter the operation wound healed, Cooper's reputation remained intact and he was rewarded with a knighthood. Almost two hundred years after the events it seems strange that a knighthood should be awarded for what is considered a very minor operation. In those days any form of surgery, without anaesthetic and proper antiseptic, was a distressingly painful risk. The king in his anguish believed a knighthood appropriate recompense.

When the Prince Regent became George IV in 1820 his medical household was expanded to include Sir Matthew John Tierney (1776–1845), who practised at the royal 'bolt-hole' at Brighton, Henry Herbert Southey (1783–1865), a specialist in pulmonary consumption, and Stephen Luke (1763–1829) as physician-extraordinary. An additional appointment was the consequence of a unique royal jaunt.

John Abercrombie (1781–1844), an Edinburgh general practitioner, was now made physician-in-ordinary in Scotland. Although several of the royal doctors in the employ of the House of Hanover had Scottish backgrounds or degrees, there was then no active royal household in Scotland. Even though many Scots noblemen like Sir Alexander Keith of Ravelston, who claimed the right to be the Hereditary Knight Marischal of Scotland, boasted such patrimonial positions at a nebulous Scottish royal court, there had been no visits to Scotland by a reigning monarch since 1650, when Charles II journeyed north to be crowned at Scone.

To the consternation of the Scots nobility and the civil servants on the staff of Robert Saunders Dundas, 2nd Viscount Melville (1771–1851), the 'Minister of the State for Scotland' (there was no Secretary of State for Scotland until 1885), George IV announced that he intended to visit his Scottish realm. Their problem was that no one knew how to organise such an event and its inherent protocols.

The king's visit developed into a fourteen-day extravaganza of 'tartanalia' from 15 August 1822, stage-managed by the enthusiastic romantic Sir Walter Scott (1771–1832). Out of his efforts grew an image of Scotland that had little to do with

---

GEORGE IV'S MEDICAL HOUSEHOLD

George IV. Born 12 August 1762. Regent, 5 February 1811; reigned 1820–30. Died 26 June 1830.

John Abercrombie (1781–1844). Physician-in-ordinary in Scotland (which the king visited in 1822).
Sir Gilbert Blane (1748–1834). Physician-in-ordinary, 1820.
Stephen Luke (1763–1829). Physician-extraordinary.
Henry Herbert Southey (1783–1865). Physician, 1823.
Sir Matthew John Tierney (1776–1845). Physician.

As Prince Regent, George IV elevated Dr Everard Home (1756–1832) – who had treated the Duke of Cumberland in the Cumberland–Sellis case – to a baronetcy and appointed him sergeant-surgeon in 1813.

George IV was attended by Sir Henry Halford and Sir Benjamin Brodie (1783–1862), in his last days and Sir Astley Paston Cooper (1768–1845) performed the post-mortem on his cadaver. Sir William Knighton (1776–1836), the king's private secretary, was appointed physician to him as Prince of Wales in 1813.

---

reality. For decades thereafter the Scots remembered the plump figure of the king, resplendent in flesh-coloured tights and an indecorously short kilt, preening at Holyrood Palace where he was invited to kiss some 400 women in an hour and a quarter.

Dr John Abercrombie joined the throng at Holyrood, but was not required to carry out any medical duties, although his expertise as a consultant specialising in the intestinal canal and the bowels might have been of some use to the royal indigestion and flatulence. In the crush at the palace, Dr Abercrombie, and the invited medics of the Royal College of Physicians of Edinburgh, were able to observe their monarch at first hand.

George IV was a sick man. Some Scots medics whispered to one another that the bloated and pasty, but perfumed and powdered monarch looked as mad as his father. Indeed, George IV sometimes expressed an anxiety that he would go insane, but in these days of 1822 he had more of a fear of death. His obsession with dying became more acute following the death of his wife shortly after his coronation. But any Scots physician or surgeon present at the levée who thought he might further his career with a word in the royal ear was soon disabused by the presence of a distinguished fellow-practitioner. Even Dr Abercrombie was made to understand that his role was purely honorary while Sir William Knighton (1776–1836) was around. Even the ubiquitous Sir Walter Scott was thwarted in his efforts to prise the king from Knighton's grasp to meet more of the people. This led to Scott referring to Knighton the 'Great Unseen' because of his influence.

By 1822 Knighton had added the roles of private secretary and keeper of the privy purse to his brief as the king's physician and was one of the monarch's closest confidants. In his early career he had been assistant-surgeon to the Royal Navy Hospital, Plymouth, and had graduated MD at Aberdeen. He was appointed physician to George IV in 1813, when he was still Prince of Wales, and his royal career had advanced from there.

One man present during the Scottish jaunt – as a guest of Sir Walter Scott – was the poet Dr George Crabbe (1754–1832), who had once practised surgery at Aldeburgh. Installed one day during the royal visit in Sir Walter Scott's parlour at Castle Street, Crabbe regaled Scott with tales of the royal doctor. Even in the best light Sir William Knighton was considered 'shady'. In court circles Knighton was known as the 'man-midwife', or '*accoucheur*', titles usually uttered with sarcastic stress. The latter term too, was usually used by those who believed him to have been an abortionist in his early days at his fashionable Hanover Street practice.

Knighton was undoubtedly a sycophant, but his embarrassing flattery of George IV won him the monarch's favour and that of Elizabeth, Marchioness of Conyngham, wife of the lord steward of the household – and the king's mistress. Knighton was widely believed in court circles to be the 'king's chief spy'; moreover it was mooted in polite circles 'that not a word was uttered at White's, or any club, that did not ultimately reach the ears of the *accoucheur*'.[9]

During the tour of Scotland Knighton had a medical problem to deal with, for the king suffered continued agony from gout; his legs swelled and no amount of cherry brandy succeeded in dulling the pain. Knighton treated him with a mixture of flattery, laudanum (to which the king was addicted), bleeding and the potions of the day. The king added to his own unhealthy aspect by enhancing his waxy pallor with increasing layers of arsenical face powder and rouge.

For Knighton the king's trip to Scotland was a boring round of levées and visits, and keeping the importuning Royal College members at bay. Writing to his wife, Knighton declared the first Sunday in Scotland was a welcome 'day of peace'. While 'the dear King' was resting, Knighton moped in his room at Holyrood Palace, watching hares on the lawn from his window, and reporting to his wife that his accommodation was haunted. The gloom of the chamber was darkened even more by a portrait of General George Monck, 1st Duke of Albemarle (1608–70), Oliver Cromwell's vandal-in-chief of the Scots campaign of 1651–2. In that very room, added Knighton in his missive, the wily Monck had signed the documents restoring Charles II to the throne.

The writer Robert Huish (1777–1850) was to supply the nation with an account of George IV's death which went beyond the bulletins issued heretofore by the royal doctors:

> The crisis was now fast approaching, yet the death of the King was not expected till Friday night, the 25th (June). The physicians, however, had been aware that it would probably be sudden, and the royal sufferer was prepared to receive the awful summons with resignation and submission. His Majesty's phrase was when this intimation was given to him a fortnight previously, 'God's will be done'. Within the last week he spoke but little, and in a tone quite faint, and sometimes almost inaudible and inarticulate. To speak so as to be heard in the chamber appeared to give him pain, and to require an effort beyond the remaining strength of his shattered constitution. Business of any kind became irksome to him, and affected his temper.[10]

The king had been seriously ill since the turn of 1830. The royal physicians had diagnosed ascites (abdominal dropsy) and logged his difficulty in breathing, hiccups and bilious attacks. The royal legs were regularly punctured to reduce the swelling and the King was lifted into 'a chair of a peculiar construction, adapted to the circumstances of the case', a gift from his brother the Duke of Sussex.

As May gave way to June the king's condition worsened and Robert Huish prepared all for the approaching end:

> The death-bed scene of a monarch is one of the most impressive lessons that humanity can be taught. It shows the nothingness – emptiness of earthly grandeur, and that a King after all is nothing more than a mere human being, subject to a common destiny as the meanest beggar of the country. Let us view George IV, in the most splendid palace of the King of England (*sic*), surrounded by elegance and luxuries unknown to his predecessors, lying on his couch of anguish. A life of prosperity was near its close; the poisonous dregs of the cup of pleasure 'gnawed his inwards' . . . A poor old man, the wreck of a fine person, loaded with more than the infirmity of age and sickness, he was the object of painful contemplation to his attendants . . . George IV had long been the envy of his people; how different were the feelings which the scene we are now about to describe was calculated to excite.[11]

Finally on 25 June, Sir Benjamin Brodie, Sir Henry Halford and the other regularly attending physicians and surgeons averred they could do nothing more. A bulletin was penned:

> From eleven to three o'clock His Majesty appeared to be suffering what is commonly called restless sleep. He opened his eyes occasionally, and when he coughed he appeared to suffer more than the usual pain, but nothing occurred until three o'clock to indicate any particular change.

The pages in attendance were beckoned by the king to move him to the Duke of Sussex's chair, and he lapsed into a fainting fit. The royal doctors were recalled to the death chamber as the pages dabbed their royal employer with eau de Cologne and held a handkerchief of sal volatile to his nose:

> At this moment His Majesty attempted to raise his hand to his breast, faintly ejaculating, "Oh, God I am dying?"; and after

two or three seconds of time, he uttered the following words, which were his last, 'This is death" – his expiring condition barely enabling him to announce the fatal sensation, so as to be heard by the page, on whose shoulders His Majesty's head had fallen.[12]

At 3.13 a.m. on Saturday, 26 June 1830, at Windsor Castle, George IV breathed his last in the presence of his doctors, his mistress's husband, and several gentlemen of the household, all bowing their head as the Bishop of Chichester intoned the prayers for the dead.

Covered with a linen sheet, George IV's cadaver was left on view until 8.00 p.m. when the post-mortem and embalming took place. The post-mortem was undertaken by Sir Astley Paston Cooper. Sir Astley's examination revealed:

The result was that His Majesty's disorder was an extensive diseased organisation of the heart; this was the primary disorder, although dropsical symptoms subsequently supervened, and in fact there was a general breaking up of His Majesty's constitution. The heart was uncommonly enlarged, but there was no effusion of water on the thorax cavity. The valves of the heart had become partially ossified, and there was a considerable degree of fatness about the organ generally. The liver was not diseased, the lungs were ulcerated, and there were dropsical symptoms of the skin in various parts of the body, but not of a nature necessarily to produce death. They appeared rather the eventual consequence of the impeded circulation of the blood, owing to the disorganisation of disease of the bones, arising from the primary disorder; indeed the debilitated circulation of the vital fluid (has) everywhere left the traces of its long existence.[13]

George IV's funeral took place on Thursday, 31 June. He was interred in the royal vault at St George's Chapel, Windsor, and the new monarch William IV and his Queen Adelaide took up residence at Windsor Castle.

CHAPTER EIGHT

WILLIAM THE SAILOR KING: ROYAL DOCTORS UNDERSTATE A DEATH

When Prince William Henry, Duke of Clarence and St Andrews and Earl of Munster, was born at Buckingham House, St James's Park, on 21 August 1765, the third child of George III and Queen Charlotte, there were few at his father's court who thought he would ever succeed to the throne. Prince William was born into a royal milieu pummelled by political and social unrest, but he was hardly aware of public affairs in the secluded nursery haven within the court. Educated by stodgy governors, the exuberant and impatient prince endured a turgid rural existence until he embarked on a naval career. At Spithead on 15 June 1779 he was received by Rear-Admiral Robert Digby (1732–1815) aboard the *Prince George* as a midshipman. In due course Prince William would rise to be Rear-Admiral of the Blue Squadron in 1790, Admiral of the Fleet in 1811, and Lord High Admiral in 1827.

Like his brothers, Prince William was to have a range of colourful gossip attached to his activities, from dalliances in the brothels of foreign ports to the *demi-mondaines* of Hanover, where his father dispatched him in 1783. To his parents' horror, one Caroline von Linsingen, daughter of Lt-Gen. Wilhelm von Linsingen, Commander of the 12th Hanover Infantry, announced that she had married Prince William at Pyrmont in August 1791. Alas for the deluded Caroline, while he was supposed to be playing a nuptial role the prince was actually in hot pursuit of the actress Mrs Dorothy Jordan (1762–1816), with whom he cohabited for twenty years until dynastic needs caused them to separate in 1812. Together the prince and Mrs Jordan had ten illegitimate children, known to society as the 'FitzClarences'.[1]

On 11 July 1818 Prince William married the 26-year-old Princess Adelaide Louisa Theresa Caroline Amelia, elder daughter of George I of Saxe-Meiningen and Princess Louise Eleanore zu Hohenlohe-Langenburg. William was now fifty-three and his health was on the slide. Already the arthritis which was to cripple his hands was present and his chronic asthma was always only a laboured breath away. Further, his 'liver was enlarged and hardened', and his ill-temper was increasing in its outbursts.[2]

Since his days as a serving naval officer Prince William's health was never totally robust. While on duty abroad he contracted several fevers, prickly heat, boils and rheumatic pains. At the end of his tour aboard HMS *Pegasus* in the West Indies, naval surgeon John Fidge reported: 'I cannot recommend it for His Royal Highness to return [to duty] where he has suffered so materially.'[3] Again the prince often drank too much and suffered the 'mercury cure' in consequence of 'a sore I had contracted in a most extraordinary manner in my pursuit of the *Dames de Couleurs*'.[4] Prince William was treated a number of times for venereal disease.

Through his intemperance and impatience Prince William was served as Duke of Clarence by a number of royal doctors from his father's court, but two medics, William Beattie (1793–1875) and Sir Andrew Halliday (1781–1839), were severally attached to his entourage. A graduate of Edinburgh and Paris, Dr William Beattie attended the prince as his physician in Hanover and he ran a successful practice at Hampstead during the years 1827–45. Like so many of his colleagues of this age, Beattie was a man of letters, who composed poetry and wrote histories. Sir Andrew Halliday was a skilled services physician with experience in the Peninsular War of 1808–14 (intermixed with Britain's second war with Napoleon 1805–15); he was present at the battle of Waterloo in 1815.

For financial and dynastic reasons Prince William was jubilant at the announcement of his wife's pregnancy in November 1818. After all, as the father of the future monarch – his elder brothers having no legitimate offspring – he could expect an increased monetary grant from Parliament. Alas, Princess Adelaide caught a cold, developed pleurisy and gave birth prematurely to Princess Charlotte Augusta Louisa, who was born and died at Fürstenhof, Hanover, on 27 March 1819. She was buried beside her great-great-grandfather George I. For a while the health of the princess caused great concern but by early August she was well enough

WILLIAM IV'S MEDICAL HOUSEHOLD
William IV. Born 21 August 1765. Reigned 1830–7. Died 20 June 1837.

William Beattie (1793–1875). Physician.
Sir Benjamin Collins Brodie (1783–1862). Sergeant-surgeon, 1832.
Sir Andrew Halliday (1781–1839). Physician.
Sir Everard Home (1756–1832). Surgeon.
James Johnson (1777–1845). Physician-extraordinary.
Robert Keate (1777–1857). Sergeant-surgeon.
William Macmichael (1783–1839). Physician-in-ordinary, 1831.
John Stevenson (1778–1846). Oculist and aurist.
Sir Matthew John Tierney (1776–1845). Physician.

During his last illness William IV was also attended by William Frederick Chambers (1786–1855), consultant physician.

or Prince William to inform the Tory prime minister, the Earl of Liverpool, that she was pregnant once more. Unfortunately, on her way home from Hanover the princess miscarried at Calais. Prince William was plunged into deep gloom.

A short while later Prince William was enthusiastically reporting his wife's new pregnancy, and Princess Elizabeth Georgiana Adelaide was born at St James's Palace on 10 December 1820, six weeks premature. Royal physician Sir Henry Halford was present at the birth and commented harshly that the mother was a 'poor wishy-washy thing'.[5] The baby survived four months, dying of 'inflammation of the Bowels' on 4 March 1821.

On his accession to the throne, at the age of sixty-five, as King William IV in June 1830, a new medical household was established at Windsor. Naval surgeon James Johnson (1777–1845) became physician-extraordinary, and the surgeon at St George's Hospital, Robert Keate (1777–1857), became sergeant-surgeon. William Macmichael (1783–1839) became physician-in-ordinary in 1831, while opthalmic surgeon John Stevenson (1778–1846), who founded the Royal Infirmary for Cataract at Little Portland Street, London, in the year of the king's accession, became the royal oculist and aurist. Sir Matthew John Tierney

(1776–1845) continued as a royal physician from his practice at Brighton. One other royal doctor was also to rise to particular academic prominence in this period.

Sir Benjamin Collins Brodie (1783–1862) was created sergeant-surgeon in 1832. Brodie had been a student of Sir Everard Home, who was continuing his royal service to William IV's court. Brodie was already a distinguished medic, having been Professor of Comparative Anatomy and Physiology at the Royal College of Surgeons from 1816, and had been consulted on an ad hoc basis by George IV.

Brodie was an astute clinician; in the year of his royal appointment he wrote on the 'Chronic Abscess of the Tibia' in *Medico-Chirurgical Transactions*. Subsequently, a condition was named after him and thus 'Brodie's Abscess' entered medical parlance. In 1840, during a lecture at St George's Hospital, where he was surgeon from 1822, he described a rare affliction which became known as 'Sero Cystic Disease of Brodie'. At the age of seventy-five, Brodie was created the first president of the new General Medical Council, a statutory body set up under the Medical Act of 1858 to maintain a register of qualified medical practitioners in the United Kingdom. The council was important in the history of British medicine, and to this day it still supervises and regulates the standards of medical education and qualifying examinations.

> 'There may be much knowledge with little wisdom, and much wisdom with little knowledge.'
> **Sir Benjamin Collins Brodie** *(1783–1863), surgeon to George IV, William IV and Queen Victoria*

During April 1837 Queen Adelaide fell ill on the return from her sister's deathbed at Meiningen. The king's worry over her condition was worsened by the death in childbirth of his illegitimate daughter (and second child) by Dorothy Jordan, Sophia FitzClarence, who had married Lord de L'Isle and Dudley. At this time too his yearly bout of asthma was particularly bad and his lack of appetite caused severe weight loss and fainting fits. His secretary, Lt-Gen. Sir Herbert Taylor (1775–1839), wrote to the Whig prime minister, Lord Melbourne:

Yesterday was a very bad day with the King, and his (natural) Daughters who are *all* here were very much alarmed, nor have they much control over their feelings . . . The Queen is the best and the quietest Nurse I ever saw and I only dread her knocking herself up, as she does not undress at night and is frequently up.

Taylor reported too that the king was a 'bad patient', with the royal doctors on duty having difficulty in getting him to cooperate with their ministrations. Taylor continued:

The fact is that He is most anxious not to be considered seriously ill, and better than He is, and this leads to his doing that which increases illness; to His sending for Numbers of Persons whose Attendance and Business is *perfectly immaterial*, to his holding a Council (*at Windsor Castle*) tomorrow . . .[6]

On 6 June the royal doctors issued a 'typically misleading' bulletin on the king's health; all but the monarch seemed to believe he was dying. Civil servants began to re-examine the files for the protocols of a royal funeral and coronation. The king's heir was clear: Princess Victoria, his niece, would succeed him and there was a general sigh of relief that a regency would not be needed as the princess was already of age; if she had not been, Victoria's mother, the difficult and querulously demanding Duchess of Kent, would have been jockeying for the position of regent.

In the presence of Queen Adelaide and the king's natural children – except for the unforgiving Lord Munster with whom he had quarrelled – William Howley, Archbishop of Canterbury, administered blessings for the dying to the king. On 16 June the king remarked to Dr William Frederick Chambers, consulting physician from St George's Hospital, who had been monitoring his 'turgid blood' on behalf of Drs Johnson and Macmichael: 'Doctor, I know I am going, but I should like to see another anniversary of the battle of Waterloo (18 June). Try if you cannot tinker me up to last out that day.'

On the morning of 18 June the king said to Chambers, 'I know

I shall never live to see another sunset'. But he was delighted to receive good wishes from the Duke of Wellington, who, the king insisted, must hold his annual 'Wellington Dinner' to celebrate the great defeat of Napoleon Bonaparte.

In a letter to his sister, Benjamin Disraeli commented: 'The King dies like an old lion.'[7] The lion lapsed into unconsciousness on the afternoon of the same day, and at 2.12 a.m. on Tuesday, 20 June 1837, the last spark of the life of William IV flickered to extinction. Thus on the morning of the longest day, 21 June, the Archbishop of Canterbury and the Lord Chamberlain, Lord Conyngham, with physician-in-ordinary James Johnson in attendance, travelled to Kensington Palace to inform the eighteen-year-old Princess Victoria that she was now monarch.

A post-mortem was performed on William IV's cadaver on the day of his death; although the report was signed by Edward Duke Moore, apothecary to Queen Adelaide, the post-mortem was probably done by Sir Astley Cooper. It confirmed that the king had died from broncho-pneumonia. Yet controversy was to rage in the medical profession for some time concerning the royal doctors' handling of the king's last days.

Each day the king moved nearer to death medical bulletins had been issued. Many medics of the day declared them mendacious, and most declared them a 'discredit to the profession'. In them the king was not declared to be gravely ill; the tone was optimistic and it was only in his final hours that the truth of his imminent death was revealed. Many people believed that the content of the bulletins had been manipulated, and the finger was pointed at William Lamb, Lord Melbourne, the Liberal prime minister who had held office since 18 April 1835. Melbourne's Liberal cabinet was divided; a general election was due and Melbourne wanted no popular sympathy for the king to be reflected in an increased Tory vote. In the event Melbourne's party won on a slashed majority (the voters of Scotland and Ireland ensuring his victory), and his administration was saved. Lord Melbourne now ingratiated himself with the young queen and acted as her adviser and secretary until his defeat at the polls in 1841.

PART TWO:

PROFESSIONAL EMINENCE

CHAPTER NINE

SCIENCE, STYLE AND SQUEAMISHNESS: QUEEN VICTORIA'S EARLY MEDICAL HOUSEHOLDS

Queen Victoria was a hypochondriac. She constantly fussed over her diet and weight, and ailments real and imagined. Nevertheless she never moderated her large intake of food. Throughout her life her courtiers continually battled with her evolving state of nervous breakdowns, hysterics and constant fear that she was going insane like her Hanoverian grandfather King George III. The medicine chest she invariably carried around with her contained a fearsome range of dangerous drugs and homoeopathic concoctions. Like her subjects, Queen Victoria avidly scoured the popular press for adverts for patent medicines and contemporary nostrums. These she avidly discussed with her two apothecaries. John Nussey (d. 1862) was her chief apothecary, inherited from William IV, and he shared his royal duties with Charles Craddock; they remained in her service until 1859 and 1862 respectively.[1]

On her desk Queen Victoria kept a copy of *Hannay's Royal Almanack*, the 1846 edition of which, for example, contained some 783 remedies for human ailments.[2] From it, with the apothecaries' advice, she chose such items as Worsdell's Vegetable Restorative Pills and Congreve's Balsamic Elixir. Before she embarked on her sea-tours she had packed a potion of Baker's Patent Antidote for the Prevention of Sea Sickness. Again, Queen Victoria was never without a dose or two of Collis Browne's Chlorodyne, which contained a mixture of chloroform, Indian hemp and morphia. In due time her name appeared in the adverts as 'patron' of such nostrums.

During Queen Victoria's reign the status and careers of her appointed physicians and surgeons developed as never

ACCOUCHEMENT OF HER MAJESTY.
BIRTH OF A PRINCESS.

(London Gazette Extraordinary.)

Buckingham Palace, Nov. 21.

This afternoon, at ten minutes before two o'clock, the Queen : is happily delivered of a Princess; his Royal Highness Prince Albert, her Royal Highness the Duchess of Kent, several Lords of Her Majesty's Most Hon. Privy Council, and the Ladies of Her Majesty's Bedchamber, being present.

This great and important news was immediately made known to the town by the firing of the Tower guns; and the Privy Council being assembled as soon as possible thereupon at the Council-chamber, Whitehall, it was ordered that a form of thanksgiving for the Queen's safe delivery of a Princess be prepared by his Grace the Archbishop of Canterbury, to be used in all churches and chapels throughout England and Wales, and the town of Berwick-upon-Tweed, on Sunday, the 29th of November, or the Sunday after the respective ministers shall receive the same.

Her Majesty and the young Princess are, God be praised, both doing well.

(From the Court Circular.)

Press report, with medical bulletin issued by Drs Clark, Locock, Ferguson and Blagden, on the birth of Queen Victoria and Prince Albert's first child, Princess Victoria. Thereafter the public clamoured for medical reports of royalty in the press. (Worcester Gazette, 28 November 1840).

before and their positions became firmly fixed within her royal household both in England and in Scotland, where she had a separate medical household. Their ranks were to include the most distinguished medical practitioners of the age, from pioneers of surgery to the most skilled clinicians. All of them contributed science, style and no little scandal to the royal court.

During the twenty years between Victoria's birth in 1819 and her coronation on 28 June 1838, medicine in Britain had taken several positive steps forward. One was in the study of the human body, using legally procured cadavers. The nation had cringed at the activities of such men as the murderers William Burke and William Hare, who smothered a number of people during 1827 and 1828 and sold their dead bodies to Edinburgh's anatomists. A year before Burke and Hare began their series of murders the merchantman *Latona*, out of Liverpool and bound for Leith, had been intercepted and was found to be carrying a cargo of eleven pickled and salted grave-robbed bodies purchased for the dissecting table. The passing of the Anatomy Act of 1838 brought this grisly trade to an end.[3]

Outside the court a number of therapeutic advances, like the successful prevention of smallpox by vaccination and the appearance of state medical services as a result of the new Poor Laws, was remoulding medical care. Nevertheless during Queen

QUEEN VICTORIA'S MEDICAL HOUSEHOLD: SOME ASIDES

Selection of Medical Household:
By Act of Parliament, 27 Henry VIII, c. 11. 1536. Under Warrant of the Lord Chamberlain, Held until death or retirement. Selected by promotion, or recommendation; had to be leaders of their profession. 57 were presidents of the various Royal Colleges; 42 members of the Royal Society. A medical household of 40–50 served Queen Victoria at various times.

Payments:
Average payments per annum were:
physician or surgeon-in-ordinary: £300
surgeon to the household: £400
apothecary to the household: £500
State surgeon Ireland: £133

Paramedics:
At various times the royal medical household included: cuppers (at Edinburgh and London); surgeon chiropodists; medical galvanists; phrenologist educationalists; and a masseuse (one of the few non-servant female posts at court – in 1883 the post was held by Madame Charlotte Nautet from Aix-les-Bains).

Locales:
Medical attendants of all types were expected to be willing to serve, call on and be attendant on the queen (often at short notice) at these specified locations; the fact that the queen visited some of them only rarely was of no consequence to her; where she was she expected her medical attendants to be:

Buckingham Palace; St James's Palace; Kensington Palace; Kew Palace; Hampton Court Palace; Windsor Castle; Osborne House; Marine Pavilion (Brighton); Claremont House; Holyrood Palace; Balmoral Castle; Dublin Castle.

A ROYAL DOCTOR ASSESSES QUEEN VICTORIA

Few royal doctors had the temerity or courage to voice an adverse opinion about Queen Victoria to her face, or even behind her back. But the Stratfield Saye manuscripts offer a glimpse behind the scenes from the *accoucheur* Sir Charles Locock. The story was recounted by Colonel Arbuthnot to the Duke of Wellington via Lady Mahon (the future Countess of Stanhope):

Locock seems to tell Lady Mahon everything (commenced Arbuthnot's particular tale). He says that having a good while ago wished to go to his Country Place in the North of England, & fearing to be called back (to the Queen's service), he told Prince Albert that he really ought to see the Queen.

This caused an interview, at the commencement of which Locock says he felt shy & embarrassed; but the Queen very soon put him at his ease.

Every Medical observation which he made, & which might perhaps bear two significations, was invariably considered by Her Majesty in the least delicate sense. She had not the slightest reserve & was always ready to express Herself, in respect to Her present situation (pregnancy), in the very plainest terms possible.

She asked Locock whether she should suffer much pain (at labour and delivery). He replied that some pain was to be expected, but that he had no doubt Her Majesty would bear it very well. 'O yes,' said the Queen, 'I can bear pain as well as other People.'

It was a subject (opined Arbuthnot) going so near the wind of delicacy, that I could do no more than listen without asking questions (of Lady Mahon). A good deal was told me by Lady Mahon to the same effect; but the results of the whole was that Locock left Her Majesty without any very good impressions of Her; & with the certainty that She will be very ugly & enormously fat. He says that Her figure now is most extraordinary. She goes without stays or anything that keeps Her shape within bounds; & that She is more like a barrel than anything else.

Victoria's infancy medical practice in the UK was still a primitive state of blood-letting, blistering and the prescribing of enemas.

The pioneering work of Dr Edward Jenner (1749–1823) into vaccination, which had caught the public eye in his *Inquiry into Cause and Effects of the Variolae Vaccinae* (1798), was monitored by Queen Victoria's parents, who had her vaccinated at three months old, on 2 August 1819, against smallpox. Later, with wry humour, Queen Victoria noted that this was her first act in setting 'a good example to the country'.[4]

For as long as there had been royal surgeons, medical science had been seeking a means of dulling pain for surgical operations. Queen Victoria's early surgeons had been trained to work speedily. All surgeons had to work with screaming patients strapped to operating tables, their screams of agony unnerving all who were present. Thus surgeons were required to amputate a leg in 120 called-out seconds, or perhaps extract a gallstone in 54 seconds. Opium and whisky were the most employed pain-deadeners, while others experimented with mesmerism. Nevertheless patients who endured surgery in 1837 faced the shocks and horrors suffered by medieval torture victims.

In 1846 the medical world was excited to read of an operation performed at Massachusetts General Hospital upon a patient who had inhaled ether vapour. The process was used in London by Robert Liston (1794–1847), Professor of Clinical Surgery at University College, and a whole raft of operations similarly conducted introduced the public to the benefits of ether anaesthesia.

In setting up her first medical household as queen, Victoria retained Sir Benjamin Brodie and Robert Keate as her sergeant-surgeons. Three other medical men were to feature during the early period of her reign. The most celebrated of the trio was Richard Bright, whom Queen Victoria appointed her physician-extraordinary in 1837.

Richard Bright had been born at Bristol on 28 September 1789. In 1808 he entered Edinburgh University and in 1819 made a visit to Iceland

> 'I have attended four sovereigns, and have been badly paid for my services. One of them now deceased, owed me nine thousand guineas.'
> **Robert Keate**
> *(served 1837–57)*

with his fellow student (Sir) Henry Holland; afterwards he published an account of the botany and natural history of that country. He graduated MD from Edinburgh in 1812 and continued to travel on the continent. In 1820 he was elected assistant physician at Guy's Hospital and began to write up his experiences walking the wards. In his day nothing was known about chronic nephritis; likewise dropsy was not considered a primary disease. Further, the connection between dropsy and urine containing albumen was not understood. Bright correlated the symptoms and his findings were given the generic name 'Bright's Disease'.

Bright entered royal circles through his reputation as one of the leading consultants of his day. He died on 16 December 1858 and his epitaph at St James's Church, Piccadilly (he was buried at Kensal Green) read: 'He contributed to medical science many discoveries and works of great value and died while in the full practice of his profession, after a life of warm affection, unsullied purity and great usefulness.'

The other two royal medics of Queen Victoria's early reign were Robert Ferguson and Sir John Forbes. Born in India, Robert Ferguson (1799–1865) studied medicine at Heidelberg and Edinburgh, graduating MD at the latter in 1823. He made a particular study of gynaecology and obstetrics and was physician to the Westminster Lying-in Hospital. In 1827 he founded the *London Medical Gazette* and four years later he was appointed Professor of Obstetrics at King's College, London. Ferguson was appointed physician-*accoucheur* to Queen Victoria in 1840.

Sir John Forbes (1787–1861) studied medicine at Aberdeen and Edinburgh, and entered the Royal Navy as an assistant-surgeon in 1807. He graduated MD at Edinburgh in 1817, building up practices severally at Penzance, Chichester and London. In 1840 he was appointed physician to Queen Victoria's household. A devotee of mesmerism and the therapeutic benefits of studying nature and art, he promoted a more extensive use of ausculation for patients. For this, he advanced the use of the stethoscope, which had been invented by René Théophile Hyacinthe Läennec (1781–1826), the French physician.

By the time she was nineteen Queen Victoria had begun her lifelong struggle with her weight. Her prime minister, Lord Melbourne, suggested that she eat less and take more exercise. Queen Victoria answered that she was always hungry and hated walking because she got stones in her shoes. Her *Journal* is bespotted with comments on her 'sick-headaches' which made her 'cross and low' and subject to days of nervous irritability. Her royal doctors noted how her anxieties about her weight, appearance and (supposed) failing eyesight were brought on by stress. She had a particularly bad spell in 1841 when Lord Melbourne was out of office after suffering defeat at the general election. Her melancholy was exacerbated at his death in 1848.

On 10 February 1840 Queen Victoria married Prince Albert of Saxe-Coburg-Gotha and a new medical household was established for the prince. Dr (Sir) Henry Holland (1788–1873) was chosen as physician-in-ordinary. A graduate of Edinburgh (MD, 1811), Holland had also studied at Guy's and St Thomas's hospitals. His interest in geology had led him to take part in an expedition to Iceland with mineralogist Sir George Steuart Mackenzie of Coul (1780–1846) in 1810, and Holland had contributed to Mackenzie's writings on Iceland. In 1814 Holland became medical attendant to Caroline Amelia Elizabeth of Brunswick-Wolfenbüttel (1768–1821), queen of George IV, while she was rattling lasciviously around Italy. He also gave evidence in her favour in 1820 during the promotion of the (aborted) parliamentary bill in the House of Lords for her divorce. Holland became physician-in-ordinary to Queen Victoria in 1852.

For his surgeon Prince Albert chose Charles Aston Key (1793–1849), who did not take up his appointment until 1847. Key had studied surgery at Guy's in 1814 and became a demonstrator of anatomy at St Thomas's Hospital and surgeon (and later lecturer) at Guy's from 1824. Key was to win a fine reputation for his operations for lithotomy. He was one of the first to use ether as an anaesthetic.

A doctor from Queen Victoria's early years, however, was to play a colourful role that was to bring her much anguish.

QUEEN VICTORIA'S MEDICAL HOUSEHOLD

Queen Victoria. Born 24 May 1819. Reigned 1837–1901. Died 22 January 1901.

During her long reign the following doctors rose to royal preferment.

Robert Adams (1791–1875). Surgeon in Ireland, 1861.

Sir James Alderson (1794–1882). Physician-extraordinary, 1874.

Neil Arnott (1788–1874). Physician-extraordinary.

William Baly (1814–61). Physician, 1859.

Thomas Barlow (1845–1945). Physician-extraordinary, 1899.

Sir Benjamin Collins Brodie (1783–1862). Sergeant-surgeon, 1834.

Sir James Clark (1788–1870). Physician to royal household.

James Begbie (1798–1869). Physician-in-ordinary in Scotland.

Richard Bright (1789–1858). Physician-extraordinary, 1837.

Sir William Henry Broadbent (1835–1907). Physician to royal family 1891.

Sir William Frederick Chambers (1786–1855). Physician (to Duchess of Kent).

Sir Philip Crampton (1777–1858). Surgeon-in-ordinary.

Sir John Eric Ericksen (1818–96). Surgeon-extraordinary.

Arthur Farre (1811–87). Obstetric physician. Physician-extraordinary.

Robert Ferguson (1799–1865). Physician-*accoucheur*. 1840.

Sir William Ferguson (1808–77). Sergeant-surgeon, 1855.

Sir John Forbes (1787–1861). Physician to royal household, 1840.

Sir William Withey Gull (1815–90). Physician-in-ordinary, 1887–90.

Caesar Henry Hawkins (1798–1884). Sergeant-surgeon 1862.

Sir Prescott Gardner Hewlett (1812–91). Surgeon-extraordinary, 1867; sergeant-surgeon, 1884; surgeon to the Prince of Wales, 1875.

Sir Henry Holland (1788–1873). Physician-in-ordinary to Prince Albert 1840. Queen Victoria 1852.

Sir William Jenner (1815–98). Physician-extraordinary then Physician-in-ordinary (and to the Prince of Wales).

Sir George Johnson (1818–96). Physician-extraordinary.

Robert Keath (1777–1857). Sergeant-surgeon.

Charles Aston Key (1793–1849). Surgeon to Prince Albert, 1847.

Peter Mere Latham (1789–1875). Physician-in-ordinary.

George Lawson (1831–1903). Surgeon-oculist, 1886.

Sir Charles Locock (1799–1875). Physician-*accoucheur*, 1840.

William Marshall. Resident medical attendant to Queen Victoria and royal household, Scotland.

James Miller (1812–64). Surgeon-in-ordinary, 1848, in Scotland.

Sir James Paget (1814–99). Surgeon-extraordinary, 1858; sergeant-surgeon extraordinary, 1867–77; sergeant-surgeon, 1877.

Alexander Profeit (d. 1897). Physician and commissioner at Balmoral.

Sir Richard Quain (1816–98). Physician-extraordinary.

Sir James Reid (1849–1923). Resident medical attendant, 1881; physician-extraordinary; 1887; physician-in-ordinary, 1889.

Douglas Argyll Robertson (1837–1909). Surgeon-oculist.

Sir Thomas Smith (1833–1909). Surgeon-extraordinary, 1895.

Edward Stanley (1793–1862). Surgeon-extraordinary, 1858.

Sir Thomas Grainger Stewart (1837–1900). Physician-in-ordinary in Scotland, 1882.

William Stokes (1804–78). Physician in Ireland 1866.

Sir William Stokes (1839–1900). Surgeon-in-ordinary in Ireland, 1861.

Benjamin Travers (1783–1853). Surgeon.

Sir Frederick Treves (1853–1923). Surgeon-extraordinary, 1900.

Sir Thomas Watson (1743–1882). Physician.

Charles James Blasius Williams (1805–89). Physician-extraordinary, 1874.

By 1887 the Medical Dept of the Queen's Household had developed thus showing patterns of title and deployment:

ENGLAND

Physicians-in-ordinary: Sir William Jenner; Sir George Burrows (1801–87); Wilson Fox (1831–87).

Physicians extraordinary: Sir Edward Henry Sieveking (1816–1904); Sir William Gull; C.J.B. Williams; Arthur Farre; G. Owen Rees.

Physician to the household: John Russel Reynolds (1828–96).

Resident physician: James Reid.

Sergeant-surgeons: Sir James Paget; Sir Prescott G. Hewett.

Surgeons-extraordinary: Richard Quain; John Eric Ericksen; Sir Joseph Lister.

Surgeon to the household: Sir Thomas Spencer Wells (1818–97).

Surgeon apothecary to Her Majesty: F.H. Laking.

Apothecary to the household: F.H. Laking.

Surgeon apothecaries to the household at Windsor: J. Ellison; W. Fairbank.

Surgeon Aapothecaries to Her Majesty at Osborne: Sir W. Carter Hoffmeister; W. Hoffmeister.

Surgeon-oculist: George Lawson.

Surgeon-dentist: Sir Edwin Saunders (1814–1901).

Dentist to the household: Edwin T. Truman (1818–1905).

Chemists and druggists in ordinary: Messrs P.W. and W.H. Squire.

SCOTLAND

Physicians-in-ordinary: William Tennant Gairdner (1824–1907); T.G. Stewart.

Surgeons-in-ordinary: George H. Baird Macleod (1828–92); Patrick H. Watson (1832–1907).

Surgeon-oculist: D.A. Robertson.

Surgeon-dentist: J. Smith.

IRELAND

Physicians-in-ordinary: John T. Banks (1815–1908).

Surgeons-in-ordinary: Sir G. Hornidge Porter (1822–95); W. Colles.

Surgeon-oculist: C.E. Fitzgerald.

Apothecary: J. Evans.

TO ALBERT EDWARD, PRINCE OF WALES

Physicians-in-ordinary: Sir William Jenner; Sir E.H. Sieveking; Sir William Gull.

Surgeons-in-ordinary: Sir James Paget; G.D. Pollock; Sir Prescott G. Hewett.

Surgeon-extraordinary: J.M. Minter.

Extra surgeon-in-ordinary: Sir Oscar Clayton.

Honorary physicians: T.K. Chambers; Sir H.W. Acland; Sir A. Armstrong; Sir Joseph Fayrer; J. Lowe.

Surgeon-apothecary to the household: F.H. Laking.

Surgeon-dentist: Sir E. Saunders.

TO ALEXANDRA, PRINCESS OF WALES
Physician-*accoucheurs*: Arthur Farre; G.T. Gream.

TO PRINCE ARTHUR, DUKE OF EDINBURGH AND SAXE-COBURG-GOTHA
Physician: Sir Joseph Fayrer (1824–1907).
Physicians-in-ordinary: Wilson Fox; G. Wilks.
Surgeon-in-ordinary: Sir Oscar Clayton.
Dentist: Charles Heath.

TO PRINCESS MARIE, DUCHESS OF EDINBURGH AND SAXE-COBURG-GOTHA
Physician-*accoucheurs*: Arthur Farre; William Smoult Playfair (1835–1903).

TO PRINCE ARTHUR AND PRINCESS LOUISE, DUKE AND DUCHESS OF CONNAUGHT
Physician-in-ordinary: Samuel Wilks (1814–1911).

On Queen Victoria's death the Medical Dept was gazetted thus:

PERSONAL HOUSEHOLD
Resident medical attendant: Sir James Reid.

MEDICAL DEPARTMENT
Physicians-in-ordinary: Sir Edward Henry Sieveking; Sir James Reid; Sir Richard Douglas-Powell (1842–1925).
Physicians-extraordinary: Sir Alfred Baring Garrod (1819–1907); Sir Samuel Wilks; Sir Henry Broadbent; J.E. Pollock; Thomas Barlow.
Sergeant-surgeon: Lord Lister.
Surgeons-extraordinary: Sir Thomas Smith; Thomas Bryant; Frederick Treves.
Physician to the household: Thomas Barlow.
Surgeon to the household: Rickman John Godlee (1849–1925).
Surgeons-apothecary to the household at Windsor: William Fairbank; William Ellison.
Surgeon-apothecary to Her Majesty and apothecary to the household: Sir Francis Henry Laking.
Surgeon-apothecary to Her Majesty and the household at Osborne: William Hoffmeister; H.E.W. Hoffmeister.

Surgeon-oculist: George Lawson.
Surgeon-dentist: Sir Edwin Saunders.
Dentist to the household: Edwin Truman.
Chemist and druggist: Peter Wyatt Squire.

TO ALBERT EDWARD, PRINCE OF WALES
Physicians-in-ordinary: Sir Edwin Henry Sieveking; Sir William H. Broadbent; Sir James Reid.
Surgeons-in-ordinary: Sir William MacCormac (1836–1901); Alfred Downing Fripp.
Surgeon to the household: Herbert Allingham.
Honorary physicians: John Lowe; Sir Dyce Duckworth (1840–1928).
Honorary surgeon-general: Sir Joseph Frayer.
Honorary deputy inspector general: A.G. Delmege.
Surgeon-apothecary: Sir Francis H. Laking.
Surgeon-apothecary at Sandringham: Alan R. Manby.
Surgeon-dentist: Sir Edwin Saunders.

TO PRINCE GEORGE AND PRINCESS MAY, THE DUKE AND DUCHESS OF YORK
Physician-*accoucheur*: Sir John Williams.
Surgeon-in-ordinary: Frederick Treves.
Surgeon-apothecary: Alan Reeve Manby.
Physician-in-ordinary: Robert W. Burnet.

TO PRINCESS MARIE, DUCHESS OF EDINBURGH AND SAXE-COBURG-GOTHA
Physician-*accoucheur*: William Smoult Playfair.

TO PRINCE ARTHUR AND PRINCESS LOUISE, THE DUKE AND DUCHESS OF CONNAUGHT
Physician: Sir Samuel Wilks.
Physician-*accoucheurs*: William Smoult Playfair; Sir Francis H. Laking.

CHAPTER TEN

WILFUL MURDER AGAINST BUCKINGHAM PALACE: THE RISE, FALL AND RISE OF SIR JAMES CLARK

It was a series of events that was to haunt Queen Victoria for the rest of her life; it was a dark scenario that brought one of her most prominent physicians to his lowest point. Both were to remember with keen penitence and blistering embarrassment the name of Lady Florence Elizabeth Hastings.

Physician James Clark and his royal employer shared a regal stage fraught with intrigue far from the little fishing town where he spent his early days. James Clark was born at Cullen House, Banffshire, on 14 December 1788. His father David Clark was butler to James Ogilvy, Earl of Findlater and Seafield. From Cullen parish school he went on to Fordyce grammar school, where he was awarded a bursary to King's College, Aberdeen, to study Arts.[1] Following his formal education he entered the office of a writer to the signet.[2]

Tiring of the law, Clark left to become an apprentice to Dr James Williamson and Dr James Smith, general medical practitioners at Banff; at the same time he attended medical classes at Edinburgh University. In 1809 he became a member of the Royal College of Surgeons of Edinburgh. Joining the medical services of the Royal Navy, he served a year as a hospital mate at the Royal Navy's Haslar Hospital, Gosport, before undertaking duty aboard several vessels in the Nova Scotia, New England and West Indies stations. At the end of the Napoleonic wars he was put on half-pay in 1815. Clark graduated MD at Edinburgh University on 1 August 1817; his thesis was entitled *De Frigoris Effectibus* (The Effects of Cold), and he later joined one of the Arctic expeditions of Rear-Admiral Sir William Edward Parry, wherein he studied climatology.

After this James Clark travelled widely on the continent

as personal physician to a patient with phthisis (pulmonary tuberculosis), and took time to study the art of percussion (diagnosis by striking) and auscultation (diagnosis from sounds within the body) from such men as the French gynaecologist Joseph Claude Recamier (1774–1852) at the Hôtel Dieu, Paris. During the period 1819–26 Clark practised as a physician in Rome, from a house in the Piazza di Spagna at the foot of the Spanish Steps. Here his roll of patients included poet John Keats.

Keats lived at 26 Piazza di Spagna (now the Keats–Shelley House Museum), attended only by his artist friend Joseph Severn. Dr Clark and his wife paid generous court to the poet and Dr Clark treated him from his arrival in Rome in November 1820 to his death on 23 February 1821.[3] He later performed the autopsy on Keats which discovered the poet's diseased lungs.[4] Analysing contemporary opinion of Clark, Amy Lowell wrote that 'he was a poor doctor, with a kindly heart and a pleasant bedside manner'.[5] Both these factors were to be apparent in royal circles.

A chance encounter at Carlsbad, where he was studying mineral springs, brought Clark into the princely milieu of Leopold, Duke of Saxe-Coburg.[6] At that time Prince Leopold was still famed as the relict of the unfortunate Princess Charlotte, the heir to the British throne who had died in childbirth.

Prince Leopold's sister was Princess Maria Louisa Victoria of Saxe-Coburg, widow of Emich Karl, 2nd Prince zu Leningen, who married King George III's fourth son Prince Edward, Duke of Kent and Strathearn, on 29 May 1818. Their daughter Princess Victoria was born on 24 May 1819. For the sake of economy the impoverished Kents rented the Gothic-style Woolbrook Cottage, Sidmouth, Devon, and there at the turn of 1820 the duke fell ill with a gastric attack. Physician Dr Wilson prescribed calomel and the popular panacea of the day known as James's Powder, but the duke's condition worsened and the Duchess of Kent sent word urgently to London for the senior royal physician Dr David Dundas to attend her husband. Alas, King George III himself was entering the final weeks of his life and Dr William George Maton (1774–1835), formerly physician-extraordinary to Queen Charlotte, was sent instead.

The Duke of Kent died on 23 June 1820 from pneumonia; some said his end had been quickened by Dr Maton's excessive bleedings. Later that year Maton became physician to the Duchess of Kent and the Princess Victoria, a post he held until his death. Subsequently Prince Leopold persuaded his sister to appoint his old friend James Clark to replace Maton. By this time Clark had established himself as a medical practitioner in London, where he practised from 1826 to 1860. He became a licentiate, then an extra-licentiate of the Royal College of Physicians, and the only public appointment he was ever to hold was as physician to St George's Dispensary. In 1832 Clark became a Fellow of the Royal Society.

On his court appointment James Clark entered the puzzling world of royal intrigue. During the late summer of 1835 the Duchess of Kent and Princess Victoria travelled to Ramsgate on vacation. This followed a tour of the north Midlands, during which Princess Victoria was unwell with headaches and a 'sore throat'. At Ramsgate they were joined by Prince Leopold, who had been elected King of the Belgians as Leopold I in 1831; he was accompanied by his wife Louise, daughter of Louis-Philippe, King of France, whom he had married in 1832. The party was completed with Queen Louise's brother, the Duc de Nemours; the Belgian ambassador to the Court of St James's, Sylvain van der Weyer; and the Duchess of Kent's household comptroller, the scheming (Sir) John Conroy and his family. King Leopold and Queen Louise were concerned about their niece's health and were perplexed by her mother's seeming lack of real concern. The reason was not hard to find – and they found it in the machinations of her comptroller.

Conroy had his eye on the main chance. Young Princess Victoria's uncle, King William IV, was failing, and Conroy wished to have himself declared her private secretary before she succeeded to the throne. This would give him pole position for future advancement under a pliable young monarch. Already he had some influence over the Duchess of Kent and he viewed Princess Victoria's 'illnesses' with some trepidation; he wanted nothing to throw any doubt on her perceived public ability to reign and looked upon any indisposition as dangerous 'from a political point of view'.[7] Conroy had dismissed Victoria's current illness as 'a slight cold' and refused permission (such was his position) for Dr James Clark to examine and treat her; thus the doctor had returned to his practice in London, accompanying Ambassador van der Weyer. When Princess Victoria went to Dover to say goodbye to her aunt and uncle prior to their return to Belgium, she collapsed in her carriage; she asked for Dr Clark but was informed by her mother that he was not available and that she was not to make a fuss.

Anxious about his niece, King Leopold insisted that Dr Clark be summoned, despite the Duchess of Kent taking Conroy's cue to minimise Victoria's symptoms. Clark diagnosed the princess's condition as an 'ulcerated sore throat' and then, with Conroy's encouragement, returned to London. King Leopold realised that Conroy was busily entrenching his position in the Duchess of Kent's entourage with an eye on the soon-to-be-vacant throne and warned him that if 'anything happens to the Princess Victoria there is of course an end to all your prospects'.[8]

Princess Victoria's condition steadily deteriorated, exacerbated by the stress of intrigue in her mother's court. The household was divided into two distinct camps: the Duchess of Kent and Conroy conspired to 'control' the princess with a view to their own positions when she was queen, while the fast-maturing Victoria was developing her own independence, a hatred of Conroy, an irritation with her mother, supported by her governess Baroness Louise Lehzen, who also loathed Conroy. Although Princess Victoria's condition continued to worsen, the duchess and Conroy still refused to call James Clark to attend her sickbed; it is clear that Conroy saw Clark as an ally of the 'Victoria camp' and wished to keep him at bay as much as possible.[9] At last the duchess became so alarmed at her daughter's illness that a local Ramsgate physician, Dr Plenderleith, was called in. He considered the princess's condition to be very serious and cared for her until James Clark was finally summoned. Clark diagnosed typhoid and stayed with her until she recovered.

Princess Victoria's confidence in James Clark increased. He had taken on great responsibility. Typhoid in those days had a high incidence of mortality, yet he treated her without consulting colleagues. The heir to the throne's attack was serious; she lost most of her hair and was three months in her recovery. Clark was diligent in his care, although his means of aiding recovery raised some eyebrows, as his own memoranda reveal. He suggested:

> . . . a drive into the country three times a week at least . . . Finchley, Harrow, Hampstead or Edgeware . . . Her Royal Highness could walk . . . Hampstead Heath . . . it will be well if Her Royal Highness would write occasionally at a standing desk. Reading aloud . . . but neither reading aloud or singing should be attempted soon after a meal . . . a warm bath every fourth or fifth night . . . the frequent use of Indian Clubs (heavy bottle-shaped wooden exercise bats to develop arm muscles).[10]

Dissatisfied by the accommodation allocated to her by her royal brother-in-law the king, the Duchess of Kent complained that her daughter needed a country residence. At last, in July 1836, the king offered her the Palace at Kew. It wouldn't do. The duchess wrote to Prime Minister Melbourne that she found the palace 'an old house quite unfit for the Princess Victoria and me to occupy, being very inadequate and almost destitute of furniture'.[11] The duchess enlisted Dr Clark to write a letter declaring the residence 'unfit'. A fanatic for fresh air, Clark deemed *every* royal building he visited to be unfit and told an incredulous Queen Victoria in years to come that Buckingham Palace needed a pump to cleanse the air.

Concerning his offer the king was adamant. It was Kew or nothing. The duchess preferred nothing, but expanded her suite to include further rooms at her abode at Kensington Palace. The king had already refused to grant permission for this expansion and was furious when he heard what the duchess had done. A rift ensued which growled on until King William IV died on 20 June 1837.

Queen Victoria's accession brought promotion for Clark; on the day of her elevation she wrote in her *Journal*: 'Saw Clark who I named my physician.'[12] On 11 November 1837 she created Clark a baronet, and gifted him in due course a copy of her portrait by the Glasgow-born painter John Partridge (1790–1872), for which she had sat at Buckingham Palace in 1840.[13] Despite all this heady promotion a dark cloud was looming for Clark in the form of Lady Florence Elizabeth Hastings.

Lady Florence, known to all as Lady Flora, was born in 1806, the eldest daughter of the soldier and statesman Francis Rawdon Hastings, Viscount Loudoun and Earl Rawdon, 1st Marquess of Hastings (1754–1826), sometime governor-general and commander-in-chief of the forces in India, and his wife Flora, *suo jure* Countess of Loudoun (1780–1840). Lady Flora became lady of the bedchamber to the Duchess of Kent in June 1834, replacing Charlotte Florentina, Duchess of Northumberland, Princess Victoria's official governess, who was becoming too 'independent'. On 30 April 1838 Lady Flora replaced Lady Mary Stopford as lady-in-waiting to the Duchess of Kent. Queen Victoria was prejudiced against Lady Flora from the start; she resented the departure of the Duchess of Northumberland and she deemed Lady Flora one of the 'Conroy set'. John Conroy's younger brother Llewellin had been *aide-de-camp* to the Marquess of Hastings, so the family ties were significant. What was more, the Hastings were Tories, and although she was to become a dedicated Conservative in her latter years the young Queen Victoria was a Whig, greatly influenced by the Whig Prime Minister Melbourne. Say nothing in front of her, the queen counselled Melbourne, for 'odious Lady Flora' is 'a spie for J(ohn) C(onroy)'.[14]

Unmarried at thirty-two, Lady Flora was an accomplished poet, and her 'graceful figure and a long slender neck supporting a neat head and delicate face' were much admired.[15] Immediately after 'coming into waiting' for her next stint on 10 January 1839, Lady Flora's state of health was seen to deteriorate; she complained of piercing stomach pains (which she attributed to ample platefuls of Christmas fare), but she consulted the Duchess of Kent's physician Sir James Clark. He diagnosed a 'derangement of the bowel' and 'a protuberance of the stomach'.[16] Clark prescribed a liniment compound of camphor soap and opium, with a dozen rhubarb and ipecacuhana pills, and from 10 January to 16 February he held consultations with Lady Flora twice weekly.[17]

To her horror Queen Victoria observed Lady Flora's 'protuberance of the stomach'. Surely it was a pregnancy? She relayed her observations to Baroness Lehzen.[18] The queen developed her opinion to aver that Lady Flora was pregnant by her *bête-noire* Conroy.[19] Had Lady Flora not travelled down from the Christmas 1838 holidays from her mother's home at Loudoun Castle, Ayrshire, with Conroy . . . *unchaperoned*?

The senior of the ladies-in-waiting, Anna Maria Russell, Marchioness of Tavistock, who acted as unofficial chaperone to the court ladies, was appalled at the gossip – 'Sir James Clark had told someone that Lady Flora appeared to be pregnant'.[20] The ladies were in uproar. Lady Tavistock believed she must do something to protect the reputation of the queen's ladies in general. Curiously, instead of interviewing Lady Flora (or even the Duchess of Kent), Lady Tavistock, who later became the mistress of court painter Sir Edwin Landseer, went straight to Prime Minister Melbourne. It seems that she was advised to do so by Baroness Lehzen, who was only too willing to blacken the name of a Conroy supporter.[21]

Lord Melbourne advised Lady Tavistock to remain silent. Was Sir James Clark wrong in his diagnosis of pregnancy? The prime minister thought the gossip serious enough to consult Clark directly. Clark agreed that he suspected pregnancy, but was not sure. All that could be done was to wait and watch the outcome. Queen Victoria was certain in her own mind and wrote in her *Journal*:

> We have no doubt that she is – to use plain words – *with child*. Clark cannot deny the suspicion; the horrid cause of all this is the Monster & demon Incarnate, whose name I forebear to mention, but which is the 1st word of the 2nd line of this page. (ie: John Conroy).[22]

As Lady Flora went about her duties 'with apparently little inconvenience to herself', the gossip in the hot-house atmosphere of the court reached new heights. Sir James Clark now grew 'pretty certain' that his patient was pregnant, but Lady Flora declined a physical examination at his promptings.

In early February 1839, Emma, Lady Portman, daughter of Henry Lascelles, 2nd Earl of Harewood – Lady Portman was second in rank to Lady Tavistock – came into waiting and met Sir James Clark with the idea of approaching Lady Flora concerning the suspicions of the court ladies. How could he do this discreetly? Say 'You must be secretly married,' Baroness Lehzen suggested to Clark via Lady Portman.[23] In due course Sir James Clark had his interview with Lady Flora, who denied any marriage. Clark suggested a second examination:

> I at length expressed to her my uneasiness respecting her size, and requested that at my next visit, I might be permitted to lay my hand upon her abdomen with her stays removed. To this Lady Flora declined to accede.[24]

The refusal suggested to Clark that Lady Flora was pregnant. She pointed out to the royal physician that her 'protrusion' had actually reduced and that she was wearing a smaller gown. Sir James Clark was not convinced and pressed for a further examination. Lady Flora was later to recount that Clark 'urged me to confess' (to marriage and pregnancy) as 'the only thing to save me'. He said that he concurred with the court ladies' gossip and that 'no one could look at me and doubt it, and remarks even more coarse'.[25] Again a physical examination was refused and Lady Portman informed Lady Flora that she should not attend the court until her virtue had been substantiated. On this Lady Flora agreed to an examination.

The examination was carried out by *accoucheur* and lecturer in midwifery Sir Charles Mansfield Clarke (1782–1857) on Sunday, 17 February, in the presence of Sir James Clark (who had little or no gynaecological experience) and Lady Portman, with Lady Flora's maid as 'indignant witness'. She was found to be a virgin, and received a certificate signed by the two doctors stating clearly:

> . . . we have examined with great care the state of Lady Flora Hastings with a view to determining the existence or non-existence of pregnancy, and it is our opinion, although there is an enlargement of the stomach, that there are no grounds for suspicion that pregnancy does exist, or ever did exist.[26]

Queen Victoria was mortified and humiliated by the blundering accusations that she had been privy to and played a part in,

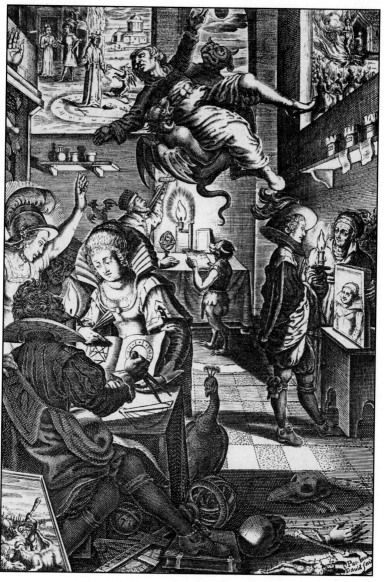

Up to late medieval times medicine and magic went hand in hand. Royal doctors were as well versed in the arcane sciences like alchemy as they were in contemporary medical thought. Thus the popular view of a doctor's consulting rooms was as a place of physic and sorcery. (Bodleian Library)

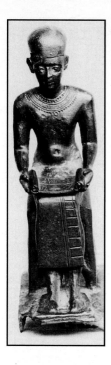

Imhotep. Egyptian physician and adviser to the 3rd Dynasty pharaoh Zoser. He flourished around 2980 BC as the prototype royal doctor. The Greeks identified him with Aesculapius, their God of Medicine. (British Museum)

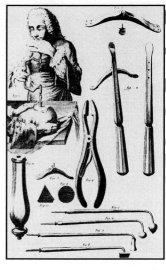

An operation to trepan a skull, with a montage of surgical instruments. Such an operation was carried out on Charles I's nephew, Prince Rupert of the Rhine. (Author's Collection)

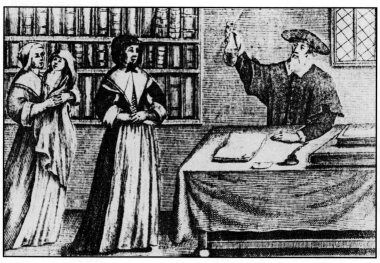

'The Doctor's Dispensary', a seventeenth-century woodcut showing a court doctor demonstrating a urinalysis to court ladies. His method is to hold the bottle up to the light for a visual examination. (Author's Collection)

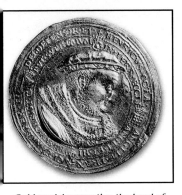

Gold medal presenting the head of King Henry VIII as 'Defender of the Faith'. As a youth he cut a dash as a vigorous sportsman, but later he became a gross bully, disabled by pain and depression, who terrorised his doctors with fits of violent temper. (National Maritime Museum)

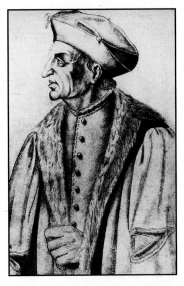

Thomas Linacre (c. 1460–1524) studied at Oxford and Padua and became physician to King Henry VIII. He was instrumental in the founding of the College of Physicians. (Royal College of Physicians)

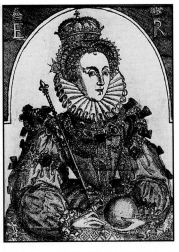

Woodcut portrait of Queen Elizabeth I, 1563. Her keen interest in magic and medicine caused her to consult the famous alchemist and sorcerer Dr John Dee. At varying times her physicians treated her for migraine, kidney inflammation and smallpox. (Huth Collection)

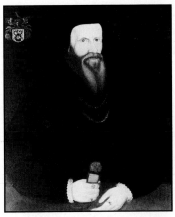

John Caius (1510–73) studied medicine under Giambattista Montano at Padua. Physician to King Edward VI and Queen Mary I, he was dismissed from serving Queen Elizabeth I as court physician because of his Roman Catholicism. (Royal College of Physicians)

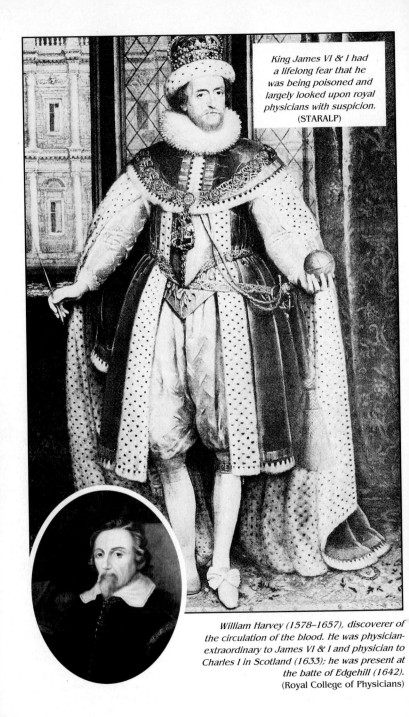

King James VI & I had a lifelong fear that he was being poisoned and largely looked upon royal physicians with suspicion. (STARALP)

William Harvey (1578–1657), discoverer of the circulation of the blood. He was physician-extraordinary to James VI & I and physician to Charles I in Scotland (1633); he was present at the batte of Edgehill (1642).
(Royal College of Physicians)

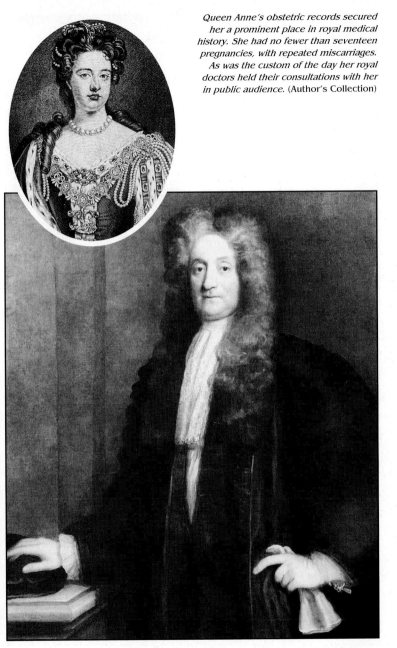

Queen Anne's obstetric records secured her a prominent place in royal medical history. She had no fewer than seventeen pregnancies, with repeated miscarriages. As was the custom of the day her royal doctors held their consultations with her in public audience. (Author's Collection)

Sir Hans Sloane (1660–1753). He attended Queen Anne and was First Physician to George II. A student of Paris and Montpellier, he is also remembered as the founder of the Botanic Garden in London. (Royal College of Physicians)

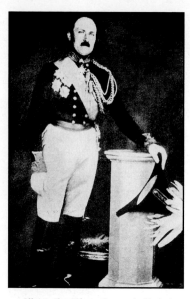

Albert, the Prince Consort, died at Windsor Castle on 14 December 1861. Lord Clarendon declared that the prince's doctors Sir James Clark and Sir Henry Holland were not 'fit to attend a sick cat'. (Purves Papers)

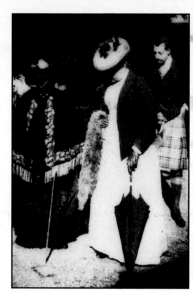

Queen Victoria walks in the garden of Abergeldie Castle, Scotland, in 1890. With her is her daughter Princess Victoria, Empress Frederick of Germany. Behind them is Prince Albert Victor, Duke of Clarence, whose name was linked with the 'Jack the Ripper' murders, as was that of the royal doctor Sir William Gull. (Purves Papers)

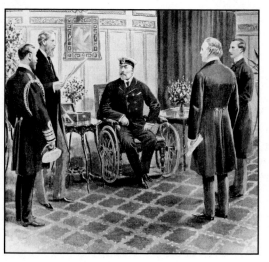

Edward VII, in a wheelchair, convalesces after his appendectomy which delayed his coronation in 1902. With him are (left to right) George, Prince of Wales, Spencer Compton Cavendish, 8th Duke of Devonshire, Lord President of the Council, Lord James of Hereford, Chancellor of the Duchy of Lancaster, royal doctor Sir Frederick Treves. (Purves Papers)

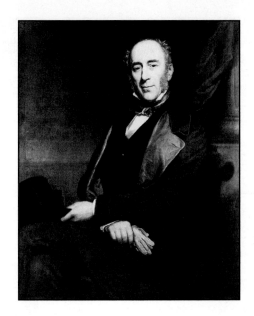

Sir James Clark (1788–1870), naval surgeon and court physician. He gained public and professional opprobrium because of his connection with the case of Lady Flora Hastings, lady-in-waiting to Queen Victoria's mother, the Duchess of Kent. (Royal College of Physicians)

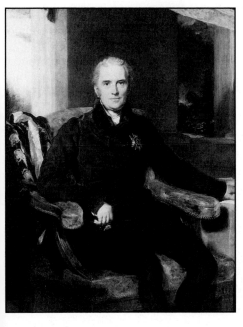

Sir Henry Halford (1766–1844) attended George IV, William IV and Queen Victoria. He was a prominent President of the Royal College of Physicians. (Royal College of Physicians)

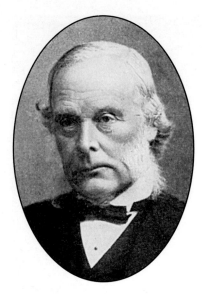

Joseph, Baron Lister (1827–1912), founder of antiseptic surgery. Surgeon-extraordinary to Queen Victoria, he used his carbolic spray while treating Queen Victoria for an abscess in September 1871. He later became sergeant-surgeon to King Edward VII. (Author's Collection)

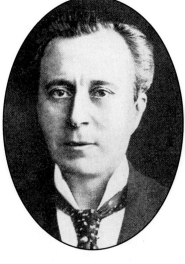

Sir Francis Laking (1847–1914), prominent court physician. He was surgeon-apothecary to Queen Victoria and physician-in-ordinary to King Edward VII. (Author's Collection)

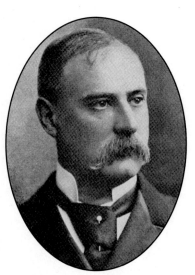

Sir Frederick Treves (1853–1923), a prominent surgical demonstrator and leading practitioner, was surgeon-extraordinary to Queen Victoria. He acquired world renown for his operation on King Edward VII for appendicitis. He was also sergeant-surgeon to Edward VII and George V. (Author's Collection)

and sent a message that she would see Lady Flora immediately should she so wish it. Lady Flora demurred. In the meantime the unfortunate predicament got worse. Neither Sir Charles nor Sir James was comfortable with their diagnosis. So agitated were they that they consulted the prime minister, who told the queen of their doubts. Victoria sent this memorandum to her mother (relations had so deteriorated between mother and daughter that they were not on speaking terms):

> Sir Clark had said that though (Lady Flora) is a virgin still that (pregnancy) might be possible and one could not tell if such things could happen. That there was an enlargement in the womb like a child.[27]

News of the scandal was spreading in society. At his country seat of Castle Donnington in Leicestershire, Lady Flora's brother George Augustus Hastings was incensed at his sister's treatment. He accused the prime minister of encouraging a Whig plot to discredit Tory ladies.

Queen Victoria began to feel bilious, and with good reason. She found out that her mother had dismissed Sir James Clark as her physician in a very strong letter of discharge, and she urged the queen to do the same. The Duke of Wellington – an unofficial royal 'troubleshooter' – advised that all sides should play down the unfortunate occurrences. Lady Flora was not attended by the Duchess of Kent's new physician, Dr William Frederick Chambers (1786–1855), the distinguished consultant physician.

By 23 February Lady Flora felt composed enough to see the queen, who granted her a swift audience. Victoria, who had not seen Lady Flora for some time, was shocked at how ill she looked and was concerned about her nervous condition. She reached for her hand, kissed her, and demonstrated real sorrow for what Lady Flora had been through. With tears in her eyes at Lady Flora's bold announcement that she had been 'treated as if guilty without a trial', the queen now hoped that all would be forgiven and forgotten. Lady Flora said that she would put the past behind her for the sake of good court relations. The queen, though, feared that trouble would bubble up again with Conroy exploiting the situation and Sir James becoming more agitated lest he be openly criticised by his professional peers.

While all this was going on Queen Victoria's nerves were being jangled by political events. For months Lord Melbourne's government had been experiencing difficulties, which led to his resignation on 7 May. The queen sent for opposition leader Sir Robert Peel to see if he could form a ministry. However, there was a problem. When a government changed it was the custom that the queen's ladies of the bedchamber changed too, so out would go her Whig ladies to be replaced by Tories. The thought of supporters of the political enemies of her beloved Lord Melbourne surrounding her at every turn – to say nothing of the Tory ladies supporting Lady Flora Hastings – caused the queen to be recalcitrant. Her ladies must stay. Under the circumstances Sir Robert Peel felt that he could not go on and form a ministry so Lord Melbourne's government limped along until August 1841. Sir James Clark prescribed for the queen's sick headaches, but was unable to do much about the storm that was brewing for himself.

Queen Victoria was already in turmoil when her worst fears concerning the Lady Flora situation became a reality. The whole case was raked over once more in the press. Who had first slandered Lady Flora? Was it Sir James Clark? If so, why was he still in court employ? If it were the court ladies, Lady Tavistock and Lady Portman, shouldn't they be dismissed? Was it one court faction trying to score over another? In the face of all this speculation Lady Flora's family decided to establish the truth, once and for all.

Lady Flora's mother, the Dowager Marchioness of Hastings (Countess of Loudoun), sent a terse letter on 7 March, via the Duchess of Kent, to the queen, regarding her daughter's treatment. She begged the queen to root out the 'criminal inventor' of the scandal and requested 'as a mark of public justice the removal of Sir James Clark'.[28]

Shortly afterwards the dowager marchioness pressed the prime minister to have Sir James Clark removed from royal office. Accusations and letters flew between the relevant parties with the queen getting more and more agitated, while the press drip-fed the public with snippets on the raging scandal. A very frank letter that Lady Flora had written to her uncle, Captain Hamilton Fitzgerald (married to her aunt Lady Charlotte Hastings), then at Brussels, saying that there were no medical grounds for accusing her of pregnancy, appeared in *The Examiner*. A re-hashing of the events was widely disseminated in the press with the queen, the prime minister, the Whigs and the royal physician all attacked for a dastardly political plot.[29]

All the while Lady Flora was becoming more emaciated. On the advice of Lord Melbourne the queen was cool towards her and 'cut' her at court. Victoria was more than willing to do this as she blamed 'that wretched Lady Flora' for the adverse press reports. Day by day the Whig and Tory ladies sniped at each other. To Sir James Clark's great discomfort, all this was further reported in the papers. Lady Flora won increased public sympathy, but the queen was criticised by name in the press and Sir James Clark lost patients. Worse still, when the queen drove up the racecourse at Royal Ascot with Lord Melbourne there were cries of 'Here come Mrs Melbourne'. And from the grandstand balcony she was 'hissed' by the Duchess of Montrose and Lady Sarah Ingrestre.[30]

On 1 June 1839 Sir John Conroy retired from the Duchess of Kent's employ and went abroad. Some whispered that Lady Flora's decline was now accelerated because she felt she had been deserted. Certainly she prepared herself and her friends with a 'Swan Song' in verse:

> Grieve not that I die young. – Is it not well
> To pass away ere life hath lost its brightness?
> Bind me no longer, sisters, with the spell
> Of love and your kind words. List ye to me:
> Here I am bless'd – but I would be *more free*;
> I would go forth in all my Spirit's lightness –
> Let me depart![31]

It was clear to all that Lady Flora's health was seriously deteriorating. Stung by her conscience, the queen resolved to do all she could for 'this unfortunate'.[32] Although she made it known that she 'would see' Lady Flora when she felt well enough, Lady Flora was too ill to seek an audience. The queen even agreed to postpone a planned ball at Buckingham Palace in accord with the Duchess of Kent's request. Charles Cavendish Fulke Grenville (1794–1865), clerk to the council, detected panic:

> (*The Queen and Melbourne*) are in great fright lest Lady Flora should die, because she is very ill, and if She should die the public will certainly hold an inquest on her body and bring in a verdict of wilful murder against Buckingham Palace.[33]

At last the queen paid a visit to Lady Flora's room:

> I found poor Ly Flora stretched on a couch looking as thin as anyone can be who is still alive; literally a skeleton, but the body *very* much swollen like a person who is with child; a searching look in her eyes, rather like a person who is dying; her voice like usual, a good deal of strength in her hands; she was friendly, said she was very comfortable, & was very grateful for all I had done for her; & that she was glad to see me look well. I said to her, I hoped to see her again when she was better, – upon which she grasped my hand as if to say 'I shall not see you again'.[34]

In her innermost thoughts it is clear that Victoria believed Lady Flora to be pregnant, and her self-delusion that she had been 'good' to Lady Flora was a significant character trait. On 5 July 1839 Baroness Lehzen woke the queen to inform her that Lady Flora had died at 2 a.m. that morning. The queen wrote in her *Journal*: 'the poor thing died without a struggle & only just raised her hands & gave one gasp . . .'[35]

Lady Flora's death sparked off another round of newspaper scandal. The medical world buzzed with the rumour that Sir James Clark had been banned by the Hastings family from performing the post mortem, or having anything to do with the cadaver. The resultant post mortem, led by old King William IV's surgeon Sir Benjamin Brodie, was embarrassing reading for Clark. It detailed how Lady Flora's uterus and ovaries were 'in a virgin state'; she had an enlarged liver and abdominal lymph nodes and gross and widespread abdominal lesions with pus in the intestines. Brodie's verdict was that Lady Flora had died of a tumour of the liver, but modern opinion suggests that Lady Flora probably died of tuberculous peritonitis.

Lady Flora was buried in her family's vault at Loudoun after a final outburst of public sympathy. As the cortège left Buckingham Palace for Scotland on 10 July, silent crowds lined the roadways to St Catherine's Wharf, despite the very early hour of 4 a.m. Behind the family carriages came the traditional empty carriages of Queen Victoria, Queen Adelaide and the Duchess of Kent.[36] As the queen's carriage passed it was stoned by the crowds. Out of the throng one man emerged shouting: 'What's the use of (the Queen's) gilded trumpery after she has killed her?'

A few months later Lord Hastings gave to the press all the information he could on the case, detailing Sir James Clark's involvement. Clark replied, defending himself, but he was attacked in medical journals such as the *Lancet*, while private individuals like Dr John Fisher Murray spread their views in pamphlets. Murray's was entitled *The Court Doctor Dissected.*[37] Dr Murray described the Whig ladies as 'viperly women', referred to Lady Flora as 'the martyred sister', and dismissed Clark as a 'medical fag'.

That was bad enough for Sir James Clark, but the 'underground press' went even further. A plethora of signed pamphlets and anonymous booklets sold widely for a few pence. A royal physician had never been so vilified and to such an extent. One such pamphlet, price one shilling, bore the title *The Dangers of Evil Counsel, By a Voice from the Grave of Lady Flora Hastings to her most Gracious Majesty the Queen*. It denigrated the queen's court in general and Clark in particular. A noble but anonymous hand turned the attack on the court and Clark into verse; part of it read:

> Strange destiny that Britain's mighty isle
> Should hang dependent on a school-girl's smile
> The court physician, with his cringing back
> And coward sneer, the leader of the pack;
> While titled beldames their assistance brought
> And the young Queen smiled blithely at the sport.

What upset Sir James Clark the most was the severe criticism of his treatment of Lady Flora voiced by Dr Chambers and Lord Melbourne. The prime minister was at his hypocritical best in this instance. His snide assessment of Lady Flora's supposed 'condition' sat uncomfortably on the shoulders of a man already cited twice as a co-respondent in divorce cases. He misguidedly fanned the flames of Queen Victoria's suspicions rather than extinguishing them, and was guilty of promoting a terrible miscarriage of justice. Sir Robert Peel would never have made such a mistake.

For Sir James Clark all this was made more humiliating by the denigrating public remarks of Sir Henry Halford, president of the Royal College of Physicians, who had also attended George IV, William IV and now Queen Victoria. In 1813 Sir Henry had published his *Account of what Appeared on Opening the Coffin of Charles I*; Sir James Clark now felt that Sir Henry was hammering nails into his.

In the Lady Flora case Sir James Clark made three serious errors. When Lady Flora had first refused a physical examination he should have withdrawn from further consultations. He should not have discussed his patient's symptoms with *anyone*, certainly not Lord Melbourne or Queen Victoria. Further, it was a very serious lapse of professional ethics to play any part in court gossip on the subject, or to ally himself with court cadres. For his errors he suffered public ignominy and his roll of patients dwindled.

Queen Victoria also acted badly in the matter. She was convinced of Lady Flora's guilt, without proof. She gossiped about it and actively pursued the calumny as a lever to oust the despised Conroy. In this matter, too, Queen Victoria proved herself a true Hanoverian; she neither learned anything nor forgot anything. In 1843 she openly accused Lady Augusta Somerset (1816–50) of being pregnant, and joined in the tittle-tattle that named her cousin Prince William George (1819–1904), Duke of Cambridge, as the purported child's father. The queen was forced to offer the Somersets a (half-hearted) apology, and the accusation was 'hushed up'.[38]

Sir James Clark retained his position as physician to Queen Victoria and somehow weathered the storms of the Lady Flora

Hastings affair, but he was well aware of the queen's penitence for her own part in the case. Some say that he settled in to his court duties too well and abused the system, as so many courtiers did, using royal carriages for private jaunts, eating at the expense of the royal household when not on duty, and so on. In particular, Clark was 'accused of always having a tradesman to recommend'.[39] Outside the court he was to play an important role in reforming medical practice and in promoting medical education; he was also deeply involved in the foundation of the Faculty of Medicine at the University of London, and organised courses at the Royal College of Chemistry and the Army Medical School. A poor researcher himself, Clark recognised research skills in others and promoted them. Yet his character and professional flaws did not smooth his path through royal service.

In late 1841 and early 1842 Clark treated Queen Victoria and Prince Albert's eldest child Princess Victoria Adelaide, 'Vicky', the princess royal, who had been born on 21 November 1840. He prescribed a diet of 'ass's milk and chicken broth'.[40] The child's lack of progress led to a furious row between the royal couple. This was exacerbated by Queen Victoria's post-natal depression following the birth of Prince Albert Edward, the Prince of Wales, on 9 November 1841. She resented her husband's criticism of the child's treatment. The queen averred that the princess's diet was at fault; Prince Albert blamed Clark's incompetence. Albert wrote:

> Doctor Clark has mismanaged the child and poisoned her with calomel and you have starved her. I shall have nothing more to do with it; take the child away and do as you like and if she dies – you will have it on your conscience.[41]

Despite this, Sir James Clark retained the good opinion of Queen Victoria although she did not always follow his advice or accept his opinions. For instance, in October 1844 the royal family took their first vacation at Osborne House on the Isle of Wight and Sir James Clark was invited to test the climate. He considered it 'not bracing enough to do children any good'.[42] Nevertheless Queen Victoria and Prince Albert purchased the property from Lady Isabella Blachford for £28,000 in 1845.

When it came to fresh air, though, Queen Victoria was a devotee of Clark. Wherever she went windows would be thrown open whatever the weather, the temperature or the inconvenience to others. During the autumn of 1848 Sir James Clark's son John convalesced on Deeside after a long illness as a guest of Sir Robert Gordon, the lessee of Balmoral Castle. He wrote to his father of the dryness and purity of the air. Indeed, while the royal party had been confined indoors at Ardverikie by rain and gales during their 1847 jaunt round the west coast of Scotland, Balmoral had basked in autumn sunshine.

At the time Queen Victoria was suffering from rheumatic pains and Sir James Clark suggested that she try the air on Scotland's Deeside. Queen Victoria's acceptance of his advice led to the leasing of Balmoral Castle in 1848 and the purchase of the estate for 30,000 guineas in 1852, and stimulated her lifelong love affair with the Scottish Highlands.

On 7 April 1853 Queen Victoria gave birth to Prince Leopold George Duncan Albert, Duke of Albany, an event which saw a new innovation in the practice of royal medicine. During her labour, Sir James Clark invited the distinguished anaesthetist Dr John Snow (1813–58) to give the queen chloroform. Snow recalled:

At twenty minutes past twelve by a little clock in the Queen's apartment, I commenced to give a little chloroform with each pain, by pouring about 15 minims by measure upon a folded handkerchief.[43]

In her *Journal* the queen was to note that Dr Snow 'gave that blessed Chloroform & the effect was soothing, quieting & delightful beyond measure'.

The pioneer of chloroform Dr (later Sir) James Young Simpson (1811–70), Professor of Midwifery at Edinburgh, received this note from Sir James Clark:

The Queen had chloroform exhibited to her during her last confinement . . . It was not at any time given so strongly as to render the Queen insensible, and an ounce of chloroform was scarcely consumed during the whole time. Her Majesty was greatly pleased with the effect, and she certainly never has had a better recovery.[44]

The use of chloroform in childbirth was controversial. Several commentators objected on moral, religious and ethical grounds. Medics wrote articles for and against the substance in learned journals, but because of the publicity associated with the queen having been given chloroform it became the norm for expectant mothers all over Britain to request its use. The queen chuckled on being told that one Scots patient of Dr J.Y. Simpson had been so taken by the procedure that she named her female baby 'Anaesthesia'.

As the smallest of Queen Victoria's children at birth, Prince Leopold was deemed 'delicate' and was so pronounced by his grandmother, the Duchess of Kent.[45] As a teenager he suffered from digestive problems, was slow to speak and had attacks of an 'epileptic character' which Dr (later Sir) William Jenner was to write about later.[46] But Leopold's life was blighted by his haemophilia. This royal scourge was passed on to several of the royal houses of Europe through Queen Victoria's line, her daughters Victoria, Alice and Beatrice being carriers, although Prince Leopold was her only child to suffer the disease. In Leopold's early life his condition was masked by his other problems.

Queen Victoria discussed her son's 'delicacy' with Sir James Clark, who came to the conclusion that Leopold needed a healthy wet-nurse – Victoria had refused to breastfeed any of her own children, being appalled at the idea that she was 'a milch-cow'. So from the Balmoral area came Gaelic-speaking Mrs Mackintosh. At first Prince Leopold thrived, but became extremely disturbed, with screaming fits. Sir James Clark was summoned to Osborne House by royal wire; he discussed the most recent events in the prince's health with local physician Dr Hoffmeister. Without any objection from Clark, who was getting more and more flummoxed by diagnoses, Hoffmeister replaced Mrs Mackintosh with Mrs Francis, 'a shipwright's wife from Cowes', and Prince Leopold began to improve.[47]

Prince Leopold had his first recorded bout of haemophilia in 1855 (when he was aged two), but as even the Royal College of Physicians did not recognise the condition until the late 1870s,

Sir James Clark (who retired in 1860) would have had little knowledge of it.

As the days of 1856 passed, Sir James Clark became more concerned with Queen Victoria's mental health. On 5 February he wrote in his *Diary*:

> I feel at times uneasy. Regarding the Queen's mind, unless she is kept quiet and still amused, the time will come when she will be in danger . . . Much depends on (Prince Albert's) management . . .[48]

In particular he warned Prince Albert that he 'felt sure if she had another child she would sink under it'.[49] Clark's fears were shared by a whole succession of Queen Victoria's physicians as she regularly suffered deflation, neurotic fits and debilitation. However, with the birth of Princess Beatrice on 14 April 1857 the queen felt better than she had done for a long time.

Despite his concern, Sir James Clark was able to take part in a happy encounter at Balmoral. When on duty at the Scottish castle Clark lodged at Birkhall, a former Gordon family property at the Deeside end of Glen Muick. In 1856 his fellow guest at Birkhall was the nurse and hospital reformer Florence Nightingale (1820–1910). The Crimean War was now five months over and Miss Nightingale was full of her future plans. Two weeks later she dined with the queen, regaling her with stories about the war and her hospital at Scutari. Eager for more, the queen later ordered up her pony cart and, unescorted, descended on Birkhall to take Florence Nightingale for a walk to hear more of her opinions on the merits of fresh air and theology. After their conversation the queen arranged for the nurse to see Foreign Minister Fox Maule, Lord Panmure, to discuss improvements in the Army Medical Service.

The parental mismanagement of the complex personality, education and recreation of Prince Albert Edward, Prince of Wales, made him a 'difficult child'. Sir James Clark, who had been present at his birth, had overseen his childhood ailments, but during the summer of 1858 the queen had a consultation with the royal physician as to the cause of the prince's 'loud interruptions to adult talk, fractious argument and sudden screaming rages'.[50] If Clark was aware of the queen and Prince Albert's severity towards the Prince of Wales – and his resultant inferiority complex – he made no allowance for it at the consultation and agreed with the queen that the problem should be tackled through a new dietary regime. Clark worked on the new diet. Wherever the Prince of Wales went, so did his diet sheets of boring blandness:

Breakfast 9 a.m.: A light one; tea, coffee, or cocoa, bread and butter; an egg if desired.

Lunch 2 p.m.: Meat and vegetables; puddings best avoided; Selzer (German mineral) water.

Dinner 7 p.m.: As light as possible; claret and Selzer water in hot weather; sherry and Selzer water in cold weather; no coffee.

Before retiring (preferably early):

A cup of tea; but Selzer water recommended.

As he got older Sir James Clark's reputation began to slide even further, as did his roll of patients. Giles St Aubyn dubbed him 'one of the worst doctors in England'.[51] Certainly Clark's comments on the health of one of Queen Victoria's grandchildren seem to bear this out.

AMUSING THE QUEEN AT TILLYPRONIE

Sir James Clark purchased the mansion house of Tillypronie, Tarland, 10 miles northwest of Aboyne, Aberdeenshire, in 1855; it was his son Sir John Clark who constructed the present house in 1867, for which the lintel was dedicated by Queen Victoria, who planted a commemorative *Abies magnifica* (blown down in the gales in 1953) on the same day.

When he was attending the royal family at Balmoral, Clark and his wife stayed at Birkhall. But the royal doctor entertained Queen Victoria many times at Tillypronie. On these occasions she was accompanied by her Highland Servant John Brown. Brown was considered (by himself and Queen Victoria) to be too grand to eat his meals with the other servants at Tillypronie, so he took his repast alone in a specially built wooden hut in the garden.

Prince Wilhelm Victor Albrecht, the first child of the eighteen-year-old Princess Vicky and her husband Fritz – destined to be Frederick III, German Emperor and King of Prussia – was born on 27 January 1859. Queen Victoria was worried about her daughter's pregnancy and sent Clark to the Palace of Potsdam with her own midwife, Mrs Innocent. The princess began her labour early and the resident physician Herr Doktor Wegner diagnosed a breech birth. During the four-hour labour Clark administered two-thirds of a bottle of chloroform. The princess suffered much pain and Clark wrote to Queen Victoria: 'My close relation to the Princess from her birth, and my affection for her made it more like the case of my own child.'[52]

Dr Wegner despaired of the princess's life and passed responsibility for the birth to the Berlin specialist Professor Edouard Martin and Clark. Alas, a traumatic birth had produced a 'shoulder-socket torn away' and Clark and Martin were blamed for the injury. Untreated, it produced a lifelong withered arm in the mentally unstable child who became Wilhelm II, 'Kaiser Bill' of the First World War.[53] In reporting the birth accident to Queen Victoria Clark remarked that 'it would all come right in the end'.

When Sir James Clark retired in 1860 he was succeeded by Dr William Baly (1814–62), erstwhile physician to Millbank Penitentiary. Although Baly's court service was to be cut short by his death, Baly was held in 'the greatest confidence' by Prince Albert.

Hardly had Clark begun to make plans for his retirement than he was called in to search for a replacement. He chose and introduced Dr (later Sir) William Jenner (1815–98), then physician to University College Hospital. They were both to be concerned with the greatest tragedy in Queen Victoria's life.

CHAPTER ELEVEN

TRIALS OF AN UNCROWNED KING: PRINCE ALBERT AND THE ROYAL DOCTORS

On 24 May 1844 Queen Victoria gave Prince Albert, her husband of four years, a present in the form of a miniature by artist Robert Thorburn. It was to remain the queen's favourite picture of him, showing him standing in medieval armour looking off to the right. He seems to gaze at infinity, and the queen wrote: 'During the fatal illness, and on the last morning of his life, he was wonderfully like this picture.'[1] She interpreted the gaze as that of a man on his deathbed, looking towards a new life; a new life she was convinced that she was to share with Albert in the hereafter – but not for forty more years.

Queen Victoria remarked that she and Francis Albert Augustus Emmanuel of Saxe-Coburg-Gotha were linked 'medically' from the first. As cousins – they shared a grandfather, Francis, Duke of Saxe-Coburg (1750–1806) – Victoria and Albert enjoyed many family connections.[2] Assisting at both their births, Victoria's on 24 May 1819 at Kensington Palace and Albert's on 26 August 1819 at Rosenau, was a remarkable woman. Charlotte Heidenreich-von-Siebold (née Heiland, 1788–1859), the daughter of distinguished medics Dr Damien von Siebold and his wife Dr Josepha Henning, studied medicine at Göttingen and qualified in midwifery at Darmstadt. She went on to be the first woman to obtain a doctorate in medicine at the University of Giessen.

On Dr Charlotte Heidenreich-von-Siebold's death the *Heidenreich-von-Siebold Stiftung* foundation was supported financially by Queen Victoria and Prince Albert, with their daughter Princess Alice of Hesse-Darmstadt as patroness.[3] This was rather ironic because Queen Victoria never really approved of young women studying medicine in the company of young men – 'Too HORRID', she opined. The advancement of women in medicine was somewhat stymied by the queen's opinion, as she would never have women doctors on her household staff.

As a child Prince Albert had not enjoyed good health. He had a weak chest, suffering recurrent inflammation of the larynx and trachea (croup) and an embarrassing proclivity to epistaxis (bleeding from the nose). He was easily tired and his family and friends got used to him dropping off to sleep halfway through his meals. By the time he met Queen Victoria for the first time at the age of eighteen he had developed into a handsome young man who charmed her despite his awkwardness in company, his lack of 'manly social sophistication' (he neither smoked nor drank alcohol) and 'weak stomach'. His constitution was strong enough, however, for, as Queen Victoria put it 'fun in bed' and he saw her through the rigours of nine pregnancies.

Despite his succumbing to feverish chills, Prince Albert, plucked by Queen Victoria from foreign obscurity, became one of the greatest figures of his generation. Worshipped by the queen, Prince Albert was never popular among her subjects, for many thought he was just another German interfering in Britain's affairs for his own and his Fatherland's ends.

In many aspects, though, Prince Albert's advice to Queen Victoria was sound and he played an important role in running the Crimean War, from the declaration of war against Russia by France and Britain on 28 March 1854 to the war's conclusion in April 1856. Prince Albert also offered good counsel during the American Civil War, 1861–65, keeping Britain away from directly supporting the Confederate Army. A keen student of contemporary industry and technology, he promoted the world's first international fair at the Crystal Palace (the Great Exhibition of 1851), and as Queen Victoria's reign advanced almost all of her instructions to her household and officials were drafted for her by Prince Albert. He also advised her on her medical appointments.

> Mankind looks grateful now on thee,
> For what thou didst in surgery.
> And death must often go amiss,
> By smelling antiseptic bliss.
> *Pundigrion on the founder of antiseptic surgery Joseph, 1st Baron Lister (1827–1912), sergeant-surgeon to Queen Victoria and Edward VII*

One of Prince Albert's recommendations was the recruitment of James Miller, Professor of Surgery at Edinburgh University from 1842 to 1864. Born in 1812 at Eassie in the old Scots county of Forfarshire, Miller studied Arts at the University of St Andrews and worked for an extra-mural medical degree. He was anatomy assistant to Robert Liston until he left for London in 1834, when Miller took over most of his private patients.

Miller won a fine reputation as the last professor of systematic surgery before Joseph Lister's discovery of the preferred use of antiseptics. Prince Albert had heard of the experiments in anaesthesia by James Young Simpson at Edinburgh and how Miller had conducted one of the earliest operations ever on a tubercular arm bone using chloroform.

The prince was greatly amused by Miller's account of how Dr Simpson and his assistants had experimented with chloroform, often to their own jeopardy. Here, in one of his many pamphlets, Miller describes one research session:

(*4 November 1847*)
Dr Simpson, with his two friends and assistants Drs (Thomas) Keith and (James Matthews) Duncan, sat down to their somewhat hazardous work in Dr Simpson's dining-room. Having inhaled several substances, but without much effect, it occurred to Dr Simson to try a ponderous material which he had formerly set aside on a lumber-table and which, on account of its great weight, he had hitherto regarded as of no likelihood (*of experimental success*) whatever. That happened to be a small bottle of chloroform.

It was searched for, and recovered from beneath a heap of waste paper. And, with each tumbler newly charged, the inhalers resumed their vocation. Immediately an unwanted hilarity seized the party; they became bright-eyed, very happy and very loquacious, expatiating on the delicious aroma of the new fluid. The conversation was of unusual intelligence, and quite charmed the listeners – some ladies of the family and a naval officer, brother-in-law of Dr Simpson. But suddenly there was talk of sounds being heard like those of a cotton mill, louder and louder; a moment more, then all was quiet and then – a crash.

On awakening, Dr Simpson's first perception was mental: 'This is far stronger and better than ether,' said he to himself. His second was to note that he was prostrate on the floor, and that among the friends about him there was both confusion and alarm.

Hearing a noise, he turned round and saw Dr Duncan beneath a chair; his jaw dropped, his eyes staring, his head bent half under him; quite unconscious, and snoring in a most determined manner. More noise still, and much motion, and then his eyes overtook Dr Keith's feet and legs, making valorous efforts to overturn the supper table.[4]

In 1848 Miller was appointed surgeon-in-ordinary to Queen Victoria and the Prince Consort, a position he held until his death on 17 June 1864.

Another addition to Prince Albert's medical household was effected in 1849. Hailed as 'the greatest surgeon of his day', Sir William Fergusson (1808–77) had studied medicine at Edinburgh, where he was a pupil of the notorious Dr Robert Knox (1791–1862), the anatomist who won public disfavour for procuring his 'subjects for dissection' from such grave-robbers as Burke and Hare. Fergusson served as surgeon to Edinburgh Royal Dispensary (1831–6) and the Edinburgh Royal Infirmary (1836–40), whereupon he became Professor of Surgery at King's College, London (1840–70). Fergusson's speed of amputation was phenomenal. Prince Albert once asked: 'Supposing I had to have my leg amputated – who is the best man to do it?' His adviser replied: 'Why Fergusson, by all means.' 'Then he shall be my surgeon,' replied the prince.[5]

Fergusson became one of the famous Victorian 'eponymous doctors' for his invention of 'Fergusson's Lion Forceps', 'Fergusson's Mouth Gag' and 'Fergusson's Speculum'. In 1855 he was appointed surgeon-extraordinary to Queen Victoria and advanced to sergeant-surgeon in 1867. He died of Bright's disease on 10 February 1877.

Two further important medical appointments were made to Queen Victoria's household in Prince Albert's lifetime, both in 1858. Edward Stanley (1793–1862) was trained as a surgeon at St Bartholomew's Hospital, London, and became severally lecturer in anatomy there and surgeon (1838–61), combining this with a professorship in human anatomy and physiology. He was given the post of sergeant-extraordinary to Queen Victoria.

Sir James Paget (1814–99) was another Victorian 'eponymous doctor' who won fame as a physiologist, pathologist, surgeon and lecturer. Following service as an apprentice to a Yarmouth surgeon, Paget entered St Bartholomew's Hospital in 1834 and qualified as a member of the College of Surgeons in 1836. For years he struggled to make a living and in 1847 he was elected assistant surgeon at St Bartholomew's.

From this point Paget's success was rapid, encompassing the Arris and Gale professorship in anatomy (1847–52). In 1858 he became surgeon-extraordinary to Queen Victoria, advancing to sergeant-surgeon in 1877, the year before he gave up operating. Paget died on 30 December 1899, and is remembered chiefly for his descriptions of 'Paget's Disease of the Nipple' and 'Paget's Disease of the Bone' (osteitis deformans).

Prince Albert lived his life at a hectic pace. He involved himself in project after project. It was almost as if he were compensating for his unpopularity. As he overworked himself on the Great Exhibition plans the royal doctors began to notice a decline in his overall health. He looked far older than his thirty-one years, his body was thickening, his gait was less steady and he began to look drawn. Queen Victoria's *Journal* regularly recorded his annual chills and fevers and the prince began to feel unwell after major functions. For instance, after the 'Camp of Instruction' military show at Chobham Heath in July 1853 he returned to his sickbed, his mind troubled by the events of Queen Victoria's eighth pregnancy – the usual post-partum hysterical crisis – and a serious fire at Windsor Castle.

Trying hard to keep his wife calm and to offer her support in the professional duties of her reign was a continual drain on Prince Albert. Despite doting on the prince she gave him *Schmerzen* (heartache). He was the battery of energy for her emotional and physical needs. Her constant need to hear his voice say: *Du liegst mir in Herzen; Du liegst mir in Sinn* (You are in my heart; you are in my thoughts) left him emotionally exhausted. When the whole family succumbed to measles, Prince Albert's overwork and lack of sleep gave him the worst repercussions of fever, delirium and a weakness that caused him to use a stick. Fussing around in his usual useless way, physician Sir James Clark saw no reason to be worried in the slightest for Prince Albert's health.

In 1858, the year after Queen Victoria had created him Prince Consort, Prince Albert was thirty-nine. He looked thirty years older, courtiers remarked; he was overweight, paunchy and took to sporting a wig on cold mornings. The physical burden of his busy life was now enormous. Queen Victoria wrote after the prince had attended the review of his proposed Volunteer Defence Force at Aldershot military camp in Hampshire:

> Monday and yesterday at Aldershot and here were really fearful. Poor dear papa had one of his stomach attacks on Monday, which made him look fearfully ill, but he remained in the field in that broiling sun the whole time and said he was all the better for it. He is however not quite right yet. He is so fagged and worked . . .[6]

His 'stomach attacks' became more frequent and fainting fits were added to his 'malaise'. His staff were alarmed – but Sir James Clark uttered his usual 'all will be well in the end'.

The court was plunged into mourning with the death of Prince Albert's stepmother, Princess Marie of Württenberg, Duchess of Saxe-Coburg, from erysipelas, while the royal family were visiting Coburg. Albert was shaken by the funeral rituals and nostalgic visits to old haunts. But worse was to follow. Queen Victoria recorded: 'Before proceeding, I must thank God for having preserved my adored one! I tremble now to think of it . . . The escape is very wonderful, *most merciful*!'[7]

It seems that Prince Albert had taken a solo ride at Coburg in a carriage and four. Suddenly the horses bolted and despite the prince's valiant attempts to rein in the beasts his carriage collided with a carrier's wagon standing at a level crossing. The prince jumped clear, sustaining only cuts and bruises. As Prince Albert rushed to the aid of the driver of the other vehicle, the unshackled horses of his stricken conveyance galloped home. The runaways were recognised and soon the new physician Dr

William Baly, who was in the suite of the royal family at Coburg, with Dr Carl Florschütz, the Duke of Saxe-Coburg's physician, rushed to the scene. The prince's old friend and mentor Baron Dr Stockmar came to his bedside after the crash: 'Here lies a man, he said to himself, incapable of fighting a severe illness.'[8]

Prince Albert rested for a few days, and before the royal couple left for England, he paid more nostalgic visits to his old haunts. It was as if he was saying a last goodbye to his Fatherland; already he had confided this to his daughter Princess Victoria in a letter: *Mein letzes Stündlein gekommen wäre* (My last hour has come).

During mid-October 1860 Prince Albert went down with a severe chill. Queen Victoria wrote an update to her daughter Princess Victoria:

> I hope by tomorrow or the next day he will be nearly his dear self again. Though of no real consequence whatever, it was the severest and most obstinate attack I ever saw him have, the more annoying as it was accompanied by violent spasms of pain; which he had both on Saturday and yesterday for two hours; he had to go to bed at three on Saturday, remaining in bed all day yesterday till ten o'clock when he got up for an hour and a half and thank God today *unberufen, unberufen* (Touch wood, touch wood) – there has been no return of pain . . . But it has been such an unusual thing to see him in bed (never except for the measles) and naturally cast such a gloom over us all, but it seems as if everything were turned upside down when dear Papa is not able to go about.[9]

It seemed as if the prince had a death wish, and the angel of death was certainly hovering over the royal family. On 2 January 1861 news was received that Princess Victoria's uncle-in-law, the insane Frederick William IV, King of Prussia, was dead; physician-in-ordinary William Baly also dropped dead after a railway accident; he was followed by the Duchess of Kent's comptroller Sir George Couper. On 16 March the Duchess of Kent died. As a result Queen Victoria suffered a nervous breakdown and the court was plunged into a kind of hysterical grief.

Prince Albert also edged slowly towards physical breakdown,

now in the care of Dr William Jenner who had replaced Dr Baly. The prince's emotional state was made no better by the news of the death from typhoid of the 25-year-old King Pedro V of Portugal and his brothers Prince Juan and Prince Frederick. Pedro, of the House of Coburg-Braganza, had been like a son to Prince Albert. Although Albert was clearly worsening, Dr Jenner assured the queen that the prince was 'much better' and averred that a physician need no longer sleep over at Windsor Castle.

His mind troubled by the outbreak of civil war in America and the worsening situation concerning Denmark's denial of Prussian claims to Holstein, Prince Albert entered a new phase of agitation. To top it all, Albert Edward, Prince of Wales, had caused a public scandal by bedding the trollop-cum-actress Nellie Clifden while he was on military duties at Curragh Camp in Ireland. It was all becoming too much. Prince Albert was losing his zest for life. He confessed to Queen Victoria: *Ich hange gar nicht am Leben; du hangst sehr daran . . .* (I do not cling to life; you cling, but I set no store by it . . .) And yet he fulfilled all the commitments he could including the inspection of the new buildings for the Staff College and Royal Military Academy at Sandhurst. The weather was dreadful and he returned home soaked and near to collapse.

The prudish Prince Albert was much affected by the Prince of Wales's perceived debauchery, and he exerted himself to have a man-to-man interview with his son, now returned to Cambridge. The Prince of Wales seemed satisfactorily contrite and Prince Albert returned to London in a calmer state of mind. There and at Windsor he would spend his last lucid days drafting papers keeping Britain's role purely 'diplomatic' in the internal affairs of America.

As he blotted the last paper on 1 December 1861 he confessed to Queen Victoria" *Ich bin so schwach, ich habe kaum die Feder halten können* (I am so weak, I have hardly been able to hold the pen). Pale and ill, with stomach pains and chills, Prince Albert spent most of his time in bed finally in the Blue Room at Windsor Castle, the *Sterbezimmer* (death chamber) of George IV and William IV.

Called out of semi-retirement, Sir James Clark was consulted to assist Dr Jenner; neither offered Albert any new medication although Jenner prepared notes on the prince's condition:

Sleeplessness is aggravated by fatigue.
Food nauseates; soup and bread causes vomiting.
Demeanour: alternating wild incoherence and normality.
Comment: No cause for concern, although a long feverish indisposition is dangerous.

Although Prince Albert was clearly worsening Queen Victoria refused to call in further medical assistance. With the help of Princess Alice she nursed and attended Prince Albert, who told all who came near him that he was a dying man. Queen Victoria continued to be reassured by Dr Jenner: 'Ma'am, there is no cause for alarm.'[10]

A 'low fever' was now confirmed and the prince's doctors remained in attendance on a 24-hour basis, with the assistance of local practitioners as required for the shifts. Jenner now thought that he saw the characteristic pink rash associated with typhoid fever. Curiously Jenner did not make much of it to Queen Victoria, and public bulletins on the prince's condition, for instance those of 11–12 December, expressed 'no unfortunate symptoms'.

Nevertheless extra physicians were called to consult; despite resentment from Clark and Jenner, physician Dr (later Sir) Thomas Watson (1792–1882) made an attendance with the equally elderly Sir Henry Holland. As neither doctor demurred at the minimal treatment given to Prince Albert, George Villiers, 4th Earl of Clarendon, erstwhile Foreign Secretary, declared the royal medics were not 'fit to attend a sick cat'.[11]

Sedated with brandy, Prince Albert was speedily failing. He was alternately burning up with fever, shuddering with chills, often delirious and took no solid food for several days. The royal doctors maintained the fantasy that the prince was getting better: Dr Thomas Watson informed the queen, 'I never despair with fever.'[12]

That 'dreadful day' – Saturday, 14 December 1861 – was to remain a constant memory for Queen Victoria for the remaining forty years of her life. That morning the doctors had Prince Albert wheeled from the Blue Room to an adjoining one. As the queen rested, Dr Watson commented: 'We are very much frightened but don't and won't give up hope.'[13]

Prince Albert continued to slip in and out of delirium, speaking French and German and expressing anxiety over the American war. He moved towards death more rapidly. *Es ist das kleine Fraüchen* (It is your little wife), Queen Victoria said as she bent over him for *ein Kuss*. With a throng of courtiers and doctors nearby, recollected Queen Victoria, the end came at 10.45 p.m.:

> Two or three long but perfectly gentle breaths were drawn, the hand clasping mine, & (oh! it turns me sick to write it) *all* was over . . . I stood up, kissing his dear heavenly forehead & called out in a bitter agonising cry: 'Oh! my dear Darling!' & then dropped on my knees in mute, distracted despair, unable to utter a word or shed a tear![14]

After receiving the condolences of her family and courtiers, Queen Victoria allowed Dr Jenner to give her a mild opiate. She wept and slept and wept again. In her heart, she would say a thousand times thereafter in letters and conversation she was 'QUITE ALONE!'

If it had been possible Queen Victoria would have had written on Prince Albert's death certificate that the primary cause of death was a heart broken by the 'disgusting details' of the Prince of Wales's debauchery at Curragh Camp. For years after, the queen averred that she could not look upon her eldest son 'without a shudder'. In the event, though, Prince Albert's death was registered by Dr Jenner on 21 December 1861. He entered the cause of death as 'typhoid fever; duration 21 days'. In spite of controversy in the *Lancet* and the *British Medical Journal* concerning the 'discrepancies' between the medical bulletins and the death certificate, there was no post mortem.[15] For good measure Dr Jenner suggested to Queen Victoria that Prince Albert had died because of 'the heart being over-strained by the Prince's heavy frame', while Sir James Clark opined that his death was due to 'exposure to chill when already weak' and overwork.[16]

The true cause of Prince Albert's death remains a matter of some dispute; modern doctors have averred that the prince may have been suffering from tuberculosis, a condition 'often difficult to differentiate' from typhoid.[17] Lord Clarendon was in no doubt as to why the prince had died: the royal doctors were high on the list of contributory factors, he wrote to the Duchess of Manchester:

> (Drs) Holland and Clark are not even average old women, and nobody who is really ill would think of sending for either of them. Jenner has had little (experience of) practice . . . Watson (who is no specialist in fever cases) at once saw that he had come too late to do any good.[18]

CHAPTER TWELVE

Battles and Blackmail at Balmoral: Royal Doctors and the Highland Retreat

The grief suffered by Queen Victoria at the death of Prince Albert was to be lifelong. She spelled out her anguish to her uncle King Leopold of the Belgians in a letter:

[Osborne House, 20 December 1861]

MY OWN DEAREST, KINDEST FATHER, – For such have I *ever* loved you! The poor fatherless baby of eight months is now the utterly broken-hearted and crushed widow of forty-two. My *life* as a happy one is *ended*! the world is gone for *me*! If I *must live* (and I will do nothing to make me worse than I am), it is henceforth for our poor fatherless children – for my unhappy country, which has lost *all* in losing him – and in *only* doing what I know and *feel* he would wish, for he *is* near me – his spirit will guide and inspire me! But oh! to be cut off in the prime of life – to see our pure, happy, quiet, domestic life, which *alone* enabled me to bear my *much* disliked position, CUT OFF at forty-two – when I *had* hoped with such instinctive certainty that God never *would* part us, and would let us grow old together (though *he* always talked of the shortness of life) – is *too awful*, too cruel! And yet it *must* be for *his* good, his happiness! His purity was too great, his aspiration *too high* for this poor, *miserable* world! His great soul is *now only* enjoying *that* for which it *was* worthy! And I will *not* envy him – only pray that *mine* may be perfected by it and fit to be with him eternally, for which blessed moment I earnestly long.[1]

More than any, the royal doctors became prisoners of the queen's grief as new rotas of them came and went. In the two decades following Prince Albert's death several doctors were prominent

Among the physicians were Sir James Allderson (1794–1882), who practised in Hull and London and was President of the Royal College of Physicians; he was appointed physician-extraordinary in 1874, the same year that Charles James Blasius Williams (1805–1889), erstwhile Professor of Medicine and physician at University College, London, was also appointed as a physician-extraordinary. Neil Arnott (1788–1874), the physician and natural philosopher, was appointed physician-extraordinary in 1837, and joined the other two as prolific writers on their subject. Dr Arnott, who graduated MD at Aberdeen in 1814, was, to use a Scottish term meaning easily recognisable, a kenspeckle character who was medical practitioner (with surgery) to the Honourable East India Company in China in George III's reign. Also in Queen Victoria's medical staff at this date was Sir Charles Locock (1799–1875), her physician-*accoucheur* since 1840, who won fame from the discovery of the efficacy of bromide of potassium in epilepsy.

Among the surgeons were Sir Philip Crampton (1777–1858) as surgeon-in-ordinary and Sir John Eric Erickson (1818–96), Professor of Surgery at University College, London, as surgeon-extraordinary in 1877, who joined Sir Prescott Gardner Hewlett (1812–91), in that role; Hewlett was also surgeon to the Prince of Wales by 1875. One of the distinguished surgical practitioners who joined Queen Victoria's household at this time was Benjamin Travers (1783–1850), who considerably raised the profile and science of eye surgery.

To represent Ireland surgeon Robert Adams (1791–1875) and physician William Stokes were appointed in 1861, while the Scottish court was represented by physician-in-ordinary James Begbie (1798–1869). Yet the Scottish court was to be given a distinctive and separate character with the appointment of several other royal doctors.

By the time of Prince Albert's death, Queen Victoria's annual presence and daily routines at Balmoral Castle were already well established. The Aberdeenshire castle was an essential part of the queen's drive to keep the memory of her husband alive. Since her first visit to Scotland aboard the royal yacht *The Royal George* in September 1842 she had kept jottings of the royal family's tours. These included the leasing of the old whitewashed castle of Balmoral from the estate of the Earl of Fife, and the ultimate purchase of the 17,500-acre estate on 22 January 1852 for £31,300, paid out of the £500,000 legacy she had received from the eccentric bachelor miser John Camden Nield (1780–1852).

The queen lovingly detailed the royal family's building of a New Balmoral, which they took official possession of during September 1855. Prince Albert had supervised the work of architect Thomas Cubitt and checked the plans of Aberdeen builder William Smith, and had paid great attention to the new castle's accessories, from bedknobs to heraldry. It became Queen Victoria's Highland heaven on earth. She wrote: 'The (new) house is charming; the rooms delightful; the furniture, papers, everything perfection.'[2]

A number of courtiers opined that her 'Highland Journal' should be published, and with the editorial help of Arthur Helps, clerk to the Privy Council, she produced *Leaves from the Journal of Our Life in The Highlands from 1848 to 1861*. Its dedication made it a personification of Prince Albert. At first the volume was for private circulation only, but it later went on sale to the public under Smith, Elder & Co.'s colophon in 1868 and became a bestseller.

For the first time the general public obtained a behind-the-scenes view of the royal family's activities at Balmoral and saw how the estate was run. Royal doctors played a prominent role in how the estate was managed. When the royal family had paid their first visit to Balmoral on Friday, 8 September 1848, George Hamilton Gordon (1784–1860), 4th Earl of Aberdeen, had asked the local Crathie physician Dr Andrew Robertson of Hopewell to make arrangements for the reception of the royal family.

Dr Robertson knew everybody and every house and bothy in the area, his medical practice having taken him, on horseback, to every corner of that part of Deeside. So well did he get on with the royal family that Queen Victoria appointed him to undertake the management of her Deeside estates as Commissioner in Scotland at Balmoral, a post he held for over thirty-three years.

Dr Robertson was to guide the royal family on regular jaunts around their new estates and deal with any medical emergencies that occurred; for his work he was given a kind of immortality in the pages of the queen's *Leaves*. On one occasion, the volume records, when they were watching 'salmon leistering' (fishing with spears) on the Dee, one of the leisterers fell in and would have drowned had it not been that Dr Robertson 'pulled the man out'.[3] Dr Robertson was to be party to an important 'secret matter' on behalf of the queen.

On 8 December 1826 Dr Robertson had delivered the second of the eleven children of Margaret Brown at the Brown family cottage at Crathienaird, not far from Balmoral. The child grew up to be the famous Highland Servant of Queen Victoria, John Brown. Brown had become a stable boy on Sir Robert Gordon's estate at Balmoral in 1842, and was one of the gillies who remained on the pay-roll when the royal family took over ownership of the Balmoral estates. The story of how John Brown became the permanent attendant to Queen Victoria – on the instigation of Prince Albert in 1851 – is well known, and after Prince Albert's death Brown was brought from Balmoral to Osborne to remind Queen Victoria of 'happier times'.

John Brown made himself indispensable to Queen Victoria; never before had she had a servant who was so painstakingly attentive to her needs and whims; his was the platonic male shoulder on which she could lean after the death of Prince Albert. In 1865 she appointed him Queen's Highland Servant at a salary of £120 and Brown's star remained in the royal ascendant for the next twenty or so years. This was the year too of Dr Robertson's 'secret matter' for the queen.

As a fine example of Highland manhood, Queen Victoria believed that John Brown must have some 'noble blood' in his veins and she directed Dr Robertson to investigate. Robertson knew perfectly well that there was no such 'noble blood'. Brown was from peasant stock and for decades his forebears had been agricultural workers on the estates of the Farquharsons of Invercauld. Robertson knew that this was not what the queen wanted to hear, so he dredged up the link between his own, and 'better', family tree and John Brown's grandmother Janet Shaw. On the strength of this, Dr Robertson overlaid his Shaw background on John Brown's ancestry and produced a four-page copper plate account for the queen's perusal.

A ROYAL DOCTOR REMEMBERED IN VERSE
At the age of twelve, in 1861, the poet William Ernest Henley
(d. 1903) developed tuberculous chronic osteomyelitis in both
ankles. His treatment followed the tough regimen of the day: his
wounds were pricked with rods of caustic, and he was taken to
a slaughterhouse and his feet plunged into the offal of a newly
slaughtered cow. Alas, in 1865 his left leg was amputated below
the knee, and thereafter he wore a wooden leg. During 1873
his condition worsened and until 1875 he was the patient of
Professor Joseph Lister at the Royal Infirmary, Edinburgh. In due
time the necrotic area of his 'good leg' was removed and he
recovered. In his *A Book of Verses* (1888) he used his hospital
experiences as inspiration. In 'The Chief' he paid tribute to Lister:

> His brow spreads large and placid, and his eye,
> Is deep and bright, with steady looks that still.
> Soft lines of tranquil thought his face fulfil –
> His face at once benign and proud and shy.
> If envy scout, if ignorance deny,
> His faultless patience, his unyielding will,
> Beautiful gentleness, and splendid skill.
>
> Innumerable gratitudes reply.
> His wise, rare smile is sweet with certainties,
> And seems in all his patients to compel
> Such love and faith as failure cannot quell.
> We hold him for another Herakles,
> Battling with custom, prejudice, disease,
> At once the son of Zeus with Death and Hell.

The account, interlarded with adjectives such as 'handsome',
'prowess' and 'noble', and descriptions as 'Highland Gentleman',
was just what the queen wanted to read. The account was copied
and circulated to members of the royal household and friends.
The Prince of Wales, who hated Brown's 'arrogance, familiarity
and influence' with a passion, tore his copy of the account to
shreds. Nevertheless Dr Robertson was off the hook and life
went on at Balmoral as before.

In 1870 Queen Victoria appointed Dr Joseph Lister as surgeon-
in-ordinary in Scotland. Joseph Lister was born at Upton Park, West

Ham, on 5 April 1827, the fourth child of seven of the Quakers Isabella and Joseph Jackson Lister. Educated at the Quaker establishment of Hitchin School and Grove House, Tottenham, he developed a bent for the sciences and did early animal dissections and wrote essays on anatomy. In 1843 he attended a class for juniors in botany at University College, London, and in August 1845, after further studies in sciences and classics, was allowed to matriculate. He graduated BA in 1847 and was permitted to carry on studies in anatomy. The pressures on him to study produced a nervous breakdown and he had a year out before re-registering for classes in 1849. In 1851 he became 'dresser' (a junior assistant) to University College Hospital's senior surgeon John Eric Erickson; thence he was Erickson's house surgeon until February 1852, the year he became a Fellow of the Royal College of Surgeons. He graduated MB in 1853.

William Sharpey, Lister's Professor of Physiology, suggested that he continue his studies at Edinburgh, where Sharpey's old friend James Syme practised. Syme was 'generally acknowledged to be the most original and thoughtful surgeon in the country'.[4] Syme was impressed by Lister's own originality in research and appointed him his house surgeon in 1854. On 21 April 1855 Lister was elected Fellow of the Royal College of Surgeons of Edinburgh. A post of assistant surgeon at the Royal Infirmary, Glasgow, in 1856 led to the Professorship of Surgery at Glasgow in 1860. Lister held the post of Professor of Clinical Surgery at Edinburgh University from 1868 to 1877.

Joseph Lister was first called to a royal consultation in October 1870. Princess Louise had developed an abscess on her leg and her medical attendant Dr Fore wanted a second opinion. Queen Victoria agreed to this and Lister was sent for, and attended on a number of occasions until the princess's recovery in November. She was married the next year.

On 3 September 1871 Queen Victoria developed a large abscess in her left armpit. Joseph Lister was sent for by Dr William Marshall, the resident medical attendant. Queen Victoria recorded the consultation:

Sir William Jenner explained everything about my arm to him, but he naturally said he could do nothing nor give any opinion till he had made an examination. I had to wait nearly half an hour before Mr Lister and Dr Marshall appeared. In a few minutes he had ascertained all & went out again with the others. Sir William Jenner returned saying Dr [sic] Lister thought the swelling ought to be cut; he could wait twenty-four hours, but it would be better not. I felt dreadfully nervous, as I bear pain so badly. I shall be given chloroform, but not very much, as I am so far from well otherwise, so I begged the part might be frozen, which was agreed. Sir William Jenner gave me some whiffs of chloroform whilst Mr Lister froze the place, Dr Marshall holding my arm. The abcess, which was six inches in diameter, was very quickly cut and I hardly felt anything excepting the last touch, when I was given a little more chloroform. In an instant there was relief. I was then tightly bandaged, and rested on my bed. Quite late saw Beatrice and Alfie for a moment, after Mr Lister had been to see me. Felt very shaken and exhausted.[5]

In her *Journal* for 4 September Queen Victoria commented:

Had a cup of coffee before the terrible long dressing of the wound took place. Dr Marshall assisted Mr Lister, whose great invention, a carbolic spray to destroy all organic germs, was used before the bandages were removed and during the dressing . . .[6]

Queen Victoria was able to witness Lister's innovative expertise. During treatment Lister noticed that the abscess was not healing and needed draining. He made drain tubes on the spot and drained the abscess which then healed rapidly. For his work Lister received no fee, but a team of horses to pull his carriage was gifted to him by the queen at a later date.[7]

From 1899 to her death Lister was sergeant-surgeon to the queen; she had created him a baron in the New Year jubilee honours list of 1897. He was the first medical man to be elevated to the peerage. When Queen Victoria died he wrote this in the address of sympathy and homage from the Royal Medical and Chirurgical Society:

I believe that I happen to be the only person who ever exercised upon her sacred body the divine art of surgery. The occasion was a most critical and anxious one, but, while she treated me with queenly dignity, nothing could exceed her kindness.[8]

In 1875, after more than three decades in royal service at Balmoral, Dr Robertson decided to retire and recommended to the queen as his successor another doctor who had become his firm friend. Dr Alexander Profeit was born on 27 October 1833, at Towie near Alford, Aberdeenshire, where his family farmed the lands of Nether Towie.[9] After elementary education at Towie parish school he entered Aberdeen grammar school and thence King's College, where he graduated MA in March 1855.[10] In 1857 he graduated as a Licentiate of the Royal College of Surgeons (LRCS) at Edinburgh.[11]

QUEEN VICTORIA WAS AMUSED BY ROYAL DOCTORS

Among the qualities Queen Victoria required of her royal doctors was that they 'be good company'. She had a great talent – contrary to public rumour – to be amused. Whereas her Hanoverian forebears had found hilarity in servants trapping their fingers in doors, Queen Victoria's pleasures were of a simpler, kinder nature and she enjoyed witty remarks.

Queen Victoria was always a ready ear for racy stories from her doctors. Sir Charles Locock had a keen wit, as did Sir William Jenner. Royal private secretary Sir Henry Ponsonby recalled how when told that two mountains were to be named in honour of prime ministers W.E. Gladstone and Benjamin Disraeli, Jenner quipped that the queen's love of Scottish mountains would produce the name 'Ben Disraeli'.

Sir James Clark usually kept Queen Victoria amused with his witticism about public figures of the day. She was amused to be told that when the Marquess of Hertford enquired of Napoleon III if he would invade England, the French Emperor replied: 'Yes, but I shall not come till I am invited by the Queen . . .'

Ever eager to please and reassure, Sir James Clark told Queen Victoria that her royal niece Princess Adelaide Hohenlohe had been thrown from her horse at Balmoral, 'she could not have fallen upon a better part of her head'. (Queen Victoria, *Journal*, 23 September 1852).

After qualifying he went to Tarland, near Aboyne, Aberdeenshire, where he met Dr Robertson, who encouraged him to take up general practice at Crathie. With Robertson's influence, Profeit was soon appointed medical resident at Balmoral. Thus on Robertson's retirement the queen confirmed Dr Profeit as her new commissioner at Balmoral and overseer of Abergeldie. An energetic, obliging and affable man, Profeit clashed with the queen's Highland Servant John Brown from their early hours together. Brown's influence was to be found everywhere on the estate, but Profeit openly opposed Brown when he thought his authority was being baulked and their rumbustious relationship continued until Brown's death in 1883.

After Brown's death, Dr Profeit would regularly carry out a tragico-comic ritual. Queen Victoria gave her particular friends and employees gold tie-pins with a miniature photograph of Brown's head set in diamonds, and expected the recipients to wear the pins at all times. Not wishing to incur a terse comment from the queen for not wearing the much-disliked John Brown's image, Profeit kept the tie-pin in his pocket, quickly pinning it in place on his cravat whenever he encountered the queen.[12]

Dr Profeit, and, after his marriage to Isabella Anderson (1840–88), his family, regularly attended the queen and the royal family, and wrought for himself the unique position as 'head of the Balmoral Highlanders'.[13] Dr Profeit involved himself in every aspect of Balmoral life and administration, as well as in the affairs of Crathie parish. His multifarious duties went far beyond the medical service he also rendered to the estate and parish, and he even helped Queen Victoria to win prizes at the shows held by the Royal Agricultural Society and the Highland & Agricultural Show, with her herd of polled Aberdeen Angus cattle, the breeding of which he had overseen.

One of his last acts as commissioner was the 'Highland entertainment' staged during the visit of Tsar Nicholas II of Russia and his wife Alexandra, Queen Victoria's granddaughter, in September 1896. Alas, the Tsar was a disastrously poor shot on the hunting trips, and described Balmoral to his mother as 'colder than Siberia'.[14]

Alexander Profeit died at his residence of Craig-Gowan (whose tenancy Queen Victoria had given to John Brown) on 27 January

1897. The Profeits had seven children: Robert became Vice-Consul at Sulima; Charles graduated in medicine and served in the Royal Army Medical Corps; Alexander took up farming; Albert banking; Leopold acting; Victoria (sponsored by the queen) took up further education; and George became a royal blackmailer.

In 1902, some five years after his father's death, George Profeit approached Buckingham Palace claiming that he possessed certain 'compromising letters' which Queen Victoria had sent to Dr Profeit concerning John Brown. Edward VII was considerably disturbed about the matter; he still remained paranoid about John Brown's memory and the public gossip and innuendoes about the supposed 'relationship' between Queen Victoria and her Highland Servant. If George Profeit published the letters, which he threatened to do if he were not paid off, an unholy scandal would break out. The letters must be suppressed. So through his private secretary, Francis, Lord Knollys, royal doctor James Reid was summoned to the palace and charged by the king to resolve the matter.

After consulting the king's sister, Princess Beatrice, as to the best way of approaching the matter, Dr Reid interviewed George Profeit. He had to have a number of meetings with George Profeit before he finally agreed the terms of the blackmail, but on 8 May 1905 George Profeit handed over a tin box containing three hundred letters. Reid described them as 'most compromising'.[15] Historians believe that the king quickly had the letters destroyed – and their content remains a mystery to this day.

CHAPTER THIRTEEN

SECRETS OF A ROYAL DOCTOR: THE CONSULTATIONS OF SIR JAMES REID

In the last two decades of her reign Queen Victoria made a variety of appointments for her 'Medical Dept'. Among the physicians were Sir William Henry Broadbent (1835–1907), an experienced fever clinician, pathologist and anatomist who conducted research into cancer, paralysis and aphasia; his advanced theory known as 'Broadbent's Hypothesis' dealt with hemiplegia. Broadbent attended several members of the royal family. Arthur Farre (1811–87), an obstetric physician and professor in the subject at King's College Hospital, was appointed physician-extraordinary, as was Sir George Johnson (1818–96), who held professorships in materia medica, therapeutics and clinical medicine. They were joined by Sir Richard Quain (1816–98), a consulting physician who was the crown nominee to the General Medical Council. In Scotland Sir Thomas Grainger Stewart (1837–1900), erstwhile Professor of Practice of Physic at Edinburgh University, was appointed physician-in-ordinary.

The surgical staff was represented by George Lawson (1831–1903), opthalmic surgeon at the Royal London Opthalmic Hospital, Moorfields, as surgeon oculist, while Sir Thomas Smith (1833–1909), surgeon to the Children's Hospital, Great Ormond Street, served as surgeon-extraordinary. Sir William Stokes (1839–1900), Professor of Surgery at the Royal College, Ireland, was appointed surgeon-in-ordinary to Queen Victoria in Ireland.

Among those medics was another 'eponymous doctor'. Douglas Moray Cooper Lamb Argyll Robertson (1837–1909) graduated MD at St Andrews in 1857, and after serving as house surgeon at the Edinburgh Royal Infirmary went on to study opthalmology in Berlin. He returned to Edinburgh to become an opthalmic surgeon at the Royal Infirmary. Robertson was one of the earliest British surgeons to become exclusively devoted to opthalmic surgery, and one of his discoveries was the 'Argyll Robertson pupil' (evidence for syphilis of the nervous system). Robertson became surgeon oculist to Queen Victoria in Scotland and later held the same position at Edward VII's court.

Another doctor of this period stands out as a remarkable courtier. The life and extant papers of Sir James Reid record what it was really like to be a royal doctor at the court of Queen Victoria.[1] Born on 23 October 1849 at Ellon, Buchan, Aberdeenshire, Reid was educated at Aberdeen grammar school before entering the University of Aberdeen as an Arts student. In 1868 he matriculated as a medical student, graduating MD in 1872. He joined the general practice of Dr William Vacy Lyle at

---

QUEEN VICTORIA ON ROYAL DOCTORS

Because of his declining popularity, Queen Victoria gave Sir James Clark rare social privileges when he was dining at court, privileges that she accorded to no others. All in all the queen looked upon her doctors as 'at least a species of upper servant', certainly not to be classed with officers in her forces. It was because of what they did that caused Queen Victoria to look upon doctors as inferior. She once told Princess Alice that the study of anatomy was 'disgusting'. This sat awkwardly with the fact that her homes were full of etchings and sculptures depicting the naked body.

Always courteous to her medical practitioners, the queen swayed from ignoring their advice and being snobbish, to being fond of them and dependent. Most royal doctors looked upon her as 'domineering'. As regards their fees and honours, the queen was meticulous in ensuring that they were promptly paid and she felt strongly that baronetcies were more fitting than plain knighthoods.

On one occasion in September 1875, Queen Victoria stifled her giggles as her new minister at Crathie, the Revd Campbell, took as his text for the sermon the woman mentioned in *Matthew ix, v20*, who had been ill for twelve years. 'Think of how she must have suffered,' Campbell intoned, 'both from nature and from physicians . . .' Sitting behind the giggling Queen Victoria, her physicians William Marshall and Andrew Robertson were livid.

Paddington, London, but in 1876 he decided to further his medical studies at Vienna, then a centre of contemporary medical advancement. Here he undertook courses in gynaecology and aural diseases. In 1877 he returned to join his father's medical practice at Ellon.

In April 1881 a great opportunity was offered to him. At the time Queen Victoria was looking for a replacement for Dr William Marshall, her resident medical attendant at Balmoral. In her usual firm manner the queen indicated that the successor must be Scottish by birth and preferably a practitioner from Aberdeenshire. Further, the candidate should be able to write, read and speak German, so that he could attend when required the hordes of German relations who regularly descended on her. Her commissioner at Balmoral, Dr Profeit, was set to work to find such a paragon. Through a local network which included Reid's uncle, the Revd George Peter, Reid's name was suggested to Profeit and in due course Reid was summoned to Balmoral. Later that day Queen Victoria recorded in her *Journal*:

[*8 June 1881*] Saw Dr Reid from Ellon, who has *the very* highest testimonials . . . He is willing to come for a time or permanently in Dr Marshall's place.[2]

Although he was acceptable to the queen, Reid had to be properly vetted by physician-in-ordinary Dr (now Sir) William Jenner. Reid passed muster and was summoned to start his medical duties at Windsor Castle on 8 July, with the title resident medical attendant.

An interesting memorandum from the Privy Purse Office sets out Reid's position, work and duties:

Dr Reid will be appointed Resident Medical Attendant on the Queen at a salary of Four Hundred Pounds (£400) per annum.

He will not be an official member of the Royal Household, but will have breakfast and luncheon with the Ladies and Gentlemen in Waiting.

He will not dine with them, unless especially invited by the Queen's orders, excepting at Balmoral, when he will always dine at the Household dinner.

He will be in constant attendance upon the Queen, and will at Her Majesty's convenience receive six weeks' leave in the Year.

He will attend the Members of the Royal Family who are residing with the Queen, if required, and will at any time visit any person whatever if directed by Her Majesty.

He is to take medical and surgical charge of all the personal attendants on the Queen (her dressers and maids) and Royal Family, of all Scotch servants, and of all other servants who may desire him to attend them.

He is to attend any lady or gentleman in the Palace who may ask for his professional assistance.

He will maintain a constant communication with Dr Ellison (surgeon apothecary to the household at Windsor), or Dr Hoffmeister (surgeon apothecary to the household at Osborne), and will report all special medical matters to Sir William Jenner.[3]

Reid's duties also included visiting hospitals at the queen's command. In particular, he had to report from time to time 'how they were getting on' at the Royal Victorian Hospital at Netley, near Southampton, which Victoria had founded in 1856.

Now aged sixty-two and mourning the death of her beloved prime minister, Benjamin Disraeli, Earl of Beaconsfield, who had died on 19 April 1881, Queen Victoria was a person of strict habits and routine. Reid's life now had to mould to the queen's pattern of a March visit to France or Germany, Windsor Castle in May, Balmoral in June, back to Windsor and from there to Osborne House on the Isle of Wight for July and August, thence back to Balmoral for September, October and November, finishing the end of the month at Windsor to prepare for Christmas and New Year at Osborne, where the royal household stayed until the end of February when the whole routine began again. For all these to-ings and fro-ings, with the occasional visit to the main cities of Queen Victoria's British realm, the new resident medical attendant was expected to be present.

James Reid quickly assessed the queen's medical needs, noting her main symptoms of indigestion and rheumatism, and what could be called her strategically brought-on 'nerves'; the latter were usually manipulated to defy, thwart or avoid those she did not like or who opposed her will, from politicians (particularly the much-disliked Liberal Prime Minister William Ewart Gladstone) to bishops.[4] Doctors she seemed to like, treating them with dignity and respect and personally overseeing their honours and advancement – even though she paid no attention to their advice.

Dr Reid soon crossed swords with John Brown, usually over the amount of alcohol consumed by the serving staff. Reid soon learned that in matters of dispute with or concerning Brown Queen Victoria invariably took her Highland Servant's part. Reid's life too was governed by the idiosyncracies and petty restrictions laid down by Queen Victoria, from her insistence of having windows wide open, even in the coldest weather, to the meticulous attention paid to the preserving of Prince Albert's memory. Reid also began to receive regular handwritten messages from the queen; one early example read:

> Let Dr Reid go out from quarter to 11 to one, unless the Queen sends before to see him, and from 5 till *near* 8. If he wishes on any particular occasion to go out sooner he shd. ask. These are the regular hours. But I may send *before* to say he is not to go out before I have seen him shd. I not feel well or want anything. This every Doctor in attendance has done and must be prepared to do.[5]

Reid was present on 2 March 1882 when the insane Roderick Maclean made the seventh and last attempt on Queen Victoria's life, firing a revolver at her as she was leaving the Great Western Railway station at Windsor for the castle. The bullet missed and Maclean was quickly seized. Reid had no need to offer first aid, and the queen seemed to suffer no ill-consequences.

From time to time the queen questioned Dr Reid's treatment. On one occasion, after she had been treated for a sore throat, Reid received a note:

> In spraying her throat with tannin before dinner, the Queen found it made the part near the right ear burn, and it is sore. She wishes to know if she had better not spray with cold water

instead? The throat does not hurt at all in swallowing but the ear still aches a little. Should the poultice be *only linseed*?[6]

Dr Reid's extant diaries vividly depict medical life at Queen Victoria's court, recalling minor incidents and matters of great importance. His duties were rigorous, and he was unable to attend his own dying father when John Brown was ill. He recorded:

25 February 1883.	Princess Alice of Albany born, daughter of Prince Leopold and Princess Helena.
17 March.	Prince Leopold sprains his leg. Queen Victoria slips on stairs, injures her knee. Attended by Sir James Paget.
25 March.	John Brown stricken with erysipelas.
26 March.	In constant attention on John Brown.
27 March.	Death of John Brown. Queen Victoria 'utterly crushed'.
28 March 1884.	Haemophilic Prince Leopold dies of haemorrhage of the throat at Villa Nevada, Cannes. (Reid attended the funeral, and was later involved in the re-coffining of the prince's body before final interment on 23 June 1885 in St George's Chapel, Windsor.) Death of Queen Victoria's dog 'Noble'. Reid prescribes during the dog's last illness and carries out the queen's detailed orders for the burial.
11 November 1885.	Reid attends Princess Beatrice during her miscarriage.
23 November 1886.	Princess Beatrice gives birth to Prince Alexander; Reid attends with *accoucheur* Dr (later Sir) John Williams.
24 October 1887.	Birth of Princess Beatrice's second child, Princess Victoria Eugenie. Reid gives chloroform; delivery by Dr Williams.

21 May 1889.	Princess Beatrice gives birth to Prince Leopold Arthur. Reid administers chloroform. Reid is appointed one of her majesty's physicians extraordinary.
3 October 1891.	Princess Beatrice gives birth to Prince Maurice at Balmoral. Reid administers chloroform; aftercare assisted by Dr William Hoffmeister. Reid attends Prince Leopold of Battenberg during bronchitis attacks. From this year Dr Reid was in 'sole charge of the Queen's health'.

As Reid became as indispensable to her as John Brown had been, Queen Victoria increasingly indulged her hypochondria. For her age (she was now seventy-two) she was in good health, with remarkable stamina and energy, but she conducted daily consultations about her imagined ailments. She was a self-confessed 'martyr' to indigestion, for which Reid prescribed the proprietary Benger's Food. Alas, the queen simply ingested it along with her large meals instead of using it as a substitute.

Reid became an expert on the queen's flatulence and 'nervous headaches', adding to his duties the developing role of 'messenger' between herself and her ministers. Even on holiday he received regular missives and memos from the queen detailing the minutiae of her health, bypassing the locum acting for Reid.

When Dr Jenner died in December 1898, Reid took his place as physician-in-ordinary to the Prince of Wales, and acted as consultant and friend to a number of the royal family, which added to his workload. Increasingly too, Queen Victoria showed Reid any letter she received concerning the health of her relatives abroad. For all of this he received the sum of £800.[7] In February 1894 this was increased to £1,500.[8] By this time Reid had become obsessed with his 'perquisites and promotion', and jockeyed for 'a Knighthood that is worth having'.[9] On 20 June 1895 he finally achieved what he wanted, being appointed Knight Commander of the Bath (KCB).

When Queen Victoria's Private Secretary Sir Henry Ponsonby

died in 1895, the queen began to rely more and more on Reid, who wrote to his mother complaining that his duties now included 'so many things to do quite apart from medical work'.[10] He was soon plunged into royal gloom once more with the death from 'Ashanti Fever' (malaria) of Princess Beatrice's husband Prince Henry of Battenberg on 20 January 1896, en route home from the Ashanti War.

The more prominent Reid became in the court hierarchy, the more he was targeted by medical interest groups seeking preferment. When the various honours lists were being prepared Reid was consulted by the prime minister and the queen's private secretary of the day as to which medical men should receive honours. It was Reid who advised the then prime minister, the Marquess of Salisbury, on the appointment of Sir Joseph Lister to the peerage.[11] Conversely, although he had dropped huge hints to obtain his own knighthood, Reid advised against honouring those who put themselves forward for honours, or those who refused a consultation fee, intimating that an honour was preferred.

Queen Victoria's selfish attitude to anything a courtier might wish to do that might inconvenience or threaten her comfort and routines was to be experienced several times by Sir James Reid. On 24 January 1899 Reid became engaged to one of Queen Victoria's maids-of-honour, the Hon. Susan Baring; she was thirty, he was fifty. The queen 'was very much astonished' and refused to allow an immediate official announcement of the engagement; her astonishment led to anger at the thought that she might lose Sir James Reid's total attention and care – in contrast to that of John Brown, who dedicated his life entirely to the queen's service. One month later Victoria relented, permitting the official announcement of the engagement, but not before she had drawn up new 'Regulations' for Reid's service:

I think it absolutely necessary that Sir J. Reid and Miss Baring should know exactly what their position will be when they are married. Sir James knows that considering my age, I cannot well allow him to leave his present post. This will entail that he must continue living in the House *wherever* we are, excepting for the fortnight and two or three days holiday in the spring, and five weeks (divided) in the autumn when he has his holiday. He must always, as now, come round after breakfast to see what I should want, and then be back before luncheon. He must also in the afternoon, before he goes out, do the same. Of course as the days shorten and in the winter, he would go out earlier and come back earlier. Sir James should always ask if he wishes to go out for longer, or to dine out, returning by eleven or half past eleven. His wife should not come up to his room here, nor to the Corridor, where some of the Royal Children live. At Windsor she might occasionally come to his room but this must not interfere with his other duties. It is absolutely necessary that they should be fully aware of these conditions so that they cannot complain afterwards.[12]

Sir James Reid was closely associated with the medical events leading up to Queen Victoria's death at Osborne House at 6.30 p.m. on 22 January 1901. The story of the deathbed scene and the secret aspects of the immediate events afterwards was first published in detail with the appearance of Reid's biography in 1987. Although Reid had been the queen's medical attendant for over twenty years he had never been permitted to make a full examination – she loathed stethoscopes and the thought of one being applied to her person, and the prospect of an examination of her intimate body was 'TOO HORRID!' As he supervised the laying out of the royal cadaver Reid noted that the queen had a ventral hernia and a prolapse of the uterus (she had borne nine children).[13]

The queen had left 'Instructions'[14] on what items were to be placed in her coffin, ranging from jewellery and handkerchiefs to plaster casts of relatives' hands and photographs. All had to be placed so that none who came to view the body would know they were there. What was perhaps most surprising to historians was that in her left hand was placed a photograph of her Highland Servant John Brown and a lock of his hair (in a case), while on her finger was placed John Brown's mother's wedding ring.[15]

Sir James Reid did not leave royal service, playing a role in the medical department of the new monarch, Edward VII, and in December 1901 was appointed physician-in-ordinary to Prince George, the succeeding Prince of Wales.

CHAPTER FOURTEEN

WHITECHAPEL WHISPERS: THE CURIOUS LOW LIFE OF DR SIR WILLIAM GULL

For many years the people who gathered at the LMS railway station at Pitlochry, Perthshire, awaiting the arrival of the morning train from Inverness to link with the express to London, regularly observed the carriage of a visiting gentleman drawing up in the forecourt. As the porters scurried to unload the luggage, the station-master, in his top hat and frock-coat, was always there to meet the gentleman and his family. Who could this important personage be, who caused such an official fuss? Local gossips were able to add that the gentleman was a '*royal doctor*', who had a holiday home overlooking the nearby Pass of Killiecrankie – where, on 27 July 1689, the royalist John Graham of Claverhouse, Viscount Dundee, won the field for James VII & II against the government veteran General Hugh Mackay. What the gossips didn't know was that the object of their curiosity, Dr Sir William Gull, was to be linked in name – and supposed action – with one of the most horrific murder investigations of all time. It was a story that would eclipse the bloody deeds at Killiecrankie.

More books, articles and theories have been published about 'Jack the Ripper' and the Whitechapel Murders than about any other unsolved crimes in the history of Scotland Yard police files. Between 31 August and 9 November 1888 five East End prostitutes were savagely done to death, their bodies 'mutilated in the most ghastly manner'.[1] Interwoven in the tangled web of the murder stories was a nexus of intrigue that cited the names of royal physician Dr Sir William Gull and Prince Albert Victor, Duke of Clarence. Their supposed involvement posed a threat to the royal family's probity for decades.

Sir William Withey Gull was born on 31 December 1816 at St Osyth Mill, Essex, one of the eight children of a barge-master.

He was pre-eminent in medical circles as a skilled clinical physician; he held teaching posts at Guy's Hospital Medical School, London, and became Fullerton Professor of Physiology. He attended the Prince of Wales during his severe typhoid illness in 1871. Gull was subsequently physician-extraordinary to Queen Victoria and physician-in-ordinary to the Prince of Wales, and was involved in a curious medical mystery surrounding Alexandra, Princess of Wales, in 1877. According to a document dated 4 May 1877, which came to public cognisance when it was sold in a bundle of papers at auction in 1990, Gull had prescribed an abortifacient to the princess, either, said professional opinion, to treat bleeding caused by a spontaneous miscarriage, or to effect an abortion.[2] No pregnancy was announced in the Court Circular at the time, and there was speculation that the princess felt the need for such a possibly induced abortion because of the 'remorse she felt over the death in April 1871 of her son John who lived only twenty-four hours'.[3] Even though she was only twenty-six, for Alexandra 'there were to be no more children'.[4]

Prince Albert Victor Christian Edward, Duke of Clarence and Avondale, Earl of Athlone, was born at Frogmore House on 8 January 1864, the eldest son of the Prince and Princess of Wales. Known to the royal family as 'Eddy', the prince was publicly considered to be educationally backward, a condition probably exacerbated by his severe deafness from otosclerosis inherited from his mother. His lifestyle was dissipated and homosexual, and his visits to male brothels scandalised the aristocracy who knew of his sexual tastes. Modern historians believe that Prince Eddy was probably bi-sexual, an opinion given more plausibility by the following tale.

Dr Sir William Gull and Prince Eddy were linked with the 'Jack the Ripper' murders as long ago as the turn of the twentieth century, but in 1970 an article by Dr Thomas Edward Alexander Stowell in the specialist magazine *The Criminologist* inferred that the prince himself was 'Jack the Ripper'.[5] Although he retracted his allegations before he died, Stowell's argument was followed up by a number of 'Ripperologists' who cited the prince in various aspects of the murders.[6]

One such 'Ripperologist' was Stephen Knight, who in 1976 published his theories in the volume *Jack the Ripper: The Final*

Solution, wherein he detailed the prince's supposed role and named royal physician Dr Sir William Gull, among others, as a willing accomplice.

The proffered story averred that the prince had fallen in love with a Roman Catholic commoner, Annie Elizabeth Crook, whom he had met through her kinsman James Kenneth Stephen, the prince's tutor at Cambridge. A homosexual and mentally unstable, Stephen was also first cousin to the writer Virginia Woolf, and was mooted as Prince Eddy's lover some time after 1883. Prince Eddy is said to have fathered a child with Annie Crook in 1885; this daughter, Alice Crook, in turn gave birth to Joseph, the natural son of artist Walter Richard Sickert 1860–1942).[7]

The story continued that the prince and Annie Crook had gone through two weddings (one Anglican and one Roman Catholic), which were, of course, proscribed by the Act of Settlement of 1701 (which forbade the heir to the British throne from marrying a Roman Catholic) and the Royal Marriage Act of 1772 (which forbade royal marriages without the monarch's consent).[8] It was, of course, only a matter of time before the prince's (canonically valid) marriage to Annie became court knowledge and Prime Minister Robert Cecil, 3rd Marquess of Salisbury, was urged to set in motion acts that would officially suppress the story.

Prince Eddy, the story went on, provided in part for his illegitimate daughter, and his money paid for a nanny, a former shop assistant, called Mary Jane Kelly.[9] According to testimony given by Joseph Sickert,[10] Prince Eddy was visiting Annie Crook one day at her home at 6 Cleveland Street, in London's bohemian area known as Fitzrovia, when two closed coaches drew up. Two men entered the property, reappearing in a few minutes to hustle Prince Eddy into a coach which soon sped away. Shortly afterwards Annie Crook was bundled into the second coach and taken off in the opposite direction.

After this Prince Eddy's movements were closely monitored by courtiers. Annie was taken to Guy's Hospital, where she was confined under the soubriquet 'Mrs Mordaunt' for some five months and was certified insane by Dr Sir William Gull. Nevertheless Gull, who diagnosed Annie as suffering from some form of paraplegia, and may even have operated on her for the condition, released her. Some said he confirmed to the royal family that in Annie Crook's mental state any ramblings about a relationship with Prince Eddy would be discounted. She died at the Lunacy Observations Ward, St George's Union Workhouse, on 23 February 1920.

Prince Eddy's daughter, baby Alice, was cared for by a nanny appointed by 'her grandmother, Princess Alexandra'[11] when her first nanny Mary Jane Kelly disappeared. Kelly sank to a life of an East End prostitute and on 9 November 1888 became one of Jack the Ripper's victims.

In his book *The Ripper and the Royals*, Mervyn Fairclough theorises on Dr Sir William Gull's purported involvement with the 'Jack the Ripper' murders on behalf of Prince Eddy. Fairclough makes this bold statement: 'Joseph (Sickert) has made it perfectly clear to me, though it was (Dr Gull) who actually killed and mutilated four of the victims, he was acting under orders, and that it was men more prominent than he, more eminent by virtue of their birthright, who were really responsible.'[12]

The five women thought to have been murdered by 'Jack the Ripper' were as follows:

Mary Ann 'Polly' Nichols, murdered 31 August 1888, aged forty-three. Killed in a coach and dumped in Buck's Row, Whitechapel. Throat cut, a few stomach mutilations; carotid artery severed. Perpetrator: (according to Joseph Sickert) Dr Sir William Gull.

Annie Chapman, murdered 8 September 1888, aged forty-seven. Probably killed elsewhere and body dumped in Hanbury Street. Throat deeply cut, stomach and genital area mutilated, some entrails removed. Perpetrator: (on say of above) Dr Sir William Gull.

Elizabeth 'Long Liz' Stride, murdered 30 September 1888, aged forty-two. Killed at Dutfield's Yard, Berner's Street. Throat cut, windpipe severed, carotid artery cut. Perpetrator: (on say of above) Dr Sir William Gull, or possibly royal coachman Joseph Netley.

Catherine Eddowes, murdered 30 September 1888, aged forty-six. Killed in Mitre Square, off Aldgate. Throat cut, severe mutilation of face and stomach. Perpetrator: (on say of above) Dr Sir William Gull.

Mary Janet (Marie Jeanette) Kelly (or O'Brien), murdered 9 November 1888, aged twenty-three. Killed at Miller's Court.[13] Perpetrator: (deduced from testimony of one George Hutchinson) Lord Randolph Churchill.[14]

George Hutchinson made a statement to the police which included a description of a man last seen in the company of Kelly. The descriptions could equally well have applied to Prince Eddy or to Lord Randolph Churchill, the manic depressive politician who was one of the prince's circle. The naming of Lord Randolph in this connection remains a part of the royal conspiracy theory surrounding the 'Jack the Ripper' murders. Churchill was a family friend of Gull, who had been summoned to give a second opinion when Jennie, Lady Churchill, suffered from typhoid in 1882.[15]

The *modus operandi* for the 'Jack the Ripper' murders was described by Melvyn Fairclough. The victims were picked up as whores and lured into a coach driven by 'royal coachman' John Charles Netley, on the pretext of paid sex to be enacted therein; once inside, they were drugged with grapes soaked in laudanum, murdered, then mutilated and their bodies left in different locations.[16] Many historians of the 'Jack the Ripper' murders make the point that the mutilations carried out on the bodies of the women showed distinct signs of the work of someone with surgical skills.

Following the first East End murder, Inspector Frederick George Abberline, former head of the Whitechapel Criminal Investigation Department, was secured by Scotland Yard to oversee day-to-day enquiries in the East End. Abberline had an unequalled knowledge of the East End and is known to have kept diaries and papers concerning the murders. It appears that for a time Abberline also acted as 'unofficial bodyguard' to Prince Eddy.[17] Further, in a diary entry composed in 1892, Abberline noted that the landlord of the victim Mary Kelly (one John

McCarthy) had received a postcard, bearing a Scottish postmark, on which was written: 'Now we've done the fourth (really fifth) one, we shall go for the mother and daughter (i.e., Prince Eddy's 'wife' Annie and her daughter Alice Crook).' Abberline believed that Dr Sir William Gull had sent the card from his holiday home at Killiecrankie.[18]

Be that as it may, in constructing his version of the Jack the Ripper story, Melvyn Fairclough avers that in his latter years (and in the year he mentions he was seventy-three) Gull exhibited a certain callousness towards the feelings of his patients and their relatives. In this he quotes Gull's biographer and son-in-law Thomas Dyke Acland, who wrote in 1896:

> (*Dr Gull*) had been attending a poor patient with heart disease, and after his death was extremely anxious for a post-mortem examination. With great difficulty this was granted, but with the proviso that nothing was to be taken away, and the sister of the deceased patient, a strong-minded old maid, was present to watch the proceedings.
>
> Gull saw that it was hopeless to conceal anything from her, or to persuade her to leave the room. He therefore deliberately took out the heart, put it in his pocket and, looking steadily at her, said, 'I trust to your honour not to betray me.' His knowledge of character was justified by the result and the heart is now in Guy's Museum.[19]

It is interesting to note that, in the case of the murder of Mary Kelly, her heart had been removed, presumably by the killer.

What might have been the motives for the Ripper murders according to the royal conspiracy theory? All the women had been told of the liaison between Prince Eddy and Annie Crook by the last Ripper victim, Mary Kelly. Blackmail was attempted by the women, news of which reached Prime Minister Lord Salisbury, who urged that they be 'silenced'. The prime minister, the theory surmises, did not intend that the women should be murdered, but others in the court circle believed that they should be permanently silenced. Thus in this version of the Jack the Ripper murders, a serious accusation against a royal physician was set out.

In his article in *The Criminologist*, Dr Stowell further avers that the Ripper (i.e., Prince Eddy) was under the care of Dr Sir William Gull, 'who treated him with such success that in 1889 (Prince Eddy) was able to take a five months' cruise during which he enjoyed some big game hunting in which he was a remarkably fine shot'.[20]

Dr Sir William Gull's papers were to reveal another curious set of details about Prince Eddy. The prince's official biography is well known to historians. In 1891 he was betrothed to Princess May of Teck. They were to be married the following year. On 7 January 1892 the prince fell ill and royal physician Sir Francis Laking diagnosed incipient broncho-pneumonia and the prince died on the morning of 14 January 1892. But that date of death was to be disputed in Gull's papers.

The first public suggestion that Prince Eddy had not died when and where the official records stated was made by Melvyn Fairclough, who had been given the startling assertion by Joseph Sickert.[21] It appears, too, that Gull's daughter Caroline, who had married Thomas Dyke Acland, her father's biographer, had invited Dr T.E.A. Stowell (of *The Criminologist* article) to review her father's private papers after his death. In the documents he discovered that Prince Eddy had not died at Sandringham House in 1892 'but in a mental hospital' nearby, from 'softening of the brain' caused by syphilis.[22]

Was all this nonsense? Many royal historians believe it was. And their reasons? Writing in *History Today*, William R. Rubinstein, Professor of Modern History at the University of Wales, concluded that Prince Eddy 'was in Scotland (Abergeldie), or Yorkshire (Danby Lodge and Cavalry Barracks, York) (and Sandringham) at the time of the Ripper murders'. He also claimed that by 1888 Dr Sir William Gull at seventy-one 'had suffered two serious strokes'.[23]

But common sense suggests that if Gull (and the other royal collaborators) had perpetrated the murders they would have disposed of the bodies without trace, instead of leaving their horrific handiwork for all to see. Much has been made of the idea that the mutilation and evisceration of the victims suggests that the murderer had surgical knowledge. Thus it was easy to tie in Gull's name. Dr Stowell, in his royal conspiracy theory, even pointed out that Prince Eddy was well versed in the flenching of deer at royal hunts. Herein he would have learned how to remove bowels, kidney, liver, heart, lungs and uterus neatly.[24] Further, the fact that there seemed to be a sado-sexual element to the Ripper murders has also been cited as a clue to Prince Eddy's purported involvement because of his own reputed sexual perversions.

Dr Sir William Gull died on 29 January 1890, after a third epileptiform attack and was buried at St Michael's churchyard, Thorpe-le-Soken, Essex. Or was he? A curious set of local traditions received a public airing in 1997 when freelance writer Kevin O'Donnell's book *The Jack the Ripper Whitechapel Murders*, based on the researches of Andy and Sue Parlour, was published. Andy Parlour is related to one of the Ripper victims.

The substance of the Thorpe-le-Soken legends and Dr Sir William Gull may be summarised thus:

1. That Gull was the 'Ripper' and that he was certified insane by 'a panel of twelve fellow doctors' and incarcerated in an asylum in Islington, London, as inmate no. 124 and using the false name Thomas Mason. To cover up Gull's disappearance, a mock funeral was staged (with a weighted but empty coffin) on 3 February 1890.

    (This story was given some credence by an article by Dr Howard in the *Sunday Times Herald*, Chicago, April 1895.)

2. That Gull was linked to the 'Ripper' murders and helped to suppress all evidence of royal involvement. Having become mentally unstable after his strokes, and thus unguardedly loquacious about his royal connections, Gull was certified insane.

    Again this version of the story is linked to a mock funeral, with Thorpe-le-Soken worthies attesting to a coffin 'containing bags of sand' being secretly buried in the Gull plot.[25]

Local tradition avers that the Gull cemetery lairs (grave spaces) were opened around 1896 and a second coffin buried in the middle of the night. Incidentally Kevin O'Donnell points out that in 1896 a pauper registered as Thomas Mason died at St

Mary's Asylum, Islington.[26] Was this Gull, now buried in secret at Thorpe-le-Soken?

Curiously, Dr Sir William Gull's will of 27 November 1888, made shortly after the fifth 'Ripper' murder, adds a further mystery. The will was certified proved on 8 January 1890. But in January 1897 it was subjected to 'double probate', a situation that arises when the original executors have died or defaulted. Had Gull's effects of £344,022 19*s* 7*d* lain *untouched* for seven years? Certainly at his supposed death his beneficiaries were alive and well, and certainly able to be in receipt of all monies and goods. Did all this remain untouched perhaps because his lawyers and executors knew Gull was not dead? Furthermore the amount certified as deathbed accumulation was a huge amount in 1890. Did it indicate that he had been in receipt of royal pay-offs for his cooperation and silence in matters the royal family wished to suppress?

Historians continue to speculate, for Dr Sir William Gull's papers are just another example of how royal medical records are not always what they appear.

CHAPTER FIFTEEN

ANXIETY AT THE COURT OF EDWARD VII: AN OPERATION MAKES HISTORY

On 9 November 1871 Albert Edward, Prince of Wales, and his wife Princess Alexandra returned to Sandringham in time for the prince's thirtieth birthday; soon afterwards he fell ill. On 23 November the royal doctors pronounced that he had typhoid. The Waleses had been staying with William Henry Forester Denison, 2nd Baron Londesborough (1834–1900), at Londesborough Lodge near Scarborough, Yorkshire. It was a house then notorious for its foul drains, and not long after the royal visit a fellow-guest, George Philip Stanhope, Earl of Chesterfield (b. 1831), died of typhoid, as did the Prince of Wales's groom. There was great anxiety that the prince would succumb himself.

By 29 November the Countess of Macclesfield gossiped that the Prince of Wales was raving in a way that was 'very dreadful, and for *that* cause the Princess [of Wales] was kept out of his room one day, all sorts of revelations of names of people mentioned'.[1] The inference was that the prince was naming those women with whom he had had a fling. The prince's condition worsened, and in early December Lord Granville informed Queen Victoria 'that there did not seem any hope left'.[2] Tension increased. The queen was frantic and stricken with gloom as the anniversary of the death of Prince Albert – 14 December – approached.

But by 15 December the Prince of Wales had begun to rally and the worst was over. The illness was a watershed in the prince's life. The trauma intensified the prince's interest in medical matters and inspired him to devote much more time and resources to medical charities and projects. In 1863 – the year of his marriage – the prince had become patron of several hospitals:

the City of London Hospital for Diseases of the Chest; the Male Lock Hospital; the London Fever Hospital; the Portsmouth, Portsea and Gosport Hospital; the Royal Orthopaedic Hospital; the German Hospital; and the West Norfolk and Lynn Hospital.[3] Now he eagerly became patron and sponsor to dozens more hospitals, and through his influence encouraged hundreds of landed gentry to follow suit. His diary bristled with engagements to lay the foundation stones of new hospitals, open new wings to existing ones and launch new medical enterprises. By the Silver Jubilee of Queen Victoria in 1887 he had supported sixty-six hospitals and a myriad of other allied institutions, orphanages and funds for 'social, moral and physical improvement'. Thus his association with royal doctors had more to do with the advancement of medicine than with his own health.

On 27 February 1898 the Prince of Wales dined at the home of his soon-to-be new mistress and her husband, the Hon. George and Mrs Alice Keppel. Included in Alice Keppel's guest list that night was Agnes Keyser (1852–1941) and her sister Fanny, the daughters of the well-to-do Jewish financier Charles Keyser.[4] A short while later Mrs Keppel and the prince took tea at the Keyser sisters' residence at 17 Grosvenor Crescent, and an important royal friendship was struck up.

On 12 October 1899 the Second South African (Boer) War broke out, an event that would greatly influence this new friendship. Agnes and Fanny Keyser were anxious to support Britain's war effort and at the next social meeting Agnes Keyser asked the prince what they might do. The suggestion came immediately that the sisters should open up their London house as a hospital. By December 1899 the small hospital at 17 Grosvenor Crescent was complete and the prince himself performed the opening ceremony. This was the origin of the King Edward VII's Hospital for Officers, which in its various forms and addresses survives today at Beaumont Street, London, its home since 1948.[5] Over the years many royal doctors were associated with the hospital and Agnes Keyser, who presided as 'Sister Agnes' – although she had no medical qualifications – at the prince's suggestion, became its life force for the rest of her days. Her friendship with the prince also encouraged her to watch over his health.

EDWARD VII'S MEDICAL HOUSEHOLD
Edward VII. Born 8 December 1841. Reigned 1901–10. Died 6 May 1910.

ENGLAND: NEW MEDICAL HOUSEHOLD
Physician-in-ordinary: Sir William Henry Broadbent (1835–1907); Sir James Reid (1849–1923); Sir Francis Laking (1847–1914).
Physicians-extraordinary: Sir Joseph Fayrer (1824–1907); Sir Richard Douglas Powell (1842–1925); Sir Edward Henry Sieveking (1816–1904); Sir Felix Semon (1849–1921); J. Lowe.
Physician to the household: Sir Thomas Barlow (1845–1945).
Sergeant-surgeon: Joseph, Baron Lister (1827–1912).
Honorary sergeant-surgeon: Sir Frederick Treves (1853–1923).
Honorary surgeons-in-ordinary: T. Bryant; Sir A.D. Fripp; Sir Rickman John Godlee (1849–1925).
Surgeon to the household: H.W. Allingham.
Surgeon apothecary to His Majesty and apothecary to the household:
  Sir Francis Laking.
Surgeons and apothecaries in ordinary to the household at Windsor: W. Fairbanks; W. Ellison.
  At Sandringham: Sir Alan R. Manby.
Honorary surgeon oculist: Sir G.A. Critchett.
Honorary surgeon dentist: Sir Henry Bell Longhurst.
Dentist to the household: Edwin T. Truman.
Honorary anaesthetist: Frederick William Hewitt.
Chemist and druggist: Peter Wyett Squire.

The medical households of the Duchess of Edinburgh and Saxe-Coburg-Gotha, Duke of Connaught and Strathearn, Prince Christian of Schleswig-Holstein and Princess Beatrice remained much as they had in Queen Victoria's day.

SCOTLAND (1902)
Physician-in-ordinary: Sir William Tennant Gairdner (1824–1907); George Balfour.
Surgeon-in-ordinary: Sir Patrick Heron Watson (1832–1907); Alexander Ogston.
Over the years leading to Edward VII's death the following doctors were appointed:

Sir Thomas Smith (1833–1909). Honorary sergeant-surgeon, 1903.

Bernard Edward Dawson (1864–1948). Physician-extraordinary 1908.

Sir Thomas Richard Fraser (1841–1929). Physician-in-ordinary, Scotland, 1908.

Sir Thomas McCall Anderson (1836–1909). Physician, Scotland, 1909.

D.W. Finlay. Physician-in-ordinary, Scotland, 1909.

Sir Anthony Alfred Bowlby (1855–1929). Surgeon to the household, 1906.

In 1910 the medical household of George, Prince of Wales, included Sir James Reid, Sir Francis Laking, Sir Richard Havelock, Sir R.W. Burnet and Samuel Jones Gee as physicians, with Sir Frederick Treves and Hugh M. Rigby as surgeons.

Agnes Keyser was never the prince's mistress, yet there developed between them an *amitié amoureuse*. He visited her often at 17 Grosvenor Crescent, where she fed him standard nursery fare – Irish stew and rice pudding – in an attempt to divert him from gorging on his favourite rich foods. Her suggestions that he smoke less and drink less alcohol fell on deaf ears. Yet he enjoyed being fussed over by her. Alice Keppel took care of the prince's other mothering and sexual needs, and between them Agnes and Alice – his two last loves – made the prince's declining years more bearable.[6] Both women were concerned when the prince, now King Edward VII, became seriously ill in 1902.

By 1 January that year King Edward VII's medical department was already in place in the royal household lists, led by physicians-in-ordinary Sir William Broadbent, Sir James Reid and Sir Francis Laking, and surgeons-in-ordinary Thomas Bryant, Sir Arthur Fripp and Sir Rickman Godlee. Baron Joseph Lister was sergeant-surgeon. They met early in 1902 to review the monarch's health.

The king's medical dossier recorded his contraction of typhoid in 1871, the painful attack of phlebitis in 1889, and his tumble at Waddesdon Manor, the lavish home of Baron Frederick de

Rothschild, at Aylesbury, Buckinghamshire, in 1898, where he fractured his kneecap. Apart from these events the prince had avoided severe illness and now, in his sixty-first year, his energy and zest for life were still remarkable. His royal doctors had to work hard to keep up with his busy schedule, from the Riviera and Paris in mid-March of each year, to Cowes in July, Germany and Austria in August and Balmoral in September. But the royal doctors noted how he drove himself to exhaustion and was troubled by the increasing occurrence of violent bronchitic coughing fits which left him purple in the face and gasping for air.

Edward VII's coronation was scheduled for Thursday, 26 June 1902, but at the beginning of that month he began to feel unwell. On the cold rainy Saturday, 14 June, he was travelling up to Aldershot for a military tattoo when he was assailed by abdominal pain. By the following morning the symptoms were worse, with the monarch's abdomen distended. Sir Francis Laking and physician to the household Sir Thomas Barlow were called.

The doctors observed the king's fevered condition with accompanying tenderness in the region of the right iliac fossa. They kept a watching brief. Soon journalists were demanding information to substantiate the rumours about the king's health. Laking was obliged to make a statement. For reasons known only to himself, he told the press agencies that the king was suffering from lumbago. Once the true story of the king's condition was released Laking suffered much press opprobrium.

Sedated with opiates, the king was moved to Windsor, with Queen Alexandra left to review the troops at Aldershot. Monitoring the monarch's condition, the two royal doctors detected a noticeable mass in the lower right abdomen. They advised an examination by a surgical consultant.

The king was adamant that nothing be done about his condition. He was determined that nothing would interfere with the preparations for the coronation. But Sir Francis Laking became as determined as the king. There followed an unprecedented confrontation between monarch and royal doctor. Laking stood his ground against the king's choleric wrath; he *must* be seen by the honorary sergeant-surgeon Sir Fredrick Treves. The king finally relented and on 18 June Treves made his examination. To the monarch's delight his appendicular inflammation seemed to disappear, as did the swelling. Feeling better, the king made ready to return to Buckingham Palace on 23 June.

Wishing to be seen by his people, the king ignored his doctors' advice and eschewed a closed conveyance once he had arrived at Paddington station; instead he rode in an open carriage with a cavalry escort to Buckingham Palace. He also insisted on attending a banquet for the crown princes of Europe. But the public and the princes could all see that the king was not well. That night his fever returned, the painful mass made its presence obvious once more and the royal doctors believed the king was gravely ill. Sir Frederick Treves was called again; so afraid were the royal household staff lest details of the king's condition should reach the press, that summonses to the royal bedside were sent via pre-arranged code telegrams. Treves consulted with sergeant-surgeon Lord Lister and physician Sir Thomas Smith and all agreed that immediate surgery was necessary.

There occurred one of the best recorded dialogues between the king and his doctors. Lister explained the graveness of the situation, but the king, a stickler for protocol and tradition, refused to have surgery. 'I must keep faith with my people,' he emphasised. 'I must go to the Abbey for the coronation.'

The doctors knew that without immediate surgery the king would die and there would be an even greater crisis. They persisted, but the king continued to refuse. At last Sir Frederick Treves took the initiative and said: 'Then Sire, you will go (to Westminster Abbey) as a corpse.' His words stunned the king, who reluctantly agreed to surgery. The royal doctors then issued this bulletin:

24 June 1902, 11.15 a.m. (Posted in Fleet Street, Strand and Piccadilly.)
The King is suffering from perityphlitis. His condition on Saturday was so satisfactory that it was hoped that with care His Majesty would be able to go through the Coronation ceremony. Yesterday evening a recrudescence became manifest, rendering a surgical operation necessary today.
(Signed): LISTER, THOS. SMITH. FRANCIS LAKING. THOS. BARLOW, FREDERICK TREVES.

Just after noon on 24 June Edward VII – dressed, to Queen Alexandra's mortification, in his scruffiest dressing gown – walked into the room at Buckingham Palace that had been prepared for the operation. Nurse Haines set all the instruments to hand ready beside the billiard table that was to serve as an operation plinth. An anaesthetic was administered by (later Sir) Frederick Hewitt. The king went 'black in the face' and began to struggle. Queen Alexandra assisted in holding him down. Treves was uncomfortable at having Queen Alexandra present. It was bad enough having to operate on an elderly obese man who was 'not a good surgical risk', without being further inhibited by the protocol that surrounded the queen's presence. He later said: 'I was anxious to prepare for the operation, but did not like to take off my coat, tuck up my sleeves, and put on an apron whilst the Queen was present.' He persuaded Queen Alexandra and her children to withdraw.

Treves's work was hampered by the king's obesity. At last a large abscess was exposed and evacuated, the wound washed out and drained. Once the wound had been packed with gauze, the procedure was logged as having taken forty minutes.[7] A series of new bulletins were issued:

24 June, 2.00 p.m.
The operation on His Majesty has been successfully performed. A large abcess has been evacuated. The King has borne the operation well, and is in a satisfactory condition.

24 June, 6.00 p.m.
His Majesty continues to make satisfactory progress and has been much relieved by his operation.

24 June, 11.30 p.m.
The King's condition is as good as can be expected after so serious an operation. His strength is maintained. There is less pain, and His Majesty has taken a little nourishment. It will be some days before it will be possible to say that the King is out of danger.

Regular bulletins continued and a few days later the royal doctors were able to post this:

28 June, noon
The King has had a good night, and his improved condition is maintained. We are happy that we are able to state that we consider His Majesty to be out of immediate danger. The general condition is satisfactory. The operation wound, however, still needs constant attention, and as much concern as attaches to His Majesty is connected with the wound. Under the most favourable conditions His Majesty's recovery must be protracted.

By this time the regal guests invited for the coronation had returned home. On 15 July Edward VII left London for Portsmouth accompanied by Queen Alexandra, all the royal doctors and Nurses Haines and Tarr, to convalesce aboard the royal yacht *Victoria & Albert*. While on board the king signed a new proclamation for his rescheduled coronation ceremony to be held on 9 August 1902. The mountains of food that had been prepared for the original celebrations were distributed among the poor. For the doctors there were state honours and Nurse Haines was appointed matron of the newly opened officers' home at Osborne House. Treves received a baronetcy, but the king's operation was to give him a higher public profile, which singles him out for special mention of his remarkable career.

CHAPTER SIXTEEN

EDWARDIAN DOCTOR EXTRAORDINARY: MONSTERS, SCANDAL AND SIR FREDERICK TREVES

The summit of Sir Frederick Treves's royal career was undoubtedly the successful appendix operation on King Edward VII, after which he became a trusted friend to both the king and Queen Alexandra. Treves was surgeon to four succeeding monarchs and also played a role in advising royalty on medical matters and relevant social policy. Apart from his surgical skills the key to Treves's success was his driving ambition, which made him one of the most remarkable doctors of any age and a polymath among his peers.

Born on 15 February 1853 at Dorchester, Dorset, Frederick Treves was the fifth child of William and Jane Treves, a family of yeoman ancestry which produced three doctors. After primary education at the Revd William Barnes's school at Dorchester, Frederick Treves moved with his family to Kennington, South London, and in 1867 enrolled at the Merchant Taylors School then at Suffolk Lane in the City. Barred by his social class from working for a position recognised by the Royal College of Physicians (who still accepted only Oxford and Cambridge graduates as members), Treves matriculated at University College, London, in 1871 for his foundation courses and chose the London Hospital, Whitechapel Road, for his practical studies.

The London Hospital was in the heart of a poor area, and its filthy consulting rooms were overseen by a matron who was 'generally the worse for drink'.[1] Nevertheless it contained the largest surgical ward in Britain and presented students with a wide range of surgical experience. Here too lectured some of the finest tutors of the day, including Sir John Hughlings Jackson

(1834–1911), a founder of modern neurology practice, Sir Jonathan Hutchinson (1828–1913), who won a great reputation as an opthalmologist and dermatologist, and Sir Andrew Clark (1826–93), a consultant physician who had the most famous panel of patients of all, from W.E. Gladstone to Robert Louis Stevenson.

The innovative techniques employed at the London Hospital, where for example Sir Morell Mackenzie (1837–92) introduced the laryngoscope to England, inspired Treves to invent surgical devices himself. He qualified as Licentiate of the Society of Apothecaries in 1874 and Member of the Royal College of Surgeons in 1875, and joined his brother William at the Royal National Hospital for Scrofula at Margate, Kent, the next year. In 1877 he married Anne Elizabeth Mason, buying a partnership interest in the practice of William Milligan at Wirksworth, Derbyshire.

Treves's sojourn in Derbyshire did not last very long. Following professional disputes with some of his colleagues, he returned to London to take on a batch of low-paid jobs. He was assistant surgeon at the London Hospital in 1879, advancing to full surgeon in 1884 and Hunterian Professor of Anatomy at the Royal College of Surgeons in 1885.

By this time Treves's career had really taken off and he was much sought after by students, who invariably packed his demonstration room. One such student was Bertrand Dawson, who was to achieve even greater fame – and some notoriety – as a royal doctor. Dawson remembered Treves operating 'in an old and well-worn coat' which, as he once boasted to Ernest Morris, was so stiff with congealed blood after many years of use that 'it would stand upright when placed on the floor'.[2]

Frederick Treves believed that the most skilled surgeon could not become so without a fundamental knowledge of anatomy; his own interest in the subject led him to be fascinated with pathology and a particular study of deformity. Most teaching hospitals had gruesome displays of congenital malformations which students of a less liberally enlightened age dubbed 'monsters'. Treves now gave lectures and presentations on such subjects as osteitis deformans (Paget's disease) and congenital coccygeal tumours. In 1884 he came across a case that was forever to be linked with his name.

In 1980 EMI-Brooks films issued the movie *The Elephant Man* starring Anthony Hopkins and John Hurt. It told the story of a penniless man, deformed by a rare illness, who was rescued by a doctor from a fairground freak-show, to become a member of fashionable society. The inspiration for the film was the unfortunate Joseph Carey Merrick, born on 5 August 1862 at Leicester; the doctor was Frederick Treves.

Treves heard about Merrick from his house surgeon Reginald Tuckett.[3] For 2*d* anyone could view the deformed Merrick as the freak 'Elephant Man' in a show run by Tom Norman in Whitechapel Road. Merrick suffered from a gross example of neurofibromatosis. This is how Treves described his first sight of Merrick in his notes on the case in 1923:

> The showman – speaking as if to a dog – called out harshly: 'Stand up!' The thing arose slowly and let the blanket that covered its head and back fall to the ground. There stood revealed the most disgusting specimen of humanity that I have ever seen. In the course of my profession I had come upon lamentable deformities of the face due to injury or disease, as well as mutilations and contortions of the body depending upon like causes; but at no time had I met with such a degraded or perverted version of a human being as this lone figure displayed. He was naked to the waist, his feet were bare, he wore a pair of threadbare trousers that had once belonged to some fat gentleman's suit.
>
> From the intensified painting in the street (a billboard had shown a drawing of a being half man, half elephant) I had imagined the Elephant Man to be of gigantic size. This, however, was a little man below the average height and made to look shorter by the bowing of his back. The most striking feature about him was his enormous mis-shapen head.
>
> From the brow there projected a huge bony mass like a loaf, while from the back of the head hung a bag of spongy, fungous-looking skin, the surface of which was comparable to brown cauliflower. On the top of the skull were a few long lank hairs. The osseous growth on the forehead almost occluded one eye. The circumference of the head was no less than of the man's waist. From the upper jaw there projected

another mass of bone. It protruded from the mouth like a pink stump, turning the upper lip inside out and making of the mouth a mere slobbering aperture. This growth from the jaw had been so exaggerated in the painting as to appear to be a rudimentary trunk or tusk. The nose was merely a lump of flesh, only recognisable as a nose from its position. The face was no more capable of expression than a block of gnarled wood. The back was horrible, because from it hung, as far down as the middle of the thigh, huge, sack-like masses of flesh covered by the same loathesome cauliflower skin.

The right arm was of enormous size and shapeless. It suggested the limb of the subject of elephantiasis. It was overgrown also with pendent masses of the same cauliflower-like skin. The hand was large and clumsy – a fin or paddle rather than a hand. There was no distinction between the palm and the back. The thumb had the appearance of a radish, while the fingers might have been thick, tuberous roots. As a limb it was almost useless.

The other arm was remarkable by contrast. It was not only normal but was, moreover, a delicately shaped limb covered with fine skin and provided with a beautiful hand which any woman might have envied. From the chest hung a bag of the same repulsive flesh. it was like a dewlap suspended from the neck of a lizard. The lower limbs had the characters of the deformed arm, they were unwieldy, dropsical-looking and grossly mis-shapen.

To add a further burden to his trouble the wretched man, when a boy, developed hip disease, which had left him permanently lame, so that he could only walk with a stick. He was thus denied all means of escape from his tormentors. As he told me later, he could never run away. One other feature must be mentioned to emphasise his isolation from his kind. Although he was already repellent enough, there arose from the fungous skin-growth with which he was already almost covered a sickening stench which was hard to tolerate. From the showman I learnt nothing about the Elephant Man, except that he was English, that his name was John (sic) Merrick and that he was twenty-one years of age.[4]

Treves negotiated a fee with Tom Norman for Merrick to be examined clinically. From his findings Treves prepared a lecture on Merrick's horrific deformities, but he met with a large degree of public revulsion. Treves persisted and wrote up new notes for the Pathological Society of London; his paper, delivered with Merrick as a live exhibit, stimulated new professional interest. With the help of interested dermatologist Dr Henry Radcliffe Crocker, the diagnosis of fibroma was reached.[5]

After Treves's lecture the police closed down the freak-show. Merrick was sold on to an Austrian freak-show but was abandoned in Brussels, his deformities being considered too gross for continental taste. Somehow Merrick returned alone to London, where the police eventually found him in a distressed condition. In his pocket was a calling card that Treves had given him. The card was Merrick's passport to the next phase of his life. Treves now helped him to cope with normal human society. Publicity about the Merrick case caused him to become 'the object of a more genteel freak show' which brought many society folk to see him.[6]

Writing in 1923 Treves reported:

The height of his social development was reached on an eventful day when Queen Alexandra – then Princess of Wales – came to (the London Hospital) to pay him a special visit. With that kindness which has marked every act of her life, the Queen entered Merrick's room smiling and shook him warmly by the hand. Merrick was transported with delight. The Queen has made many people happy, but I think no gracious act of hers has ever caused such happiness as she brought into Merrick's room when she sat by his chair and talked to him as to a person she was glad to see.[7]

Joseph Merrick died of asphyxia on 11 April 1890 in the room Treves had acquired for him at Bedstead Square, opposite the gardens of the London Hospital. His skeleton still rests in the Museum of the Anatomy Department of the Medical College of London Hospital, and the story of the 'monster and the royal doctor' still captures the imagination today.

During the next few years Frederick Treves did much to enlarge the practice of British surgery. As his biographer wrote, he devised and perfected 'operations for conditions previously held to be either untreatable by surgery, or to be attended by very great risk to life'.[8] He had achieved much; he had risen to be 'the leader of English surgery'.[9] Yet still he craved adventure and influence.

Frederick Treves's connection with the royal family began in 1897 when he was appointed surgeon-in-ordinary to Prince George, Duke of York. This was the beginning of the 'influence' he sought; his desire for 'adventure' was to be satisfied through the South African (Boer) War of 1899. That November the Duchess of Bedford, wife of the 11th Duke, placed money at Treves's disposal so that he could form his own surgical team to follow General Sir Redvers Henry Buller's Natal Army.

On 10 November Treves was invited to Marlborough House for the Prince of Wales to wish him well in his enterprise. With a medical team and surgical kit of his own device, Treves served (in a private capacity) with the No. 4 Field Hospital and was present at the battles of Colenso, Spion Kop and Spearman's Hill. Just before the British broke through to Ladysmith, Treves suffered an attack of dysentery. Although the Second Boer War was not concluded until the Peace of Vereeniging, signed on 31 May 1902, Treves came home to a hero's welcome in 1900 where, despite the euphoria and jingoism, the South African War was something of an embarrassment. Queen Victoria's great empire had been challenged by an army of Boer farmers in a far-flung corner of Africa, producing a bloody conflict. Once back home Treves became involved in the growing criticism of the activities of the Royal Army Medical Corps in South Africa. The whole brouhaha developed into a public scandal as Treves abandoned his derogatory, independent opinions of the RAMC and instead began to actively support the establishment position. It was a stance that was to win him royal favour.

Following Edward VII's appendicitis operation, Treves's name was regularly mentioned in royal gossip regarding the rescheduling of the coronation. One aspect of this was to cause him embarrassment. The king had decided the coronation should be on 9 August 1902. In conversation Treves mentioned this to Queen Alexandra. To his surprise she uncharacteristically exploded with anger. Her biographer Georgina Battiscombe describes the scene:

> By some oversight, this was the first that Queen Alexandra had heard of the matter. Her indignation astonished Treves, who had come to regard her as a paragon of gentleness. The ceremony, she protested, concerned her almost as much as it concerned the King; she was to be crowned too, and she had every right to be consulted. To fix a date whilst King Edward still lay very sick was, she considered, to fly in the face of providence, and she would have them all remember that such matters did not rest in the hands of men but of God. She expressed herself so strongly on the subject that instead of an official announcement of the date, a very cautious bulletin was issued stating that if the King were sufficiently recovered it was hoped that the Coronation would take place some time between 8 August and 12 August.[10]

Treves endeavoured to pour oil on troubled waters; he certainly would never make such a mistake again.

Treves accompanied the king and queen on a convalescence cruise aboard the royal yacht *Victoria & Albert* in July 1902. To the delight of his doctors, and no little embarrassment to himself, the king had lost some six inches of flabby waist, and the bracing air of the cruise soon had him back to his former energetic and enthusiastic self. Treves allowed the king back to his royal state papers boxes, but carefully monitored his royal patient's increased depression about foreign affairs. Republicanism was gaining ground in Europe and the king feared that his throne would not survive the inevitable reign of his son Prince George.

Frederick Treves was made a baronet as Sir Frederick Treves of Dorchester in 1903. In June 1904 he decided to retire from private practice, although he kept up his own interest in developing medical practice and encouraged the king to do likewise in the many medical charities. In 1908 Treves visited Paris to view the Radium Institute, and was enthusiastic about the idea of setting up such an institution in Britain. The king was keen too; he had been treated with radium for an 'ulcer' between his right eye and his nose in 1907. In 1908 Treves announced that a radium institute would be founded in London with himself as chairman.

Treves enjoyed his retirement at the grace and favour house of Thatched House Lodge in Richmond Park, which the king had granted him. He was still a part of the king's private entourage, and went on trips which included bridge playing and shooting at Balmoral. Treves loathed shooting, yet he basked in his enhanced social prominence and valued his academic honours.

In March 1910 Edward VII put aside his everyday political and constitutional worries and heeded his royal doctors' advice that he should take a holiday. Accompanied by his mistress, Mrs Alice Keppel, he made his way to his favourite French resort of Biarritz, calling at Paris en route. But his depression was never far away. At Paris he attended the Théâtre de la Porte St Martin, taking in a performance of Edmund Rostand's new allegorical verse drama *Chantecler*. He was unimpressed, and left the theatre muttering 'stupid' and 'childish'.

The theatre had been hot and the king suffered a few bronchitic splutterings; the shortness of breath exacerbated his indigestion and he had a sharp pain in the heart region. His physician in the entourage, Sir James Reid, advised bed rest. The king refused but agreed to stay in his room at the Hôtel du Palais, entertained by Alice Keppel and his old friend, the Portuguese minister in London, Luis, Marquis de Soveral (d. 1922).

Edward VII fretted continually about the political situation at home and his health continued to trouble him. Queen Alexandra wired him to join her on the Mediterranean cruise she was enjoying and get away from that 'horrid Biarritz' (i.e., the queen's code for Alice Keppel).[11] By 1 April the weather had deteriorated, and snow, wind and rain persistently interrupted the royal pleasure. Yet for the king the Mediterranean had no attractions to compare with those supplied by Alice Keppel.

On 26 April the local authorities in Biarritz staged a musical and fireworks spectacular outside the Hôtel du Palais for the king's delectation. Before he returned to Britain on 27 April the king strolled out on to his balcony and said to no one in particular: 'I shall be sorry to leave Biarritz. Perhaps it will be for the last time.'[12]

On his return the king undertook an exhausting round of opera visits, state and private audiences and paperwork, retiring for the weekend to Sandringham. Back in London by 2 May the king took time for an evening of dinner and fussing from Agnes Keyser at 17 Grosvenor Crescent; she feared the onset of another severe bronchitic attack. When the king had left her house she sent a note to Sir James Reid requesting his attendance at Buckingham Palace that night. When Reid arrived he found the king having difficulty breathing. He prescribed '15mil.Tr.Chlor.et.Morph BP 1885' and linctus, and penned a report for physician-in-ordinary Sir Frederick Laking.[13]

The king was coughing even more when Reid and Laking attended him next morning, but he refused to give up his huge cigars. Although his usually voracious appetite had vanished and exhaustion from coughing slowed his steps, the king insisted in giving audiences and carrying out his duties. During his audience with John Dickson-Poynder, Governor of New Zealand, he had a violent fit of coughing which left him black in the face. His doctors realised it was the beginning of the end.

By now the king's last medical team of doctors were in attendance: Sir Francis Laking, Sir James Reid, Sir Douglas Powel, Dr Bertrand Dawson and throat specialist Dr St Clair Thomson. The queen was sent for from her cruise to Corfu. On the way she received regular reports on the king's health from Sir Francis Laking. She was shocked to see her husband looking so ill. The royal doctors wished to issue a public bulletin on the king's health but he refused to give consent. At length, having been persuaded that his people would be worried by his non-appearance at the station to welcome the queen home, he reconsidered and a bulletin was issued at 7.30 p.m. on 5 May 1910; it read that the king was suffering from bronchitis and that his condition 'caused some anxiety'.

Edward VII pushed himself to continue his daily routines as he had always done, but even his favourite cigars now gave him no pleasure. On 6 May, feeling 'wretchedly ill', he insisted on dressing properly (in frock coat) to receive his old friend and financial adviser Sir Ernest Cassell. Sir Francis Laking and Queen Alexandra cautioned Sir Ernest to make his visit brief and to prevent the king from talking too much. When Sir Ernest had gone the king rose from his chair and walked across the room to look at his caged canaries. Suddenly he collapsed.

The king now suffered a series of heart attacks. The royal doctors knew they could do nothing other than administer oxygen to ease his laboured breathing and inject him with strychnine and tyramine. Refusing to go to bed, the king sat up in a chair. He complained weakly: 'No, I shall not give in (to death); I shall go on; I shall work to the end. Of what use is it to be alive if one cannot work?'

The last coherent phrase the king uttered was a reply to Prince George, who told him that his horse Witch of the Air had won the 4.15 race at Kempton Park. 'I am very glad,' the king wheezed. Soon after he lapsed into a coma. He died at 11.45 p.m. on 6 May 1910. Sir James Reid prepared reports for the *British Medical Journal* and the *Lancet*, and Sir Frederick Treves signed the death certificate. Both doctors then went on to a new chapter of royal service.

CHAPTER SEVENTEEN

'ENGLISH PHYSICIANS KILL YOU . . .': THE MEDICAL HOUSEHOLDS OF GEORGE V AND QUEEN MARY

William Lamb, Viscount Melbourne, Queen Victoria's Whig prime minister and early mentor, was outspoken about English physicians in general and royal doctors in particular. Among his papers was found the remark 'English physicians kill you; the French let you die'. His words were to be remembered by many in court circles when one king in particular came to die.

Prince George Frederick Ernest Albert chose the title George V for his reign name. He was crowned at Westminster Abbey by Randall Davidson, the Archbishop of Canterbury, on 22 June 1911. Born at Marlborough House on 3 June 1865, Prince George had married Princess Victoria Mary Augusta Louise Olga Pauline Claudine Agnes, the ex-fiancée of his dead brother Albert Victor, at the Chapel Royal, St James's Palace, on 6 July 1893. She was crowned with her husband.

Within the new royal medical household were two new positions: (Sir) Milsom Rees (1866–1952) became laryngologist and Harold Robert Dacre Spitta (1877–1954) bacteriologist. By the end of the reign Lt-Col. W.H. Lester McCarthy (1885–1962) would join as coroner to the royal household.

Sir Francis Laking survived only three years into the new reign. He was to be long remembered in court circles for treating royal knock-knees. A man of slight stature, George V passed on to his children a congenital malformation of the knees, and Sir Francis Laking devised leg splints in which the unfortunate royal brood were obliged to sleep.[1]

Sir James Reid also played a role in court circles, mostly at Balmoral, where he was once summoned to cut the queen's corns.[2] Reid also accompanied his royal employers to Germany and France. Only three weeks after the outbreak of the First World War Reid received a letter from Sir Frederick Treves with the news that Prince Albert (later King George VI) had been struck down with appendicitis while serving aboard HMS *Collingwood*. The prince's appendix was removed on 9 September 1914 by Sir John Marnoch (1867–1936), Professor of Surgery at Aberdeen University, who was to become extra-surgeon to the Scottish household. Reid was present at the operation and wrote the official bulletin.

Reid's final royal event was Prince Albert's marriage to Lady Elizabeth Bowes Lyon at Westminster Abbey on 26 April 1923. The royal doctor died on 28 June 1923, to be followed by his fellow Buckingham Palace stalwart, Sir Frederick Treves, on 7 December. Treves died of peritonitis at the Clinique de Rosemont at Lausanne. Two years later came the death of physician-in-ordinary Sir Richard Douglas Powell, who had been with the court for thirty-eight years.

On the death of Sir Francis Laking, the post of king's physician-in-ordinary went to Sir Bertrand Edward Dawson, who was to be the physician to four kings. He was the only royal doctor to be created Viscount. Dawson is known to have kept a file of medical notes about the royal family, which was handed to King George VI's private secretary Clive Wigram at Dawson's death. The notes list the following royal patients:[3]

King Edward VII
King George V
King George VI
Queen Alexandra
Queen Elizabeth
Queen Mary
Princess Elizabeth
Princess Margaret Rose
Princess Mary, Princess Royal
Prince Edward, Prince of Wales
Prince Arthur of Connaught (Queen Victoria's son)
Princess Helena Victoria and Princess Marie Louise (Queen Victoria's grandchildren)

King George of Greece (Queen Alexandra's brother)
Dowager Empress Marie of Russia (Queen Alexandra's sister)
Queen Maud of Norway (King George V's sister)
King Leopold III of the Belgians (Cousin of George V)

Bertrand Edward Dawson was born at Croydon on 9 March 1864, one of the seven children of Henry Dawson, architect. Educated by a governess, at a preparatory school and at St Paul's School, he matriculated at University College, London, in 1882. Dawson graduated BSc in 1888 and took up studies at the London Hospital where he qualified MB in 1890. By 1896 he was assistant physician there, and he was to remain as physician at the London Hospital from 1906 to 1945. During the First World War he was a consultant physician in France with the acting rank of major-general.

In July 1907 Dawson entered royal service as physician-extraordinary to Edward VII. Dawson had made friends with Sir Frederick Treves and Sir Milsom Rees and had already met the king. Furthermore, his private patients already included Edward VII's private secretary Sir Francis Knollys and his family so Dawson's appointment was no surprise. While Dawson considered his promotion an honour of which he could 'conceive of no greater',[4] the position was then no great social plum. The titles 'apothecary' and 'doctor' were of no real status at court. Although present, he was to play no critical role in Edward VII's final illness. Dawson continued in his role of physician-extraordinary to the new King George V, and in 1911 he was knighted for his services to the royal family.

For many years Dawson had considered it important for all doctors to involve themselves in the promotion of good national health and during 1919 and 1920 he was chairman of the Ministry of Health Consultative Council on Medical Services. The report of this council foreshadowed the national Health Service Act which became law in 1946 (but did not come into operation until 5 July 1948). On being made a baron in 1920, Dawson assumed the role of spokesman for the medical profession in the House of Lords.

In the medical file that he kept on George V (as Prince of Wales and king), Dawson noted that in 1891 he had suffered from

GEORGE V'S MEDICAL HOUSEHOLD
George V. Born 3 June 1865. Reigned 1910–36. Died 20 January 1936.

ENGLAND: ROYAL MEDICAL HOUSEHOLD AS AT 1911
Physicians-in-ordinary: Sir Francis Laking (1847–1914); Sir James Reid (1849–1923); Sir Richard Powell (1842–1925).
Physicians-extraordinary: Sir Thomas Barlow (1845–1945); Sir William Allchin (1846–1911); (Sir) Bertrand Dawson; Sir Alan Manby (1848–1925).
Physician to the household: Sir Robert Burnet (1851–1931).
Sergeant-surgeon: Sir Frederick Treves (1853–1923); Sir Richard Charles (1858–1934).
Honorary Surgeons-in-ordinary: Sir Rickman Godlee (1849–1925); (Sir) Anthony Bowlby (1855–1929); Sir William Cheyne (1852–1932); Sir Albert Fripp (1865–1930).
Surgeon to the household: (Sir) Hugh Rigby (1870–1944).
Surgeon apothecary to the household: Sir Francis Laking.
Surgeons apothecary-in-ordinary at Windsor: W. Fairbanks; W. Ellison.
Surgeon apothecary-in-ordinary at Sandringham: Sir Alan Manby.
Surgeon oculist: Sir George Critchell (d. 1925).
Laryngologist: (Sir) Milsom Rees (1866–1952).
Bacteriologist: Harold Spitta (1877–1954).
Dental surgeon: Charles Truman.
Anaesthetist: (Sir) Frederick Hewitt (1857–1916).
Chemist and druggist: (Sir) Peter Wyatt Squire (1847–1919).

There were medical households for Queen Alexandra; the Duke of Connaught; Prince Christian; and Princess Beatrice.

SCOTLAND, 1911:
Physicians-in-ordinary: Sir Thomas Fraser (1841–1920); D.W. Findlay.
Surgeons-in-ordinary: (Sir) Alexander Ogston (1844–1929); (Sir) William MacEwan (1848–1924).
Surgeon apothecary at Balmoral: (Sir) Alexander Hendry (1867–1932).
Surgeon apothecary at Holyrood: W.B. Alexander.
Surgeon oculist: (Sir) George Berry (1853–1940).
Surgeon dentist: John Smith.

typhoid which had laid him low for six weeks of bed rest. The notes also revealed a series of minor ailments which included a manifestation from around 1908 of chronic indigestion (dyspepsia) 'that was almost certainly due to frayed nerves'.[5] Royal doctors attributed George V's gloomy and bad-tempered character to this condition.

King George made four visits to the British Expeditionary Force in France. His last was during July and August 1917, along with Queen Mary. On 28 October 1915 (during his second visit) King George arrived at Hesdigneul by car and mounted a chestnut mare provided for him by General Douglas Haig, Commander of the 1st Army Corps. As he rode towards the lines of the 1st Wing, Royal Flying Corps, the horse reared twice and the king was thrown. In the 1930s Dawson wrote his recollections of the accident:

When the King's horse, frightened by the sudden outburst of a military band, reared and fell backwards in the greasy mud of Flanders, the King was underneath the horse in the mud. The injuries were more serious than could then be disclosed. Besides widespread and severe bruising the pelvis was fractured in at least two places and the pain was bad, the subsequent shock considerable and convalescence tedious. The callus which formed at the sites of injury could be felt as irregular bony nodules for the remainder of the King's life, and his movements were henceforth somewhat limited and stiff and even at times painful. How well I remember the insistent urging of G.H.Q. that we should get the King to England before the Germans had time to bomb the house, indifferently sheltered in a small wood, and how we insisted we must wait till there had been some recovery from the shock and time enough to know that there were no hidden internal injuries. And then the Channel crossing when we did go – the worst possible. The seasickness with that injured and bruised frame meant bad pain for him and anxiety for us. When we reached London (Sir Frederick) Treves met us and took control. Considering the gravity and circumstances of the accident recovery was good, for the bladder might easily have been ruptured and the result have been fatal.[6]

The king was confined to his room for six weeks. A man of abstemious habits, he was persuaded by the royal doctors that he might put aside his total abstinence from alcohol (for the duration of the war) and for his health 'take a little stimulant daily during his convalescence'.[7] These words were enshrined in a bulletin on the king's health.

In the New Year's honours list of 1920 Dawson's name appeared as a new peer. Dawson's name had been entered by Lloyd George in the Birthday honours list of 1919, which caused the king some perturbation. With the exception of Joseph Lister in 1897, this would be the first peerage for the medical profession. The king was not objecting to Dawson's elevation as an individual but rather 'that senior doctors might feel they had been passed over, that surgeons might be thought to have a higher claim than physicians' and so on.[8] Lloyd George temporarily removed Dawson's name but told the king that he saw merit in having 'in the House of Lords some real authority in public health'.[9] All demurrings were withdrawn and the royal physician was gazetted as Baron Dawson of Penn.

Dawson now embarked on a busy programme of public health enquiry along with his medical consultancies and royal position. For the public, though, his profile would be further expanded. During the evening of 21 November 1928 a medical bulletin was issued, signed by (Sir) Stanley Hewitt and Dawson of Penn. It read: 'His Majesty the King is suffering from a cold with some fever, and is remaining in bed.' It was the prelude to a protracted royal illness.

At Buckingham Palace the king had no premonitions of a long illness, entering in his diary under the same date: 'Feverish cold they call it, and I retired to bed.'[10] Dawson and Hewitt made an initial diagnosis of a blood infection and sent a blood culture to Sir Lionel Ernest Howard Whitby, a pathologist at the Bland Sutton Institute. Whitby was a leading authority on haematology and was later Regis Professor at Cambridge. Whitby left this record of his summons to Buckingham Palace:

My services were required at the palace about 9 p.m. but I could not be located. I was, in fact, out to dinner, and for once (never again!), had failed to leave my whereabouts. When I returned home about midnight, after a good dinner, Lord Dawson's chauffeur was patiently waiting at my door. He had been there for two hours. Needless to say I was at the palace in record time, to be received by an unperturbed Lord Dawson (though I have no doubt he was storming with impatience) who said: 'I'm so glad you have come. I have had a job to avoid sending for somebody else but I said you were the only man I wanted.' And then I was taken to the King, whose first words, when he saw I was lame (ill and tired as he was at one in the morning), have also always remained in my memory: 'Have you lost your leg? Well, it's very good of you to come and see me at this time of night.'

And so the drama developed which all the world knows. As and when he required them Lord Dawson sought and used the advice of various specialists whom he knew and trusted, and brought to a successful conclusion one of the most hazardous cases it has ever been my lot to see. During those anxious months I have never admired a man more. He was never rattled, and his timing and judgement were perfect . . .[11]

The blood culture examined by Whitby exhibited a growth of streptococcus, providing a further diagnosis of septicaemia.

By 23 November the streptococcus manifested as small clots of blood in the sputum and closer care was advised. From the Westminster, London and St Thomas's hospitals came Sisters Nellie Purdie, Catherine Black, Rosina Davis and Elizabeth Gordon to nurse the king – 'representatives of the nursing profession from England, Scotland, Wales and Ireland'.[12]

Dawson and Hewitt now identified 'some congestion' on one of the king's lungs, and an X-ray examination (by portable apparatus) was carried out by Dr H. Graham Hodgson, diagnostic radiologist at King's College Hospital. This was the first recorded instance of X-rays being used outside a controlled hospital environment. Hodgson's X-ray films confirmed a right lung lobe pneumonia. In those pre-sulphonamide and pre-antibiotic times the struggle against pneumonia was a very serious business.

On 25 and 26 November the following bulletins were issued:
The King has had a disturbed day due to an increase in the fever.

The temperature is now 101.6°, but the pleurisy has not extended further, and the strength is maintained.

The next bulletin also contained the name of the eminent clinician and pathologist Sir Humphrey Davy Rolleston (1862–1944), dubbed 'the last of the scholar-physicians'.[13] For the next few weeks the medical bulletins tracked the decline in the king's health, with the royal physicians concerned about the effects of the illness on the king's heart. For fellow medics the following information was published in the *British Medical Journal*:

As early as practicable in the illness a blood culture was taken and a positive result obtained. The infection was coccal in character. Blood counts have shown a leucocytosis of the polymorphonuclear variety. Radiology has been useful, and the clear pictures obtained confirmed the clinical evidence that the lower two-thirds of the right lung was the area involved . . . Therapy directed against the infection has taken the form of chemical antidotes, the raising of immunity and the promotion of leucocytosis.[14]

Two days later the royal doctors wrote:

During the week there was great anxiety due to the fact that the infection involved the whole of the system. Now the physicians are dealing with a localized infection . . . Both the needle exploration and the X-ray examination carried out on Friday (7 December), show there is no appreciable pleural effusion, and therefore there is no object in any operation . . .

(10 December) The fever persists, due to some return of the general infection.[15]

When the Prince of Wales arrived at his father's bedside from game shooting in Tanganyika on 11 December he found the king 'barely conscious'.[16] Although the king's right lung was now punctured to drain off 'purulent fluid', Dawson realised that an urgent operation was necessary. *The Times* published this bulletin:

(Thursday, 13 December 1928: 8.45 p.m.) An operation on the King for the drainage of the right side of the chest has been successfully performed this evening. The condition of His Majesty is satisfactory.

The operation had been performed by surgeon-in-ordinary Sir Hugh Rigby with Francis Shipway as anaesthetist and Dawson, Farquhar Buzzard, Rolleston and Hewitt in attendance.

As the king began to rally after his operation, on Saturday, 15 December two doctors were seen by the assembled crowds to drive into Buckingham Palace. Dr Robert Stanton Woods was physician-in-charge of the Department of Medicine and Electrology at the London Hospital, while Dr Frederick Dutch Howitt was physician-in-charge of the Department of Physiotherapy and Massage at the Prince of Wales's General Hospital, Tottenham. They had been summoned by Dawson. Soon after they left the palace a medical bulletin was posted on the railings: 'It has now been decided to employ ray therapy as part of the treatment.'

By the end of January 1929 some one hundred bulletins had been issued, and on 9 February the king was taken to recuperate at Sir Arthur du Clos's home of Craigweil House, near the seaside resort of Bognor, West Sussex. Beforehand Dawson had subjected the property to a finicky overhaul, having the water supply checked, the drains examined, the carriageway to the house levelled and new glass inserted in the windows to increase the 'health-giving properties' of the rooms. At Bognor the king was allowed his first cigarette after his operation by medical attendant Hewitt. His illness, however, was not over.

> 'Middle-aged people may be divided into three classes: those who are still young; those who have forgotten they were young; those who were never young.'
> **Lord Dawson of Penn**
> *(1864–1945),*
> *physician to Edward VII and George V*

All the time the king was ill the nation was in a state of agitation, desperate for news. What would Lord Dawson report next? Professionally, though, he came in for some rather unkind comments. In their clubs doctors retold 'Dawson tales'. One said that Dawson had treated a patient for jaundice for several weeks before noticing that he was Chinese. And the prominent Leeds General Hospital surgeon Baron Berkeley George Andrew Moynihan (1865–1936), who had crossed swords with Dawson over the treatment of a junior royal, riposted with this jingle:

> Lord Dawson of Penn
> Has killed lots of men
> So that's why we sing
> God save the King.[17]

During the week of convalescence an abscess formed on the site of the king's operation. On 15 July an operation was performed at Buckingham Palace in which two ribs were partially removed in order to drain and treat the abscess. The procedure was carried out by Wilfred Batten Lewis Trotter (1872–1939) of University College Hospital, later sergeant-surgeon to the king, assisted by Sir Hugh Rigby and Dr Francis Shipman as anaesthetist. On 23 July the royal doctors were able to report: 'Purulent discharge from the abscess cavity has now ceased'.

Wilfred Trotter, by the by, was now given a higher public profile by the press. A surgeon, physiologist and philosopher, as well as being an outstanding teacher and the leading brain surgeon of his day, Trotter was a 'frail-looking, quiet, soft-spoken (man) . . . stooping as a result of a childhood disease'.[18] He contributed much to dealing with the delicate problems of cancer of the larynx and pharynx. Of his work it was written:

It was perfect joy to watch him remove a simple appendix, the knife handled as (Johannes) Vermeer must have wielded his brush, the needle with the skill of an embroidress, and above all, the surpassing gentleness of his manipulation.[19]

In all, thirteen doctors had been consulted during the king's illness of 1928–9 and the result was hailed 'a triumph of teamwork'.[20]

Former Harley Street specialist and consultant otolaryngologist Dr
R. Scott Stevenson averred:

> Whether (the thirteen doctors) were all necessary is another
> matter, and whether they all really helped to bring about
> recovery may be doubted. Lord Dawson, a charming and
> kindly man, was a medical diplomat of distinction rather than
> a physician of any scientific standing – the family doctor *in
> excelsis* . . .
>
> When a King is the patient the inclination is always to
> spread the responsibility. The calling in of Sir Humphrey
> Rolleston and Sir Farquhar Buzzard . . . did no more than
> this. X-ray and bacteriological examinations were, of course,
> necessary, but ultra-violet light treatment was a waste of time
> when further surgery was clearly indicated. Sir Hugh Rigby was
> a pleasant personality, a careful, rather diffident surgeon and
> he obviously was not drastic enough when he operated on
> King George's empyema.
>
> After drifting on for six months with a discharging sinus, the
> empyema wound was cured in a week when Mr Wilfred Trotter
> treated the King as he would have done any other patient in
> hospital. As (Trotter's) brother-in-law Ernest Jones wrote in
> his autobiographical *Free Associations* (Hogarth Press, 1959).
> 'With Trotter rank, authority, veneration counted for nothing.'[21]

At the end of it all the royal medical team received state
honours in the Birthday honours list of 3 July 1929. Wilfred
Trotter, though, refused a baronetcy. Yet even the king's place
of recuperation was remembered: thereafter Bognor was known
as Bognor Regis.

Public reaction to the king's illness was remarkable and a new
trend was noticed. Dozens of people sent remedies and medical
advice to Buckingham Palace. These ranged from a chest
protector (an old-fashioned woollen garment) knitted by an old
Scots woman who had sewn into it dried herbs 'guaranteed to
draw out the worst inflammation', to a cough-mixture whose
recipe dated back to the days of Elizabeth I.[22]

More seriously though, Dawson had to field criticism from

the public and professionals alike on the king's treatment and the perceived lack of detailed reports on his progress. Although numerous, the bulletins issued by the royal medics were seen by some as 'deceiving' the public. Not since the reign of George III had royal doctors been subject to after-the-event criticism.

But the king had survived a serious illness and was able to play a key role in the Silver Jubilee celebrations of his reign in 1935. After his efforts he relaxed for a while at Eastbourne and though continually tired he resumed the familiar royal round of visits between Cowes, Sandringham, Windsor and Balmoral. Dawson monitored his patient continually and noted 'a narrowing and rigidity of the cerebral vessels and the gradually failing force of the myocardium, weakened by the valvular affection of long standing'.[23]

Ever since his 1928–9 illness Sister Catherine Black had nursed the king, administering oxygen when needed. There was a steady decline to be noted in the king's energy and his interest in life. International affairs were also disturbing his peace of mind and he became particularly agitated when the Italian Expeditionary Force began its invasion of Ethiopia on 2 October 1935. Nearer home, the king was rocked with personal tragedy.

King George was very close to his second eldest sister, Princess Victoria Alexandra Olga Mary. Born at Marlborough House on 6 July 1868, Princess Victoria was another of Lord Dawson's patients, and when she was not at court she would telephone her brother each day. She never married, and died at her home at Coppins, Iver, Buckinghamshire, on 3 December 1935. The shock of her death was severe, and the king was still deeply depressed when the royal family spent their Christmas holidays at Sandringham. All those who listened to the king's fourth and last Christmas broadcast were aware of his weakening voice.

On 7 January 1936 Sister Black reported that the king was becoming more breathless. Alarmed, Dawson hurried to Sandringham. He realised that there was little he could do and left the king in the care of the two 'Sir Fredericks', Hewitt and Willans. Sister Black was now supported by Sister Robina Davis.

On Friday, 17 January Queen Mary sent for the Prince of Wales. Dawson, realising the king was dying, did not reassemble

GEORGE V'S MEDICAL HOUSEHOLD
ENGLAND, 1936:

Physicians-in-ordinary: The Lord Dawson of Penn; Sir Edward Buzzard (1871–1945).

Physicians-extraordinary: Sir Thomas Barlow; Sir Humphrey Rolleston (1862–1944); Sir Maurice Cassidy (1880–1949).

Physicians to the household: John Alfred Ryle.

Serjeant-surgeon: Wilfred Trotter (d. 1939).

Honorary sergeant-surgeon: Sir Richard Charles.

Honorary surgeons: Sir Hugh Rigby; Sir Thomas Dunhill (1876–1957).

Surgeon to the household: Sir James Walton.

Surgeon apothecary to the household: Sir Frederick Hewitt.

Surgeon apothecary to the household at Windsor: Sir Henry Martyn (1888–1947).

Surgeon apothecary to the household at Sandringham: Sir Frederick Willans (d. 1949).

Surgeon oculist: Sir Richard Cruise.

Surgeon oculist to the household: Col. Sir William Lister.

Laryngologist to the household: Sir Milsom Rees.

Surgeon dentist: Guy Birt.

Surgeon dentist to the household: Francis Donovan (1894–1948).

Coroner to the king's household: Lt. Col. W.H. Lester McCarthy (d.1962).

SCOTLAND, 1936:

Honorary physicians: Sir Robert Philip (1857–1939); J. Cowan; Sir Ashley Mackintosh (1868–1937).

Honorary surgeons: John Fraser; Sir John Learmonth (1895–1967).

Extra surgeons: Sir Harold Stiles (1863–1941); Sir John Marnoch (1867–1936).

Surgeon apothecary at Balmoral: Sir George Proctor Middleton (1905–87).

Surgeon apothecary at Holyrood Palace: Norman Carmichael (1883–1951).

Honorary surgeon dentist: Leslie Broughton-Head (d. 1961).

Extra Surgeon oculist: A.H. Sinclair.

During his 26-year reign George V also consulted other physicians. For instance, in 1923 he appointed the heart specialist and pioneer in the promotion of general practice Sir James Mackenzie (1853–1925) as consulting physician to the king in Scotland.

the medical team which had treated the king in 1928–9. Instead he contacted the heart specialist Sir Maurice Cassidy, and issued the first of six medical bulletins that would record the last days of King George V. The BBC broadcast the first bulletin at 6.30 p.m. and at midnight, it reported: 'The bronchial catarrh from which His Majesty the King is suffering is not severe, but there have appeared signs of cardiac weakness which must be regarded with some disquiet.'

His heart growing steadily weaker, the king drifted in and out of consciousness, and lost the use of his right arm. Only shakily was he able to pen two crosses which were accepted as representing GRI on the document appointing a Council of State to act for him in the constitutional duties he could no longer accomplish. On 18 January Dawson issued bulletins at 10.15 a.m., 3.30 p.m. and 10 p.m., and at 11 a.m. and 7.15 p.m on 19 January. Thus the nation was slowly prepared for the worst.

Dawson stood by the king's bedside and observed his condition: 'Evening, cyanotic – recumbent flat in bed. Slowly progressive myocardial failure – no obvious lung congestion, but cerebral thrombosis and almost venous stasis . . .'[24]

As the king moved from sleep to stupor to coma, Dawson left his bedside to pen his most famous bulletin: 'The King's life is moving peacefully towards its close.' The words were broadcast to the nation by the BBC five minutes after Dawson wrote them at 9.25 p.m.

At 11.15 p.m. on Monday, 20 January Sir Frederick Willans advised the Archbishop of Canterbury, Dr Cosmo Gordon Lang, to say his last prayers over the king: 'Go forth, O Christian Soul' and a final Benediction.[25] Forty minutes later the king was dead. Fifty years later Dawson's biographer Francis Watson revealed the details of the fatal dose of morphine and cocaine that the doctor had administered to the king (see pp. 1–2).

Queen Mary was to survive her husband by almost twenty years. For most of this time she was in the care of the homoeopathic physician Sir John Weir (1879–1971). A graduate of Glasgow, Weir studied homoeopathy at the Chicago clinic of Dr James Tyler Kent. On his return he set up practice in London and was on the staff of the London Homoeopathic Hospital by 1910. His devotion to homoeopathy was lifelong. He was appointed first

SANDRINGHAM, NORFOLK.

The King's life is moving peacefully towards its close.

Frederic Willans

Stanley Hewett.

Dawson of Penn

Jan: 20
9.25 p. m

as physician-in-ordinary to the Prince of Wales in 1923, and also included Queen Mary, George VI, Queen Elizabeth (the Queen Mother) and Queen Elizabeth II among his patients.

Following the funeral of King George VI on 15 February 1953 Queen Mary, now almost at her eighty-fifty birthday, focused her declining energies on her granddaughter's coronation, which was set for 2 June. Queen Mary knew that she was dying. At Buckingham Palace she made it quite clear that if she were to die in the interim the coronation should not be postponed. But it was not as easy as that – a lengthy court mourning was prescribed by protocol following the death of a crowned consort. Should her death be hastened too, as it was suggested her husband's was? Certainly this was put forward in a television programme in July 2000.[26]

Did Sir John Weir perform the same service as Lord Dawson is supposed to have done in 1936? Weir treated Queen Mary 'on careful Homoeopathic principles' and was a dour principled Scot of the old school. It seems incredible that he would contemplate regicide. Certainly we are unlikely ever to know for sure. Queen Mary died on 24 March 1953 after drifting into a coma.

CHAPTER EIGHTEEN

THE DARK SIDE OF A KING: EDWARD VIII AS KING AND IN EXILE

Prince Edward Albert Christian George Andrew Patrick David was born at White Lodge, Richmond Park, on 23 June 1894. On the accession of his father George V he was granted the royal dukedoms of Cornwall and Rothesay, and was created Prince of Wales on 2 June 1910. He ascended the throne as King Edward VIII on 20 January 1936, but his was to be a short, troubled reign in a lifetime of dark personal shadows that would earn him the name of traitor to his country and betrayer of his generation. Long before his abdication royal doctors had spotted the character flaws that would lead the kingdom to anguish and despair.

Edward VIII's medical household was to remain largely unchanged from that of his father's reign except for the addition of six new men. Thomas Jeeves Horder, 1st Baron Horder (1871–1955), became physician-in-ordinary. During the period 1921–36 Horder was senior physician at St Bartholomew's Hospital and was widely regarded as the most outstanding clinician of his time. Sir William Stewart Duke-Elder (1898–1978), became the new surgeon-in-ordinary. Duke-Elder had a varied career as a demonstrator severally in physiology and anatomy, becoming honorary consulting surgeon to St George's Hospital and Moorfields Eye Hospital. A prominent opthalmologist, he operated on Prime Minister James Ramsay MacDonald for glaucoma in 1932. Like Horder he was to have a long period of royal service.

Into the new royal post of manipulative surgeon came Sir Morton Warrack Smart (1877–1956). A pioneer in manipulative surgery and an authority on rehabilitation, during the Second World War he was consultant in physical medicine to the RAF. He was joined on the royal staff by (Sir) Arnold Stott (d. 1958) as physician to the royal household and Frank Anderson Juler

(1880–1962) as surgeon oculist to the royal household, with (Sir) Alexander Greig Anderson (d. 1961) as physician in Scotland.

> 'Many Britons a hundred years ago were bursting with good health and the remarkable thing was that they knew nothing of vitamins.'
> **Thomas, Lord Horder**
> *(1871–1953)*

From toddler-hood Prince Edward – David to his family – showed physical courage and great energy.[1] It seemed, noted all who had a care for his health, that physical exertion was necessary for his well-being, and the more violent the better. He suffered from a lifelong restiveness, which often led to physical and mental exhaustion – and no little danger. An early hobby was point-to-point horse-racing, wherein he showed a great talent for falling off his mount. He took a particularly bad fall in the winter of 1924 in a race for the Earl of Cavan's Cup at the Army point-to-point at Arborfield Camp. Royal doctors diagnosed concussion and kept him in a darkened room for a week, with bed rest for nearly a month.[2] At length his parents forbade him the sport as 'too dangerous for the heir to the throne'.[3]

Prince Edward and his siblings were brought up largely out of the public eye, but during the First World War the public began to see the prince's courage, energy and enthusiasm for life, although the royal doctors continued to monitor his somewhat shifting personality. The prince had a contradictory nature and, like his grandmother Queen Victoria, could present opposite sides of his character within seconds, from self-assuredness to diffidence, and from self-confidence to tongue-tied silence.

Medical records show that Prince Edward suffered from mumps and measles twice; the second time was as a naval cadet at Dartmouth in 1911; he convalesced at Newquay, in north Cornwall.[4] More seriously in terms of the nation's welfare, royal practitioners noted three distinct features of Prince Edward's health and nature: his proclivity to mortification of the flesh; his depression, melancholia and dark moods; and his arrested development.

Back in 1913, prompted by royal physicians, George V had admonished his son for smoking and exercising too much, and eating and resting too little. The prince 'dismissed the

EDWARD VIII'S MEDICAL HOUSEHOLD

Edward VIII. Born 23 June 1894. Reigned 20 January–10 December 1936. Died 28 May 1972

In 1936 the royal medical household of Edward VIII was as for King George V with these alterations:

Physician-in-ordinary: The Lord Horder (1871–1955).
Physician-extraordinary: John Alfred Ryle (1889–1950).
Surgeon: Sir James Walton (1881–1955).
Surgeon oculist: Sir Stewart Duke-Elder (1898–1978).
Consulting surgeon oculist: Col. Sir William Tindall Lister (1868–1944).
Manipulative surgeon: Sir Morton Smart (1877–1956).
Physician to the household: (Sir) Arnold Walmsley Stott (d. 1958).
Surgeon oculist to the household: Frank Anderson Juler (1880–1962).

Additional member for Scotland:
Physician: (Sir) Alexander Greig Anderson (d. 1961).

QUEEN MARY'S HOUSEHOLD (1936)
Physicians-in-ordinary: Dawson of Penn; Sir John Weir (1879–1971).
Surgeons: Baron Alfred Edward Webb-Johnston (1880–1958); Sir James Walton.
Surgeon-anaesthetist: Sir Stanley Hewitt.
Surgeon oculist: Sir Francis Richard Cruise (d. 1946).
Surgeon dentist: Guy Capper Birt (1884–1972).

There were medical households for the Duke and Duchess of York, the Duke and Duchess of Kent, the Duke of Connaught and Princess Beatrice.

injunctions of the royal doctors as the vapourings of the King's hired lackeys'.[5] His own diary gives examples of how he mortified his flesh. On one occasion he rose at 6 a.m. after the ball given by Lord Londesborough, was up at 7 a.m. after the Duke of Portland's Ball and at 7 a.m. after the Marquess of Salisbury's Ball: 'I've had only 8 hour's sleep in the last 72 hours,' he wrote.[6]

During the First World War Prince Edward subjected his constitution to a 'ferocious battering', noted one biographer, with visits to the trenches, field hospitals and as near to the front line as he thought he could get away with. In March 1915 he came under shellfire at Givenchy while visiting the 1st Battalion of the Grenadier Guards. A worried and furious George V was counselled by royal physicians that his son's behaviour derived from obvious feelings of inadequacy. What George V made of this is not known; he had been a distant father to his children and when in his presence the offspring were subjected to his stern querulousness.

As to the feelings of depression and melancholy that assailed the prince for most of his life, his diary of the First World War shows how he slipped in and out of dark moods. He was obviously frustrated that his position as Prince of Wales kept him out of front-line warfare and from playing a significant role. He even spoke of committing suicide in his, perhaps over-dramatised, misery. Yet, as the royal physicians pointed out, the Hanoverian 'melancholia gene' had been passed on by fellow-sufferer Queen Victoria.

This was the period when many noted Prince Edward's 'arrested development'. His erstwhile private secretary, and later severe critic, (Sir) Alan Frederick 'Tommy' Lascelles (1887–1981), averred: 'For some hereditary or physiological reason [Prince Edward]'s mental and spiritual growth stopped dead in his adolescence, thereby affecting his whole consequent behaviour.'[7]

As confirmed by the Declaration of Abdication Act, Prince Edward as King Edward VIII renounced the throne of Great Britain for himself and his descendants on 10 December 1936. On 8 March 1937 he was created Duke of Windsor. The story of his marriage to the twice-divorced Wallis Warfield Simpson at the Château de Cande in France on 3 June 1937 – and their sybaritic descent to death – is the stuff of decades of truth and legend.

In 1939 the Duke of Windsor suffered another psychological collapse which mirrored the one that he had endured during the Abdication Crisis. Having relinquished his royal medical household on his abdication, the Duke of Windsor usually 'flew in' any medics he might need. In 1937, for instance, he sent for

Dr Sumner Moore, from his Wimpole Street practice, to the royal lodgings at St Wolfgang, Salzkammergut Lake, Austria, to treat a bad tooth.[8] And while in Austria he continued treatments for a 'bad ear' by Professor Heinrich Neumann, who had treated him already in 1936.[9]

In 1958 the Duke of Windsor, at sixty-four, suffered a protracted, painful and prostrating attack of shingles. Psychologically he prepared himself for a non-hyperactive old age. This was the year too, that the duke underwent orthodontic surgery in New York for an ulcerated jawbone.[10] He continued to have no royal doctor in his entourage. He took treatments when he needed them from a range of doctors who prescribed medicaments to treat a range of problems from gastro-enteritis to his lumbago attack in Paris in 1952.

In early December 1964 the duke went to the Houston Methodist Hospital, Texas, to have an aneurysm removed from his abdominal aorta. There he consulted the heart surgeon Dr Michael E. DeBakey, Professor of Surgery at Baylor University College of Medicine, about the aneurysm, which had begun to enlarge in about 1960. DeBakey was to become an unofficial 'royal doctor' in his subsequent lifelong friendship with the Windsors. Charles Higham, Regents Professor of Commonwealth Literature at the University of California, described DeBakey thus in 1988:

Often up at dawn, he was known to be at the operating table for as many as twelve to fourteen hours in the course of a day, and he was capable of performing as many as forty-five operations a week. He would run many of the young and athletic members of his staff completely off their feet. He was a delightfully comical figure, racing along the hospital corridors, bent forward, his long legs loping away, in his shapeless surgeon's scrub suit that flapped around his ankles, looking, according to the *New York Times* reporter, 'like Groucho Marx without a moustache'. He talked sharply and rapidly, earning his nickname of 'The Texas Tornado'. Nobody really believed that he slept at all. He seemed like a man possessed, and the human cardio-vascular system was completely familiar to him. His zany genius enthralled the Windsors.[11]

The 67-minute operation took place on 16 December. Dr DeBakey excised the aneurysm, which he described as about 'the size of a small canteloupe or a large grapefruit'; four inches of dacron tubing replaced the aneurysm. A few days later the Duke and Duchess of Windsor flew to New York with Dr Arthur Antenucci as 'personal physician' in attendance.

Soon after retiring to France the duke was in hospital again, this time in England at the London Clinic for the repair to a detached retina. Here his treatment was supervised by Sir Stewart Duke-Elder, after an operation performed by James Hudson. Slowly the Duke of Windsor withdrew from public activities; his arthritic hip, which caused him to use a walking-stick from 1968, deprived him of his hobby of gardening.

His health slowly deteriorated. On 17 November 1971 he underwent a biopsy which confirmed that he had a small tumour in his throat; it was malignant and inoperable. He underwent 41 days of deep therapy with cobalt treatments, beginning on 30 November. By 12 January 1972 his doctors knew that the treatment had not worked. During February 1972 he was operated on for a double hernia at the American Hospital at Neuilly, Paris.

It was clear that the Duke of Windsor was dying of cancer. He knew it, but French medical ethics forbade his surgeon Dr Jean Thin from telling him so.[12] He agitated to go home from hospital: 'I want to die in my own bed,' he remarked.

In accord with her proposed visit to Paris in connection with the UK government's decision to enter the Common Market, Queen Elizabeth II arranged to meet her uncle the Duke of Windsor at 4 p.m. on Thursday, 18 May 1972, at his home in the Bois de Boulogne. At the request of the British Embassy in Paris, Dr Thin supplied bulletins on the former king's health twice a day in the period leading up to the planned visit. The bulletins showed that the duke was steadily weakening. Dr Thin describes how he prepared for the royal visit:

He was bedridden, and depended on an intravenous drip that had to be kept going twenty-four hours a day. I asked him if he had any instructions to give me in connection with the visit of the Queen to his bedside. He replied that it was out of the question that the Queen should see him wearing his bedclothes. She was his sovereign, and the least he could do was receive her, properly dressed, in the adjoining sitting room which separated his room from the Duchess's. I tried to object that this was impossible because he could not be deprived of his drip, but he only answered: 'That's your problem.'

It was indeed a difficult problem but, thanks to the ingenuity of Dr Françoise Jacquin, we found a solution. This was to hide the drip underneath the Duke's shirt and attach it to a long tube, which would emerge from the back of his collar and lead to the fluid flasks, which could be concealed behind a curtain near which the Duke would be sitting.

With much patience from the Duke, we managed to set all this up about an hour before the Queen arrived. When she entered the room, however, something happened which none of us had anticipated. Showing an effort of will that was remarkable, he rose slowly to his feet and gave the traditional bow from the neck. We were all terrified that the apparatus would come apart before our eyes. Fortunately it held in place, and I don't think anything was noticed.[13]

Queen Elizabeth had a fifteen-minute interview with her uncle before retiring to take tea with the duchess. Soon after, the Duke of Windsor was visited by his 'personal physician', Dr Arthur Antenucci from Roosevelt Hospital, New York, but it was clear that he could do nothing for his old royal friend.

By 27 May the duke had lapsed into a coma. He never regained consciousness and died around 1.23 a.m. on Sunday, 28 May 1972, a few weeks before his 78th birthday. His cadaver was transported by the RAF from Paris to RAF Benson, Oxfordshire, for onward cortege to the nave of St George's Chapel, Windsor, where he would lie in state within sight of the tomb of his parents. He was buried on 5 June in the royal private burial ground at Frogmore.

Postscript

Following ten years under the supervision of her lawyer Maître Suzanne Blume (d. 1994), plagued with arthritis and haemorrhaging from stomach ulcers, the Duchess of Windsor died at her home in the Bois de Boulogne, Paris, on 24 April 1986, in her ninetieth year. She had been bedridden since her intestinal haemorrhage of 13 November 1975. Bizarre rumours still circulate concerning her medical treatment in her final years.

After a funeral service at St George's Chapel, Windsor, she was buried privately beside the Duke of Windsor in the royal burial ground at Frogmore. In her latter years the duchess had been attended by Dr Jean Thin, who had treated her husband, and Dr Thomas Hewes, senior physician at the American Hospital at Neuilly, Paris.

CHAPTER NINETEEN

THE LITTLE PRINCE THE NATION FORGOT: DR MANBY DRAWS THE CURTAIN

The surgeon-apothecary at Sandringham House, Norfolk, Sir Alan Reeve Manby (1848–1925) penned the date and location – 18 January 1919, Wood Farm – on a sheet of Sandringham House notepaper and prepared the following medical bulletin for the Court Circular and the national press:

> HRH Prince John, who has since infancy suffered from epileptic fits, which have lately become more frequent and severe, passed away in his sleep following an attack this afternoon at Sandringham.

Prince John? Who was he? Half the nation had forgotten he existed, while the other half had never heard of him.

Prince John Charles Francis had been born at 3.05 a.m. at York Cottage, Sandringham, on 12 July 1905, the sixth and last child of Prince George and Princess Mary of Teck, the future King George V and Queen Mary. John was 'a surprise, so unexpected', wrote Princess Caroline Augusta, Grand Duchess of Mecklenburg-Strelitz, to her niece Queen Mary, who was plunged once more into 'the penalty of being a woman'.[1]

The birth was a difficult one, attended by Dr Sir John Willans, who recorded that the child had early respiratory problems. The prince was named after his father's second brother, Prince Alexander John Charles Albert, who was born at Sandringham on 6 April 1871 and died the next day. It was an ill-omened gesture. Soon after the birth Prince George and Princess Mary boarded the battleship HMS *Renown* for a state visit to India; they did not return until April 1906.

With them on that trip was Dr Alan Reeve Manby, by now

a friend of the family, and father-in-law of Dr Willans. Manby was created physician-extraordinary and surgeon-apothecary to Sandringham by King Edward VII in 1885. He had studied at Guy's Hospital, London, and became an obstetrics resident after qualification in 1869. He had then gone into the family practice in Norfolk, where his father and grandfather had been medical practitioners, taking time off to study for (and gain) an MD from Durham in 1888; he was created FRCS in 1918.[2] Manby was to play a key role in the Prince John story.

It is a well-known historical cliché that Queen Mary was a neglectful mother. Her eldest son, when Duke of Windsor, wrote to the Earl of Dudley after her death: 'I'm afraid the fluids in her veins have always been as icy cold as they now are in death.'[3] While jumping to her defence, Mabell, Countess of Airlie (1866–1956), Queen Mary's loyal lady-in-waiting for over fifty years, openly agreed that the queen 'had no interest in her children as babies'.[4]

The royal doctors' reports on her children's mental and physical welfare were hardly encouraging. They all exhibited the characteristic oddities and health characteristics of the House of Hanover. Prince Edward, Prince of Wales, suffered from deafness inherited from his grandmother Queen Alexandra, and was also a severe depressive, with the 'Hanoverian melancholia gene' of his great-grandmother Queen Victoria. Prince Albert, Duke of York, later King George VI, had a distressing stutter and congenitally malformed knees. He would fly into uncontrollable rages. Prince Henry, Duke of Gloucester, had unfathomable fits of tears interlarded with episodes of nervous giggling. He was declared 'mentally backward' and developed a number of eccentricities. Prince George, Duke of Kent, howled whenever he came into his mother's starched presence. He was a 'frenetic character' who was to be absorbed into a milieu of homosexuality and drugs. Princess Mary, later the Princess Royal, suffered from a crippling shyness, but had to be removed from her brothers' schoolroom for being a 'disruptive influence'.[5] Prince John showed early signs of mental retardation. At the age of four he began to suffer from fits, which the royal doctors diagnosed as epilepsy originating after conception (genetic epilepsy). His fits, however, rendered him violent. When the royal children were out in the hills above Balmoral, Prince John had to be roped to his nanny as a precaution.

Whereas his siblings were 'presentable' to the outside world, Prince John was not. The Prince of Wales considered his brother a 'regrettable nuisance',[6] while Reginald Baliol Brett, 2nd Viscount Esher, noted Prince John's increasing unpredictability in his diary entry for 21 August 1910. On one occasion at lunch with the king and queen at Balmoral, wrote Esher, Prince John continually ran round the dining table 'all the while they ate'.[7] He also had a predilection to slip from his nanny's notice to appear impromptu at his parents' official gatherings and make a scene. As Prince John's behaviour became more eccentric, his parents realised that he was not controllable as 'normal' children are, but things were to become worse.

It appears that King George and Queen Mary were concerned that Prince John might have a fit in public. Thus it was thought risky for the prince to attend their coronation in June 1911. Cynics said they feared that their reputation and public image would be damaged. King George was always worried about republicanism and was hypersensitive about anything that might be used by the enemies of monarchy to denigrate the institution. Thus, said the gossips, Prince John was packed off to a cottage on the Sandringham estate to be largely out of the public eye.

Prince John now spent most of his life in the care of Mrs Lalla Bill, the royal nanny. As his condition worsened it was decided that he should be removed from any public contact whatsoever. Consequently he was 'hidden away' from society, aged eleven, at Wood Farm with the devoted Lalla Bill and two male attendants to cope with him when he had his violent fits.

In this way Prince John became the forgotten member of the royal family. He met few strangers and hardly appeared in family portraits for public consumption; perhaps the last family photograph of him was the one taken by the Prince of Wales at Balmoral in 1912, wherein Prince John is pictured riding in a metal toy car and sporting a white sailor suit. Writing in 1998 Ross Benson noted:

Queen Mary quite simply cut her son out of her life. She would occasionally write to him. But not once, in the years he lived (at Wood Farm), did she ever make the short drive from (Sandringham House) over to the farm . . .[8]

It seems that Prince George showed some interest in Prince John, offering him 'kindness and affection'. The Prince of Wales hardly knew him, and scarcely mentions him at all in his ghosted autobiography *A King's Story* (1951). But Queen Alexandra, Prince John's grandmother, showed him a degree of compassion. Despite her crippling deafness and rheumatism, she would sometimes send her car to Wood Farm to bring the 'dear and precious little boy' to her at Sandringham for afternoon tea, music and games.[9] She was distressed when, in 1917, the king and queen decided that the time had come for Prince John to be shut away at Wood Farm.

Dr Sir Alan Manby was called to Prince John's bedside during the early morning of 18 January 1919. His condition had deteriorated through the night and he succumbed to 'a severe seizure' that afternoon.[10] In her 'Sandringham Diary' his mother – who, it was rumoured, had not seen him for years – wrote:

At 5.30 Lalla Bill telephoned to me from Wood Farm, Wolferton, that our poor darling little Johnnie had passed away suddenly after one of his attacks. The news gave me a great shock, tho' for the poor little boy's restless soul, death came as a great release. I broke the news to George & we motored down to Wood Farm. Found poor Lalla very resigned but heartbroken. Little Johnnie looked very peaceful lying there.[11]

In a letter of 2 February 1919 to her friend Miss Emily Alcock she added:

For him it is a great release as his malady was becoming worse as he grew older, & he has thus been spared much suffering. I cannot say how grateful we feel to God for having taken him in such a peaceful way, he just slept quietly into his heavenly home, no pain, no struggle, just peace for the poor little troubled spirit which had been a great anxiety to us for many years, ever since he was four years old – The first break in the family circle is hard to bear but people have been so kind & sympathetic & this has helped us much.[12]

On the death of his brother, Prince Edward wrote to Queen Mary a letter of 'chilling insensitivity'.[13] Queen Alexandra, on the other hand, expressed genuine grief. She wrote to the queen, 'now our two darling Johnnies lie side by side'.[14] Prince John was buried in the churchyard of St Mary Magdalene, Sandringham, next to his baby uncle.

Assessing the information in the public domain, some historians have criticised King George and Queen Mary for being 'cruel' to Prince John in keeping him incarcerated without family companionship in order 'to keep up royal appearances'. Others have attributed this apparent ruthlessness in 'safeguarding their reputation and public image' to the advice of royal doctors, particularly physician to the household Sir Robert Burnet and Sir Alan Manby. It is likely that Prince John had the best care as prescribed by the medical and social criteria of the time. It is the modern interpretation of these criteria, eighty years on, that makes it seem an embarrassing chapter in royal medical history.

CHAPTER TWENTY

GEORGE VI AND THE KING-SIZED KILLER

Prince Albert Frederick Arthur George, Duke of York, ascended the throne as King George VI. Born at York Cottage, Sandringham, on 14 April 1895, he was crowned at Westminster Abbey on 12 May 1937 with his consort Elizabeth, whom he had married in 1923. On 22 June 1948 he relinquished his title of Emperor of India.

By 1938 his new medical household was in place, with Lord Dawson of Penn as, perhaps, the royal doctor best known to the public. This was largely because of the media coverage of the death of George V and Dawson's public works, from the Radium Trust to the Fitness Campaign which (through the Physical Training and Recreation Act) sponsored *inter alia* the training of physical training instructors and holiday camps for children.

During the Second World War Dawson was involved in the Emergency Medical Service but continued with a busy private practice which included such patients as David Lloyd George.[1] In 1938 Dawson lost one of his royal patients in Queen Maud of Norway (the daughter of Edward VII and Queen Alexandra), and in 1942 he lost Prince Arthur of Connaught and Strathearn (third son of Queen Victoria). Dawson's last official contact with the royal court was his letter to Sir Ulick Alexander, Keeper of the Privy Purse, urging the king to contribute to the Royal College of Surgeons Restoration and Development Fund. He died the next day, 7 March 1945.[2]

Among the other 'stalwarts' was Sir John Weir, who became the foremost expert in homoeopathy in Britain. Weir was to play a prominent role in royal circles, attending the births of all four of the children of George VI's daughter, Princess Elizabeth, as heir and queen. In court circles he had the reputation of being strict with his royal patients – he rationed the Duke of Windsor to four cigarettes a day – and always recommended vigorous walks as a recuperative measure. A rare anecdote to come from royal provenance concerns Weir. On one occasion his patient, Queen Mary, gave him a huge bunch of flowers to take back to the homoeopathic hospital with him. These were distributed around his wards. On his rounds later he noticed that some of the flowers had been placed next to one of his six-year-old cockney patients. 'Aren't they lovely?' remarked Weir. 'Wasn't it kind of the Queen to send them to you.' The boy answered: ''Ow did she know I was 'ere?'[3]

The 'new faces' among George VI's medical household included such as Sir George Frederick Still (1868–1941), the prominent paediatrician who, as physician for diseases of children at King's College Hospital from 1899, established the occurrence of a chronic rheumatoid arthritis peculiar to children. Still joined the household as an extra physician. Sir Lancelot Edward Barrington-Ward (1884–1953) became a royal surgeon; he too had consulted at the Great Ormond Street Hospital for Sick Children, where Still was physician.

In Scotland Professor (later Sir) John William McNee (1887–1984) joined as physician as well as being consultant physician to the Royal Navy. And an extra physician was appointed in Professor Sir Robert William Philp (1857–1939), who had won public distinction in opening a tuberculosis dispensary at Edinburgh in 1887.

All his life Prince Albert – 'Bertie' to his family – was plagued with digestive problems, which several of the royal doctors attributed to his nervous temperament. Royal doctor Sir Francis Laking, in an attempt to mollify with fresh air the effects of a series of 'severe colds', advised that Prince Albert be sent to his own house at Broadstairs in 1909, under the care of Sister Edith Ward. The prince's most recent chill there developed into whooping-cough. Thereafter the prince was sent to the royal lodge at Alt-na-Guithasach, near Balmoral, to convalesce.

In September 1913 Prince Albert joined the battleship HMS *Collingwood* as a midshipman and was destined for a life in the Royal Navy. Public records released in September 2000 show that during his service he battled with endless seasickness.[4] A recurrence of gastric troubles led to Sir James Reid being summoned by Sir Frederick Treves to go to Wick where Prince Albert was ill aboard the hospital ship *Rohilla*. Reid and Fleet Surgeon Lomas diagnosed a grumbling appendix. The condition worsened and Prince Albert underwent surgery on 9 September 1914 at the Northern Nursing Home in the care of Professor John Marnock. Thus the prince spent the early months of the war in convalescence; he returned to duty in February 1915.

The Navy Medical Board had delayed his fitness clearance which, it seemed to royal doctors, was a sensible decision. During May 1915 Prince Albert fell ill again. Prone to anxiety and hysteria he became depressed and lost much weight. By July 1915 royal doctors recommended that he leave his ship, and diagnosed 'a mucal disturbance of the stomach caused by muscle weakness'.[5] He was given a strict regimen of a carefully monitored diet and 'daily stomach pumps'.[6]

It was a period of national war hysteria and George V was anxious that his second son did not appear to the general public to be lacking in courage. Captain Ley of the *Collingwood* had promised that if the vessel were called into action Prince Albert would be recalled to duty. But Ley informed the king that on medical advice he had considered Prince Albert 'unfit for sea-going service'. So a suffering Bertie was thus informed while on the hospital ship *Drina*; he was placed on sick-leave with convalescence at Abergeldie. Physician Sir Frederick Treves opined that the prince should never go back to sea.

Nevertheless public records show that in May 1916 Prince Albert returned to *Collingwood*. Alas, he went down with food poisoning following a meal of soused herring.[7] However, he roused himself from his sickbed to take part in the action at the battle of Jutland on 31 May 1916. Thus he became the last British monarch to see action in war. By July 1916 he was back on the sicklist and was treated at the Aberdeen Naval Hospital. Royal doctors diagnosed a duodenal ulcer on his return to Windsor. After a slow recovery he returned to duty aboard the battleship HMS *Malaya*.

Notes written at this time by royal doctors reflected Prince Albert's character traits of 'a bland, underdeveloped character . . . moulded chiefly by circumstances', his unstable temper – some said it was inherited from his ancestors the dukes of Teck –

GEORGE VI'S MEDICAL HOUSEHOLD
George VI. Born 14 December 1895. Reigned 1936–52. Died 6 February 1952.

ENGLAND, 1938:
Physicians: The Viscount Dawson of Penn; The Lord Horder; Sir John Weir; Sir Maurice A. Cassidy.
Extra physicians: Sir E. Farquhar Buzzard; John Alfred Ryle; Sir George Frederick Still (1868–1941); (Sir) Henry Letheby Tidy (1877–1960).
Serjeant surgeon: Wilfred Trotter.
Surgeons: Sir Thomas Peel Dunhill; Sir James Walton; Sir Launcelot Edward Barrington-Ward (1884–1953).
Surgeon oculists: Wilfred Trotter; Sir Stewart Duke-Elder.
Consulting surgeon oculist: Col. Sir William T. Lister.
Manipulative surgeon: Sir Morton Smart.
Surgeon dentist: Charles Sculthorpe Morris (1875–1949).
Surgeon apothecary to His Majesty and apothecary to the household: Sir Stanley Hewitt.
Physicians to the household: Arnold Stott; (Sir) David Thomas Davies (1899–1966).
Surgeon to the household: F.A. Juler.
Surgeon dentist to the household: Francis D. Donovan.
Surgeon apothecary to the household at Windsor: Sir Henry L. Martyn.
Surgeon apothecary to the household at Sandringham: Sir Frederick Jeune Willans.
Coroner to the king's household: Lt. Col. W.H.L. McCarthy. (1885–1962).

There were separate medical positions in the households of Queen Mary, the Duke and Duchess of Kent, the Duke of Connaught and Princess Beatrice.

SCOTLAND, 1938:
Physicians: J. Cowan; A.G. Anderson; (Sir) John William McNee (1887–1984).
Extra physician: Sir Robert William Philip (1857–1939).
Surgeons: Sir John Farmer; J.R. Learmonth.
Surgeon oculist: A.H.H. Sinclair.
Surgeon dentist: L.C. Broughton-Head.
Surgeon apothecary to the household at Balmoral: George Procter Middleton.
Surgeon apothecary to the household at Holyrood Palace: N.S. Carmichael.

shyness, limited intelligence and nervousness.[8] Most of these traits went unnoticed by the general public, but few could fail to be aware of another lifelong disability. Unfit for public duty, and unprepared for kingship, Prince Albert's undoubted patriotism, courage and persistence were of no use in controlling his nervous stammer. His biographer John Wheeler-Bennett noted that some royal doctors believed that Prince Albert's being forced to write with his right hand (although left-handed) had produced a psychological condition known as misplaced sinister, which affected his speech.[9] On the other hand, courtier Mabell, Countess of Airlie (lady-in-waiting to Queen Mary), averred that Prince Albert stammered long before he was forced to write right-handed.[10] She, and others, presumed that the treatment he had received from callous nannies had undermined his confidence. Nevertheless the stammer marred his progress in the schoolroom, in the Royal Navy and in his public service, wherein speechmaking was a nightmare. Often newsreel film would edit out the worst moments when he was addressing public gatherings.

Prince Albert underwent various forms of therapy for his stammer, which resisted all attempts at a cure. Tradition has it that his wife Elizabeth encouraged him in 1926 to consult the speech therapist Lionel Logue. Inspired by Logue's successful methods, Prince Albert visited him every day for two months, sometimes accompanied by his wife, who studied the treatment exercises Logue recommended so that she might assist her husband once they had returned home. Although never completely cured, Prince Albert became more confident in trying to control his stammer when having to speak in public. He even improved in the presence of his father George V who heretofore had reduced him to stuttering incoherence on many occasions,[11] with asides of '(you) really must pull (yourself) together.[12]

The health of Prince Albert, as King George VI, was to be greatly impaired by 'a king-sized killer'. He was to enter history as the fourth British monarch to be killed by smoking. His grandfather Edward VII had done much to popularise the smoking of cigars and cigarettes in society. Edward's devotion to the noxious weed was in part a defiance of his mother Queen Victoria's distaste for the habit. His biographer Sir Philip Magnus-Allcroft averred:

'He rationed himself strictly to one small cigar and two cigarettes before breakfast, but he smoked thereafter a daily average of twelve enormous cigars and twenty cigarettes.'[13] Hints by royal doctors Laking and Reid that this was too much were ignored, so their warnings of recurrent bronchitis because of smoking began to be realised when Edward was in his forties.

During the reigns of the four monarchs from Edward VII to George VI, Benson & Hedges – 'Purveyors of Cigars and Cigarettes to His Majesty' – won great publicity from their royal warrant; they even named one of their pipe tobaccos 'Prince of Wales's mixture'. Royal patronage sustained the company's financial turnover and bolstered the personal fortune of William Hedges, whose 'Cairo Citadel' cigarette was based on a mixture given to Hedges by Edward VII as Prince of Wales. Edward introduced the fashion of smoking cigarettes 'immediately after dinner', so Alfred Hedges was encouraged by him to produce cigarettes suitable for society women; thus the miniature 'Cigarette Turc' came into being.

Like his father, George V was a heavy smoker; he also suffered from severe bronchitis that plagued him for the rest of his life. It was not surprising, then, that Edward VIII and George VI began to smoke when they were thirteen and twelve respectively at the naval training school at Osborne House, Isle of Wight. Royal tradition has it that George VI smoked 40–50 cigarettes per day – they were to be his 'king-sized killer'.

Not long after the Second World War ended in 1945, George VI showed signs that he was suffering from 'severe arterial impairment'.[14] Royal physicians feared that gangrene might develop in the sovereign's right foot, necessitating amputation. Further his doctors noticed that he suffered from 'intermittent claudication' and privately discussed the possibility of Buerger's disease which caused pain when walking.

On 23 November 1948 it was announced at Buckingham Palace that the king was to visit Australia and New Zealand early in 1949; this trip would never take place. By March 1949 surgery was necessary to alleviate the king's worsening condition. (Sir) James Learmonth, Regius Professor of Surgery at the University of Edinburgh and a leading expert in peripheral vascular disease, and Professor (Sir) James Paterson Ross of St Bartholomew's

Hospital performed a right lumbar sympathectomy to allow the blood vessels to dilate and the circulation improve.

The king's doctors had saved his leg and a good recovery was made by the royal patient, who undertook a series of public engagements in 1950. By 1951, though, it was clear to all that the king's health was rapidly deteriorating. On 1 July 1951 the royal physicians Sir David Thomas Davis, Sir Horace Evans, (Sir) Geoffrey Marshall and Sir John Weir issued this bulletin:

> The King has been confined to his room for the past week with an attack of influenza. There is now a small area of catarrhal inflammation in the lung, but the constitutional disturbance is slight.[15]

The public remarked how ill and thin the king looked. A further announcement followed on 4 June:

> The catarrhal inflammation in the King's lung has not entirely disappeared, though His Majesty's general condition has improved.
> A period of complete rest will be essential to His Majesty's recovery, and on the advice of his doctors he has reluctantly decided to cancel all his public engagements for at least four weeks.

Convalescence followed at Balmoral, but the king's physicians saw no real improvement. More X-rays were taken, followed by a bronchoscopy, and a sample of tissue was taken for pathological examination. A further bulletin was issued on 18 September:

> During the King's recent illness a series of examinations have been carried out . . . These investigations now show structural changes to have developed in the lung. His Majesty has been advised to stay in London for further treatment.

The observant public would see new names added to the bulletin, including Dr Peter Kerley, radiologist at Westminster Hospital, and (Sir) Clement Price-Thomas (1893–1973) senior surgeon at Westminster and surgeon at the Brompton Hospital for Diseases of the Chest; Price-Thomas was a member of the 'small group of pioneers who established the science and art of thoracic surgery'.[16]

These doctors collaborated on a new bulletin issued on 21 December:

> The condition of the King's lung gives cause for concern. In view of the structural changes referred to in the last bulletin we have advised His Majesty to undergo an operation in the near future. This advice the King has accepted.

To the general public there was as yet no real hint of what the royal physicians suspected ailed the monarch; to the knowledgeable, reading between the lines gave a clear clue. It was lung cancer.

A flurry of activity now broke out at Westminster Hospital and Buckingham Palace where an operating theatre had to be set up. The operating theatre staff were led by theatre superintendent Sister Sarah Minter, with Sister Vera Ream, Staff Nurse Audrey Patterson and Staff Nurse Hilda Ross. They created at Buckingham Palace an exact replica of Price-Thomas's operating theatre at Westminster. Then the surgery team was assembled. Price-Thomas was to be assisted by his two senior resident surgeons, Charles Drew and Peter Jones. Anaesthetists Robert Mackray and Cyril Scurr were joined by haematologist Joseph Humble. During the morning of Sunday, 23 September 1951, they performed surgery on George VI, wherein sections were removed from two of the monarch's ribs so that they could view the extent of the diseased tissue. Thereafter they removed the whole of the left lung, which was badly diseased (pneumonectomy).

Medical anecdote recalls that Price-Thomas insisted that he would only operate on the king if court protocol was set aside; he would treat the king like any other patient. It is said, too, that when the operation was over Price-Thomas left the closing of the wound to his assistants, with the words: 'I haven't stitched up a chest for twenty years and I'm not going to start practising on the King.'[17] Incidentally, as Price-Thomas was driving out of Buckingham Palace, his work done, he collided with another vehicle. The police declined to prosecute.[18]

GEORGE VI'S MEDICAL HOUSEHOLD
ENGLAND, 1952:
Physicians: Sir John Weir; Sir Horace Evans; Sir David Thomas Davies.
Extra physicians: The Lord Horder; Sir Henry Letheby Tidy.
Serjeant surgeon: Brigadier Sir Thomas Dunhill.
Surgeons: Sir Launcelot Edward Barrington-Ward; Sir Arthur Espie Porritt; Sir James R. Learmonth.
Extra surgeon: Sir James Walton.
Surgeon oculist: Sir Stewart Duke-Ellis.
Extra manipulative surgeon: Sir Morton Smart.
Orthopaedic surgeon: Sir Reginald Watson-James (1902–72).
Aurist: John Douglas McLaggan
Surgeon dentist: Alan Macleod.
Extra surgeon apothecary: Sir Stanley Hewitt.
Physician to the household: Ronald Bodley Scott.
Extra physician to the household: Sir Arnold Walmsley Stott.
Surgeon to the household: Ralph Marnham.
Surgeon oculist to the household: F.A. Juler.
Apothecary to the household: J. Nigel Loring.
Surgeon apothecary to the household: E.C. Malden.
Surgeon apothecary to the household at Sandringham: J.L.B. Ansell.
Coroner to the king's household: Lt-Col. W.H.L. McCarthy.

SCOTLAND, 1952:
Physicians: A.G. Anderson; Sir John McNee; Professor L.S. Davidson.
Surgeon: George G. Bruce.
Surgeon oculist: A.H.H. Sinclair.
Surgeon dentist: R.C.S. Dow.
Surgeon apothecary to the household at Balmoral: George Procter Middleton.
Surgeon apothecary to the household at Holyrood Palace: N.S. Carmichael.

There were also medical appointments to the households of Queen Mary, and Princess Elizabeth, Duchess of Edinburgh.
The following were appointed *Honorary Physicians to the King* (Civil appointments):
Dr S. Barron, Medical Officer of Health for Belfast.
Dr W.E. Chiesman, Medical Adviser to HM Treasury.
Dr S.W. Fisher, Principal Medical Inspector Mines Dept. Ministry of Fuel and Power.
Dr A. Massey, Chief Medical Officer, Ministry of National Insurance.
Professor R.H. Parry, Medical Officer of Health, Bristol.
Dr H.J. Rae, Medical Officer of Health, Aberdeen and Counties of Aberdeen and Kincardine.

On the evening of the operation the public were assured that 'His Majesty's immediate post-operation condition is satisfactory.' The king made a steady, unanxious recovery, and was able to record his Christmas broadcast for the BBC as usual, despite a troublesome cough.

As biographer Sir John Wheeler-Bennett remarked: 'A great sense of well-being returned and (the king) looked forward to a period of years during which he could devote himself to training Princess Elizabeth in the art of statecraft.' It was an intention he would be unable to fulfil. Pronounced fit by physicians the king was at Sandringham in February 1952, relaxing with a day's shooting after waving off Princess Elizabeth and Prince Philip on the tours of Africa, Australia and New Zealand which he had hoped to fulfil himself. On 5 February he retired to bed as usual; the next morning a valet bringing a cup of tea found him dead in bed. The declared cause of death was coronary thrombosis. The nation believed the king had died from smoking.

TOWARDS A MODERN PRACTICE

Royal medical practitioners are not what they were. The terms murderer, charlatan, freeloader and embezzler have all been used to describe royal doctors. But at the court of Queen Elizabeth II they tend to keep a low profile. Few holding positions in the royal medical household are recognised by sight, and even fewer are known by name to the general public. Gone are the days when royal physicians and surgeons were easily identified as they strutted the pavements of London with emblematic gold-topped canes and a *bouquet des herbes* held under the nose to dispel the aromas of the nation's unwashed bodies and open drains.

Once crowds would gather at royal palace gates to read bulletins on the royal health, details of which are now given a wider comment in the media. And because of the public's not-always-kindly interest in royal activities today's royal medical practitioners are more tight-lipped than they used to be.

The modern medical household of Queen Elizabeth II comes under the remit of the Lord Chancellor's office at Buckingham Palace and consists of twenty members for England and Scotland, namely:[1]

Head of the medical household and physician to the queen: Richard Paul Hepworth Thompson, DM, FRCP. (Physician to the royal household, 1982–93.)

Physician: William Davey, MD, LRCP, FFHon, AKC. (Since 1986.)

Physician to the household: John Cunningham, DM, FRCP. (Since 1993.)

Surgeon oculist: Timothy Ffytche, LVO, MB, FRCS, FRCOphth. (Since 1980.)

Sergeant-surgeon: Barry Trevor Jackson, MS, FRCS. (Since 1991.)

Orthopaedic surgeon: Roger Vickers, BM, CCh, FRCS. (Since 1992.)

Surgeon dentist: Nicholas Sturridge, CVO, LDS, BDS, DDS. (Since 1975.)

Surgeon-gynaecologist: Marcus Setchell, FRCS, FRCOG. (Since 1990.)

Surgeon to the household: Adam Lewis, MB, FRCS. (Since 1991.)

Surgeon oculist to the household: Jonathan Jagger, MB, BS, DO, DRCS, FRCOphth. (Since 1999.)

Apothecary to the queen and to the household: Nigel Ralph Southward, CVO, MB, BChir, MRCP. (Since 1975; and to the queen mother since 1986.)

Apothecary to the household at Windsor: Jonathan Holliday, MB, BS, MRCGP, DCH, DRCOG, DFFP. (Since 1997.)

Apothecary to the household at Sandringham: Ian K. Campbell, MB, BS, D.Obst, RCOG, FRCGP. (Since 1992.)

Coroner to the queen's household: John D.K. Burton, CBE, MB, BS, MRCS, LRCP, FFARCS.

Medical officer to the queen abroad: Surgeon captain David Swan, LVO, MB, ChB, FRCA, RN. (Since 1993.)

The queen's medical household for Scotland is gazetted thus:[2]

Physician: Anthony Douglas Toft, CBE, FRCPE. (Since 1996.)

Surgeons: Jetmund Engeset, ChM, FRCS. (Since 1985.)

Iain Melfort Campbell Macintyre, MD, FRCSE, FRCPE. (Since 1997.)

Apothecary to the household at Balmoral: Douglas J.A. Glass, MB, ChB. (Since 1988.)

Apothecary to the household at the Palace of Holyrood: Jack Cormack, MD, FRCPE, FRCGP. (Since 1991.)

Because of protocol and the rights of patient privacy, only circumspect bulletins and reports on the health of the royal family are issued. Of the kings and queens since the accession of George II (1727) up to 1952 four monarchs, and one crowned consort, have undergone what the royal doctors described as 'serious operations'. In their day the operations stood out as remarkable and attracted great public interest and concern.

For instance, in 1737 Queen Caroline of Ansbach, consort of George II, was operated on for a strangulated umbilical hernia by Serjeant-surgeon John Ranby. This was perhaps the first case of royal illness to stimulate great public interest since the death of Charles II. In 1820 George IV was operated on by Sir Astley Paston Cooper for a sebaceous cyst on the scalp. Public reaction was mixed, depending if you were for or against the man they had called 'Prinny'.

Queen Victoria had an axillary abscess that was drained by Joseph, Baron Lister, opening a new area of public interest about the everyday events of royalty. By the time that Edward VII was operated on for an appendiceal abscess by Serjeant-surgeon Sir Frederick Treves in 1902 public interest in both royal doctors and royal patients had begun to grow. In 1928 George V was operated on for empyema by Serjeant-surgeon Sir Hugh Mallinson Rigby and newspaper interest in the matter further widened the audience for such royal events. Public concern reached new heights in 1949, when George VI underwent a right lumbar sympathectomy, carried out by Professor James Learmonth and Professor James Paterson Ross, and again in 1951 when he had a pneumonectomy performed by Sir Clement Price-Thomas.

Although royal doctors have carried out operations at Balmoral and Buckingham Palace, in more modern times royal patients are usually treated at the King Edward VII's Hospital for Officers, Beaumont Street, London, as was the Princess Royal in 1992[3] and Queen Elizabeth the Queen Mother on various occasions, including the operation for an appendicitis in 1964 and a hip replacement in 1997.[4]

Since Edward VII's serious illness of 1871 deepened his interest in medical matters and medical charities, members of the royal family have played a role in medical eleemosynary encouraged by royal doctors. A public profile in these fields has come to be expected by the general public, who were satiated by the regular presence in hospitals and clinics of the late Diana, Princess of Wales. In history, not to show an interest caused public offence. To give an example of a particular snub, on Wednesday, 23 September 1936, Edward VIII sent the Duke and Duchess of York to open new Royal Infirmary buildings at Aberdeen. Criticised for not attending himself, Edward VIII averred that he had already told Edward Watt, the Lord Provost of Aberdeen, that he could not attend as his court was still in mourning for George V. But court mourning had not stopped him sporting in the Mediterranean with his mistress Mrs Ernest Simpson, whom he met personally at Aberdeen railway station on the very day he could have been opening the hospital buildings. The late issue of the Aberdeen *Evening Express* that day juxtaposed a photograph of the Duke and Duchess of York opening the hospital buildings with the headline 'HIS MAJESTY IN ABERDEEN – SURPRISE VISIT IN CAR TO MEET GUESTS'. Aberdonians never forgave him this blunder, and royal medical staff were offended.[5]

Homoeopathy, the medical system of treating diseases using small quantities of preparations that excite symptoms similar to those of the disease suffered, was introduced to Britain by Frederick Harvey Foster Quin (1799–1878), the first homoeopathic physician in the country. A graduate of Edinburgh (MD, 1820), Quin was physician to the wife of the Lord President of the Council, W.G. Spencer Cavendish, 6th Duke of Devonshire. After practice at Naples he was converted to homoeopathic principles in 1826 and returned to England as physician to Queen Victoria's uncle Prince Leopold of Saxe-Coburg. Denounced as a quack by several of his peers, he founded the British Homoeopathic Society in 1844 and the London Homoeopathic Hospital in 1850.

Homoeopathic physicians have appeared from time to time in the royal medical households. One such was Sir John Weir (1879–1971), *inter alia* Professor of Materia Medica of the Homoeopathic Society, who treated such eminent figures as Queen Mary, George VI, Queen Elizabeth the Queen Mother and Queen Elizabeth II. Perhaps the best-known homoeopath of modern times was Dr Marjorie Grace Blackie (1898–1981), who was physician to the royal household from 1969.

An interest in homoeopathy and 'alternative' medicine – often dubbed 'new age' medicine – has been maintained and supported by Charles, Prince of Wales. In November 2000 he 'secretly challenged' the Labour government to spend millions of pounds on alternative medical research.[6] In 1996 the prince set up the Foundation for Integrated Medicine to promote the campaign for alternative medicine. His opinions though run counter to the findings of a House of Lords Select Committee on Science and Technology, which concluded that several therapies, from Ayurvedic Medicine (mind–body–spirit interaction, employing herbs to stimulate and aid relaxation) to Naturopathy (diet, herbs, exposure to sunlight and fresh air), have a lack of scientific backing to sustain their effectiveness.[7] In November 2000 the British Medical Association called for a greater regulation of the 50,000 practitioners of alternative medicine in Britain.[8] Royal personages, certainly since the days of Henry I, while employing medics at their courts, have been selective in what advice to follow. The situation remains the same in the twenty-first century.

Over the centuries royal doctors have formed a special relationship with members of the royal family. Their professional role renders them rather different from other members of the court. Sometimes the relationship has tipped over into friendship in personal life. One example may be cited. Sir George Middleton (1905–87), who graduated in medicine in 1926 from Aberdeen University, became assistant to Sir Alexander Hendry in general practice at Ballater, the little Aberdeenshire town a few miles from Balmoral Castle in the heart of royal Deeside. In 1932 he succeeded Sir Alexander as surgeon apothecary to the royal household at Balmoral Castle, a post he held for four decades, attending George V, Queen Mary, Edward VIII, George VI, Queen Elizabeth the Queen Mother and Queen Elizabeth II and their families. As his obituary noted: 'A shrewd doctor, he took a deep interest in people. He was also an accomplished *accoucheur* and once reckoned he had delivered over 1000 babies – equal to the entire population of Ballater.'[9] In 1986 Queen Elizabeth the Queen Mother attended a special service at the church at Glen Muick to dedicate a stained-glass window to Sir George's wife Margaret, who died in 1964.

Health, royalty and medicine still make news. The press were in constant attendance, for instance, outside the King Edward VII's Hospital for Officers in early 2001, to monitor the deteriorating health of Princess Margaret, Countess of Snowdon. Increasingly an examination of royal health, relationships with royal doctors and royal attitudes to medicine reveal long-ignored aspects of great importance to the nation's history. Each diagnosis, medical error and success, accident and disease, has played a part in shaping the outcome of royal history, but only now is the importance of the royal doctor in dynastic history being acknowledged.

Similarly, but very differently in practice, the history of the employment of doctors in America to attend succeeding presidents and their families mirrors the changing aspects of American medical practice. More than in Britain, because the President of the United States is a political appointment by the people, different pressures confront US doctors when treating a president. Does the White House physician, for instance, have first loyalty to the president, or to the people of the United States? This is just one conundrum a physician has to face. To date there are no set protocols to select a White House physician. Presidents generally choose their own physicians based on a variety of criteria from expediency and convenience to friendship and location.

Only in 1967, with the adoption of the 25th Amendment to the Constitution, was a procedure laid down to cope with the issue of presidential disability. As stated, when the president is unable to 'discharge the Powers and Duties' of the presidency, then those duties fall to the vice-president until such time as 'the Disability be removed, or a President shall be elected'. The 25th Amendment has never been invoked. Constitutional lawyers point out that neither the Amendment nor the Constitution defines 'Disability'. Thus if it were left to the White House physician to define on the spot, the history of the United States of America could be changed in a moment.[10]

ROYAL MORTALITY

The glories of our blood and state
Are shadows, not substantial things;
There is no armour against fate;
Death lays his icy hand on kings:
Sceptre and crown
Must tumble down,
And in the dust be equal made
With the poor crooked scythe and spade.

James Shirley (1596–1666),
The Contention of Ajax and Ulysses, I.iii.

From the Middle Ages chroniclers were more likely than royal physicians to record the death details of a monarch. With modern research medical historians have been able to expand the death notices of monarchs. Here I have taken the opportunity to contrast what chroniclers and historians recorded on the deaths of British monarchs alongside a modern assessment:

William I, The Conqueror (1066–87)
'Burst bowels' (William of Malmesbury).[1]
'(From) the changeable autumn warmth (the king) contracted a disease'; 'burst the bowels'. (Matthew Paris).[2]
Rupture of the urethra. Extravasation of the urine (incontinence). Uraemia (kidney failure).

William II, Rufus (1087–1100)
Hunting accident in the New Forest; arrow wound. (William of Malmesbury).[3]
Probable murder.[4]

Henry I, Beauclerk (1100–35)
Food poisoning; 'devoured lampreys'. (Henry of Huntingdon).[5]
Perforated duodenal ulcer. Peritonitis. Paralytic ileus.

Stephen (1135–54).
'The King was suddenly seized with pain in the iliac region along with an old discharge from haemorrhoids.' (Gervase of Canterbury).[6]
Acute appendicitis. Peritonitis.

Henry II, Curtmantle (1154–89).
'Henry plunged into the depths of despair . . .' (Matthew of Westminster).[7]
'From great sadness he derived a fever . . .' (William of Newburg).[8]
Manic depressive syndrome. Bronchopneumonia.

Richard I, Coeur de Lion (1189–99)
'Bertram de Gourdon wounded the king in the arm . . .' (Roger de Hovedene).[9]
Arrow wound in the left shoulder; septicaemia.

John, Lackland (1199–1216).
'He fell into despondency . . . (he was) seized by a disgusting gluttony . . . he greatly increased his feverishness.' (Matthew Paris).[10]
Perforated peptic ulcer. He may have been murdered by poison in the meal mentioned by Paris.

Henry III (1216–72).
'The King returning to St Edmund's Shrine (at Bury St Edmunds Abbey) began to wax somewhat craxie but having a little recovered he called a cousin there. But his sickness again renewed . . . so increased upon him that finally he departed this life at Westminster . . .' (Raphael Holinshed).[11]
Cerebral haemorrhage.

Edward I, Longshanks (1272–1307).
'The King began to be troubled with dysentery and gave up hope of living longer.' (Thomas Walsingham).[12]
Carcinoma of the rectum.

Edward II (1307–27)
Murdered at Berkeley Castle, Gloucestershire, by the orders

of (or at the hands of) Sir John Maltravers and Sir Thomas Gournay.[13]

'Cum veru ignito inter celando confossus ignominiose peremptus est' (he was ignominously slain with a red-hot spit thrust into the anus). (Ranulph Higden).[14]

Traumatic perforation of the rectum: peritonitis.

Edward III (1327–77).

'(The king) fell into a weakness not of the kind that is believed to be usual in old men, but which is said to attach itself for the most part to youth given to lechery. But the cure of that disease is far more difficult in an old man than in a young one, for the different reasons of the old man's chilliness and the young man's heat. And, therefore the Lord King was weakened the more because the natural fluid and nutritive heat in him were now exhausted, and his virility failed.' (Thomas Walsingham).[15]

Cerebral thrombosis. Bronchopneumonia.

Richard II (1377–99)

Deposed by his first cousin Henry, Duke of Hereford (later Henry IV).

Murdered (supposedly) at Henry's fortress of Pontefract Castle, West Yorkshire.

Some accounts say he was suffocated, or died of starvation. (Thomas Walsingham).[16]

Raphael Holinshed avers he was 'felled with a stroke of a poleaxe'.

Probably murdered by poison.

Henry IV (1399–1413)

'. . . as the common opinion, from (1404) until his death, he was a leper and even fouler and fouler'. (John Capgrave).[17] It is unlikely the king died of leprosy, as an examination of his cadaver in 1832 proved.[18]

Ureamia. Chronic pemphigus (a skin condition). Chronic nephritis.

Henry V (1413–22)

'The King from having an old distemper, which he had

contracted from excessive and long-continued exertion, meanwhile fell into an acute fever with violent dysentery. This his physicians did not venture to treat by any internal medication, but forthwith gave up hope of his life.' (Thomas Walsingham).[19]

'He was attacked by a cancerous disease which the peasantry called St Fiacres Ill.' (John de Fordun).[20]

Carcinoma of the rectum. Bronchopneumonia. Pleurisy.

Henry VI (1422–61 and 1470–1)

Murdered (supposedly) in the Tower of London on the orders of Edward, Duke of York (King Edward IV).

An examination of his presumed cadaver in 1910 purported to detect blood-matted hair and skull fragments.[21]

Edward IV (1461–70 and 1471–83).

'(The king was) neither worn out with old age, nor yet seized with any known kind of malady.' (Croyland Chronicle).[22]

Pleurisy. Pleural effusion. Bronchopneumonia.

Edward V (April–June 1483)

See p. 27.

Supposed murder.

Richard III (1483–5)

Slain at the battle of Bosworth Field.

Henry VII (1485–1509)

'The King began to be diseased (1509) of a certain infirmity which thrice a year, but especially in the spring time sore vexed him. The sickness which held the King daily more and more increasing he well perceived that his end drew near. He was so wasted with his long malady that nature could no longer sustain his life . . .' (Raphael Holinshed).[23]

Uraemia. Pulmonary and renal tuberculosis.

Henry VIII (1509–47)

'Henry, long since grown corpulent, was becoming a burden to himself and of late lame by reason of a violent ulcer in his leg,

the inflammation whereof cast him into a lingering fever which, little by little, decayed his spirits.' (Thomas Goodwin).[24]
Uraemia. Chronic nephritis. Leg ulcers. Cushing's syndrome. Amyloid disease.

Edward VI (1547–53)
Serious attack of measles and smallpox (1552).
Pulmonary tuberculosis.

Jane (10–19 July 1583)
Beheaded.

Mary I (1553–8)
'(The departure of Philip II, her husband) is not the greatest wound that pierced my oppressed mind . . . when I am dead and opened, you will find Calais lying in my heart.' (Raphael Holinshed).[25]
Ovarian tumour.

Elizabeth I (1558–1603)
'At the beginning of her sickness (1603) the almonds of her jaws began to swell and her appetite . . . failed her . . . a kind of denumbness seized upon her with a deep melancholy . . . she would sit silently, refrain her meat . . . her speech failed . . .' (Sir Richard Baker).[26]
Carcinoma of the stomach. Myxoedema. Bronchopneumonia. Suppurative parotitis.

James VI & I (1603–25)
Possible poisoning. (See p. 41.)
Bronchopneumonia. Pulmonary tuberculosis.

Charles I (1625–49)
Beheaded.

Charles II (1660–85)
'He fell sick of a tertian fever . . .'. (Sir Richard Baker).[27]
Uraemia. Chronic nephritis. Syphilis.

James VII & II (1685–8)
Chroniclers aver that the king died of 'piety'.[28]
Cerebral thrombosis. Hypertension. Syphilitic vascular disease.

Mary II (1689–94)
A mid-eighteenth-century assessment was that the queen died of smallpox.[29]
Modern assessments confirm this.

William III (1689–94 and 1694–1702)
Contemporary historians make much of the fall from his horse.
Pulmonary embolism. Deep venous thrombosis. Bronchopneumonia.

Anne (1702–14)
See p. 51.
Uraemia. Chronic nephritis. Hypochromic anaemia. Lupus erythe matosus.

George I (1714–27)
See pp. 54–5.
Cerebral haemorrhage. Hypertension.

George II (1727–60)
'. . . the ventricle of his heart had burst'. (Horace Walpole).[30]
Rupture of the ventricle. Syphilitic aortitis.

George III (1760–1820)
See pp. 104ff.
Terminal dementia. Porphyria. Bronchopneumonia.

George IV (1820–30)
Royal doctor Sir Astley Cooper averred: 'The immediate cause of His Majesty's dissolution was the rupture of a blood vessel of the stomach.'[31]
Gastric haemorrhage. Portal hypertension. Hepatic cirrhosis. Aortic and mitral valvular disease. Diverticulum of the bladder. Calculus.

William IV (1830–7)

'On the left side of the heart, the mitral valves were found to be ossified . . .'[32]

Bronchopneumonia. Aortic and mitral valvular disease. Myocarditis. Syphilis.

During 1837 official registration of death took place for England and Wales. Thus the death certificates for British monarchs from this time on were on record.[33]

Victoria (1837–1901)

Cardiac failure. Senility.

Edward VII (1901–10)

Cardiac failure.

George V (1910–36)

Progressive myocardial failure. See also pp. 1, 237 and 239.

Edward VIII (January–December 1936)

Carcinoma of the throat.

George VI (1936–52)

Carcinoma of the bronchus.

From the Norman Conquest to 1952 there were forty-one monarchs, including Jane Grey, of whom a few were purportedly kicked into eternity by royal physicians. Here is a breakdown of their causes of death: 28 died of what might be called natural causes; 7 were probably murdered; one died by accident; one was slain in battle; 2 were executed; one is thought to have succumbed to iatrogenic regicide; and one's death was 'hastened' by a physician.

THE ROYAL HOUSE OF SCOTLAND

> For lords or kings I dinna mourn; *do not*
> E'en let them die – for that they're born.
>> Robert Burns (1759–96)
>> *Elegy on the Year 1788.*

The causes of death recorded by historians for the royal house of Scotland until the forced abdication of Mary, Queen of Scots, 24 July 1567, begin in the ninth century:

Alpin, King of Kintyre (834). Killed in battle with the Picts in Galloway.

Kenneth I Macalpin (844–59). Probably died of natural causes at Abernethy, Perthshire.

Donald I (859–63). Described by the Gaelic bards as of *dhreachruaid* (ruddy complexion). Died at Balachon, causes unknown.

Constantine II (863–77). Killed in battle with the Danes at the Black Cave, Angus.

Aedh Whitefoot (877–8). Probably murdered at Strathallan, Perthshire, by regent Giric of Strathclyde.

Eahaid (878–89). Deposed. Mode of death unknown.

Donald II Dasachtach (889–900). Mode of death unknown.

Constantine III (900–42). Abdicated. Mode of death unknown.

Malcolm I (942–54) Murdered by the men of Moray at Fetteressoe, Kincardineshire.

Indulf (954–62). Slain by Norse invaders, near the Bay of Cullen, Banffshire.

Dubh (962–7). Murdered by the men of Moray at Forres, Morayshire.

Cuilean (967–71). Murdered by Riderch of Strathclyde.

Kenneth II (971–95). Murdered at Fetteressoe.

Constantine IV (995–7). Murdered by Kenneth III at Rathinveramon.

Kenneth III (997–1005). Killed in a skirmish at Monzievaird, Perthshire.

Malcolm II (1005–34). Died of (probable) natural causes at the hunting lodge of Glamis, Angus.

Duncan I, The Gracious (1034–40). Murdered by Macbeth at Bothnagowan (modern Pitgaveny), Morayshire.

Macbeth *Ard Righ na h'Alba* (High King of Scotland) (1040–57). Killed in battle at Lumphanan.

Lulach, The Simple (1057–8). Murdered by the agents of Malcolm III.

Malcolm III (1058–93). Killed in a skirmish at Alnwick, Northumberland, by Sir Morel de Bamborough.

Donald III Bane (1093–4 and 1094–7). Eyes put out by his nephew Edgar; died at Rescobie, Forfarshire.

Duncan II (May–November 1094). Murdered by agents of his half-brother Edmund and uncle Donald III Bane.

Edgar (1097–1107). Died of natural causes at Edinburgh Castle.

Alexander I, The Fierce (1107–24). Died of natural causes at Loch Tay.

David I, The Saint (1124–53). Died of natural causes at Carlisle.

Malcolm IV, The Maiden (1153–65). Died of natural causes at Jedburgh, Roxburghshire.

William I, The Lion (1165–1214). Died at Stirling Castle of old age and exhaustion.

Alexander II (1214–49). Died of fever on the Island of Kerrera, Bay of Oban.

Alexander III (1249–86). Killed in riding accident at Kinghorn, Fife.

Margaret 'The Maid of Norway' (1286–90). Drowned in storm.

The First Interregnum 1290–2.

John Baliol 'Toom Tabard' (Empty surcoat) (1292–6). Died at his castle of Helicourt, Bailleul-on-Gouffern, Normandy.

The Second Interregnum 1296–1306

Robert I, The Bruce (1306–29). Dies at Cardross Castle, Dumbartonshire, of leprosy.

David II (1329–71). Died of natural causes at Edinburgh Castle.

Robert II, Stewart (1371–90). Died of old age at Dundonald Castle, Ayrshire.

Robert III (1390–1406). Died at Dundonald, demoralised at the capture of his heir by English buccaneers.

James I (1406–37). Murdered at Perth by his uncle Walter, Earl of Atholl.

James II 'of the Fiery Face' (1437–60). Killed when a bombard exploded at the siege of Roxburgh.

James III (1460–88). Killed in a skirmish following the main battle of Sauchieburn. Tradition has it that he was murdered in a cottage at Milltown, near Bannockburn.

James IV (1488–1513). Killed at the battle of Flodden, Northumberland.

James V (1513–42). Died at Falkland Palace, demoralised by the defeat of the royal army at the battle of Solway Moss.

Mary, Queen of Scots (1542–67). Executed.

Union of the Crowns of England and Scotland, 24 March 1603

From the ninth century the forty reigning monarchs of Scotland escaped largely unscathed by the ministrations of royal physicians and surgeons. Nevertheless, only 11 were known to have died from natural causes; 10 were murdered; 9 were killed in battles or skirmishes; 6 died of unknown causes (i.e., the court chroniclers were silent about their mode of death); only 2 had known terminal diseases; one was drowned; and one was executed.

Royal Death Certificates

No death registration records for monarchs exist in the usual official form at the General Register Office. When the Births and Deaths Registration Act 1936 was brought into being the sovereign was excluded, but not other members of the royal family. Even though the 1836 Act has been amended by the Acts of 1874, 1926 and 1953 the sovereign is still excluded from the legal requirements of registration.[33]

GLOSSARY

Apothecary: A medical practitioner (of an inferior branch of the profession), who often kept a shop selling drugs and herbal potions. In recent times it is still a legal description for Licentiates of the Society of Apothecaries (LSA). The Society is one of the London City Guilds (Livery Companies) and has its Hall at 14 Blackfriars Lane, London, EC4V 6EJ.

Specific royal appointment since the days of Edward II, as Prince of Wales.

Apothecary to the person: Position from the reign of George I, started 1714.

Apothecaries to the royal household: Appointments since 1714.

Apothecaries to the queen and her household: Appointments from Queen Anne (1723) to Queen Adelaide (1849).

Apothecaries to the Prince of Wales, later Prince Regent and George IV: 1782–1820. George IV had his own defined chemists and druggists.

Apothecary-extraordinary: From the reign of George IV.

Extra-apothecary: From the reign of George IV.

Spicer-apothecary: specific royal appointment since the reign of John Lackland.

Yeoman-apothecary: From the reign of Elizabeth I.

Queen Victoria had various apothecaries in her household from 1837 to 1901; some like her physician Sir Francis Henry Laking, held the title *apothecary to the household* and later (1880) *surgeon apothecary*. She also had apothecaries specified at Windsor Castle and Osborne House.

During the period 1901–52 apothecaries were specifically designated for the royal households at Windsor and Sandringham, and from 1911 at Balmoral and 1909 at Holyrood Palace.

The current royal households retain the position of apothecary.

Cirurgicus Regis/Surgeon to the King: A title noted as early as 1233. The Household Ordinances of Edward II define the rewards of the royal physicians and surgeons thus: 'the surgeon shall have his diet every day in the Hall (of the castle wherever the monarch was residing), if he is not hindered by some business certified before the Steward and Treasurer. And then he shall have his livery as a Knight of the Household, whether he be well or ill, that is to say, two *darres* of bread, one pitcher of wine, two *messes de gros* from the kitchen, and one mess of roast. And shall take every day for his chamber, one pitcher of wine, three candles, one *tontis*, litter all the year and fuel for dinner time, of the Usher of the Hall. He shall have twelve pence a day wages until he be advanced by the King and two robes yearly in cloth, or 8 *marks* in money. For things medicinal he shall have forty shillings by the year'.

Doctor of the king's body: A term used, for instance, in the reign of Richard III.

Domestic-physician: Title used in George III's time in the household of his son Prince William Henry, Duke of Clarence.

First (king's) physician: A title used in the reigns of William III and Queen Anne. Uniquely used for John Hutton while on service in Ireland.

Garciones: Attendants/apprentices of barbers/surgeons.

General medical attendant: Title used in the household of Queen Victoria's mother, the Duchess of Kent.

Magister: A general title in medieval documents to denote a Doctor of Medicine.

Mediciner: A term (with various spellings) used in Scotland from the fourteenth to the seventeenth century to describe physicians. From the late sixteenth century it was the title (with a capital letter) of the Professor of Medicine at King's College, Aberdeen.

Medicus regis: General term in monastic and court records for *phisici* (physicians) and *cirugici* (surgeons) employed at the royal court, or within the convent. A variation, *Regis medicus*, is a form which first appears in the early eleventh century when assumed by the Cluniac medical monk Ranulf.

Physician-in-ordinary: Consultants to the monarch, quite often acting as general practitioners. Usually served for ten to twelve years. The senior physician-in-ordinary served as the head of the medical department in Queen Victoria's court.

Physician-extraordinary: Retired or specialist physician, who could be called to the court *ad hoc*.

Physician-accoucheur: Title used in Queen Victoria's reign.

Principal physician: A seventeenth-century term in Scotland for the chief royal physician.

Second physician: After 1714 a Scottish term for an 'ordinary physician' of Scottish extraction at the court.

Physicus regis: king's physician. Title noted from the court rolls of Edward I.

Protomedicus: chief court physician. Term used in various reigns, mostly sixteenth century. Used as the title of John Baptist Boerio at the court of Henry VII.

Socii: Term used in medieval texts to identify associate helpers of court medics.

Surgeon-in-ordinary: Consultants to the monarch. Usually served ten to twelve years.

Surgeon-extraordinary: Retired, or specialist surgeons, who could be called to court *ad hoc*.

Sergeant-surgeon: This title appears in 1253 as an Anglo-Norman translation of the Latin *serviens* (servant). After this date the prefix 'serjeant' or 'sergeant' became more common for many royal appointments, for instance, sergeant of hounds, sergeant-at-arms. In the reign of Richard II the title was expressed as *serviens noster* (our servant/surgeon). In 1513 Henry VIII promoted Marcellus de la More to the post of serjeant of the king's surgeons. The inference from the title was that the surgeon accompanied the monarch on military engagements.

The last royal surgeon to do so was John Ranby during the War of the Austrian Succession (1740–8) in the reign of George II.

Extra surgeon: A twentieth-century post, usually for retired surgeons who had directly served the royal household as surgeon or serjeant-surgeon.

Groom-surgeon: A title settled upon Thomas Bekbank, as cited in the 'Proceedings of the Privy Council of King Henry VI' for 1454.

Surgeon-in-ordinary-of-the-person: A title settled on Richard Wiseman at the court of Charles II.

Surgeon-aurist-in-ordinary: A title settled on William Wright in the household of Queen Charlotte.

Yeoman-surgeon: A title settled upon John Marchall and cited in the 'Proceedings of the Privy Council of King Henry VI' for 1454.

Surrigicus Domini Regis: surgeon to (our) Lord King. Title used at the court of Edward III.

Valetti: Used in medieval texts to identify junior assistants of court medics.

NOTES

PROLOGUE

1. Kenneth Rose, *King George V*, p. 402. Bertrand Dawson qualified as a doctor in 1890 and became a Fellow of the Royal College of Physicians in 1903, of which college he was President during 1931–8. In 1907 he was appointed to the medical household of Edward VII, and subsequently administered to George V, Edward VIII and George VI. He was the only royal doctor ever to be made a viscount.

2. Michael Thornton, *Sunday Express*, 24 May 1992, p. 35. Christabel Aberconway (d. 1974), spouse of the 2nd Baron Aberconway, was the daughter of Sir Melville Macnaughten, Assistant Chief Constable, Scotland Yard.

3. Melvyn Fairclough, *The Ripper and The Royals*, p. 209.

4. Ibid., pp. 187–96.

5. J.J. Keevil, *The Stranger's Son*, pp. 123–31.

6. *See* T. Whitmore Peck and K. Douglas Wilkinson, *William Withering of Birmingham*.

7. J.B. Atlay, *Henry Acland – A Memoir*, pp. 259–61.

8. George Whitfield, *Royal Physicians*, p. 4.

9. *The Concise Dictionary of National Biography*, 1992, p. 2468.

10. *See* C.R. Hone, *The Life of John Radcliffe*.

11. A. Aspinall, *The Correspondence of George, Prince of Wales, 1770–1812*, Vol. IV.

12. Ibid., letter, Carlton House, 27 September 1800.

13. Michaela Reid, *Ask Sir James*, p. 110.

14. Sir James Clark's *Diaries*, December 1865.

15. Kenneth Rose, *Kings, Queens and Courtiers*, p. 38.

16. Ida Macalpine and Richard Hunter, *George III and the Mad-Business*, p. 241.

17. *The Life and Times of Henry Lord Brougham by Himself*, Vol. 2, p. 332.

18. A. Aspinall, *Letters of King George IV*, Vol. 2, p. 212.

19. Baron E. von Stockmar, *Memoirs of Baron Stockmar*, Vol. 1, p. 70.

20. Richard B. Fisher, *Joseph Lister 1827–1912*, p. 178.

21. Correspondence between the author and the secretary of the Lord Chamberlain's Office, February 2000.

INTRODUCTION

1. Named after the American Egyptologist who acquired it; now in the collection of the History Society of New York.

2. Discovered in a tomb at Thebes in 1862 by Professor Georg Ebers, and now in the library of the University of Leipzig.

3. Dr E.T. Withington, *Medical History from the Earliest Times*, p. 14.

4. E. Meyer, *Geschichte des alten Aegyptens*, Vol. II, p. 95.

5. Jameson B. Hurry, *Imhotep: The Vizier and Physician of King Zoser*, p. 29.

6. Ibid., p. 45.

7. Ibid., p. 170.

8. Ibid., p. 172.

9. Ibid., p. 169.

10. Z. Iskander and A. Badawy, *Brief History of Ancient Egypt*, pp. 34–4.

11. A.E. Weigall, *Guide to the Antiquities of Upper Egypt*, p. 298.

12. General overview of the subject in Chi Min Wang and Lien-Teh Wu, *History of Chinese Medicine*.

13. Leonard Mosely, *Hirohito: Emperor of Japan*, p. 3.

14. Ibid., p. 100.

15. E.M. Bick, 'The Cult of Asklepios', *Annals of Medical History*, Vol. IX, p. 327.

16. E.T. Withinton, 'Background Study', in ibid. As dissection of the human body was not permitted in Greece or Rome, a doctor trained at Alexandria was perceived to have greater academic skills as there anatomy was taught by human dissection.

17. Background study in E.G. Browne, *Arabian Medicine*.

18. *See* biographical entry in: C.H. Talbot and E.A. Hammond, *The Medical Practitioners in Medieval England*.

19. Ibid., pp. 231–2.

20. Ibid., pp. 63–5.

21. Ibid., pp. 192–3.

22. Edward J. Kealey, *Medieval Medicus*, p. 57.

23. Ibid., pp. 62–3.

24. J. Stevenson (ed.), *Chronicon Monasterii de Abingdon*, Vol. II, p. 44.

25. W. Stubbs (ed.), *The Historical Works of Gervase of Canterbury*.

26. Matthew Paris, *Chronica Majora*, ed. H.R. Luard, Vol. ii, p. 668.

27. Henri de Mandeville, *Chirurgia* ed. Julius Leopold Paget, 40, p. 668. The *Chirurgia* follows what people in the Middle Ages learned about physicians and surgeons from the classics. In Ancient Greece physicians were healer-priests who were deemed supernatural intermediaries between the patient and the gods and devils who were the mysterious causes of disease. Surgeons were non-religious-based private practitioners. Thus physicians were deemed intellectuals and surgeons illiterate functionaries.

28. *Calendar of Patent Rolls* (*CPR*), 12 May 1233. 17 Henry III, 1233.

29. *CPR*, 1241. 23 Henry III, 1241. *Escheat*: Property which fell to a feudal lord, or to the Crown, for want of an heir, by forfeiture or plunder. In this case the land had fallen to the Judiciary of Ireland.

30. *Calendar of Close Rolls* (*CCR*), 1243. 27 Henry III, 1243.

31. *CCR*, 1248. 32 Henry III, 1248.

2. *CPR*, 1251. 35 Henry III, 1251.

3. *CPR*, 1253. 37 Henry III, 1253. Herein is an interesting instance of cash payment as fee instead of land or incumbency.

4. *Calendar of Documents Relating to Ireland*, Vol. I, p. 3106, 1250–1.

5. Ibid., note 22.

6. British Museum. MS. Royal 12 B. xii, fol. 181r.

7. For details of Thomas de Weseham's career in royal service see *Calendar of Charter Rolls* (*CChR*), 1255. 27 Henry III, 1255; *CPR*, 1256. 40 Henry III, 1256; and *CPR*, 1260. 44 Henry III, 1260. A known example of de Weseham's coins bears the legend *Henricius Rex III* with stylised crowned portrait on the obverse, and a voided long cross and the legend *Thomas on Lund* on the reverse.

8. *See* Edward's campaigns in *Liber Quotidianus Contrarotulatori Garderobae*, Society of Antiquities, 1787.

9. Thomas Rymer and Robert Sanderson, *Foedera*, Vol. II, pp. 999ff.

0. Edward I's first wife Eleanor of Castile had her own physician in Nicholas of Montimer (*c*. 1283) of the Spanish court.

1. *Calendar of Documents Relevant to Scotland*, Vol. III, 1887, p. 142.

2. Medieval physicians believed that the human body was made up of the four mystic elements of Earth (cold and dry), Water (cold and wet), Fire (hot and dry), and Air (hot and wet). Diseases were thought to result from an imbalance of these elements.

43. Aesculapius, Hippocrates and Galen were all well-known medics of history. Dioscorides was a Greek physician of the first century. Hali, Serapion and Avicenna were Arabian doctors of the tenth and eleventh centuries, Averroes a Moorish practitioner of the twelfth century, and Rhazes a Spanish Arab doctor of the tenth century. Rufus may refer to Ruffinus of Lincoln who practised *c*. 1276. Constantine remains unknown. Bernard (Gordon) was Professor of Medicine at Montpellier around 1300, and Gilbertine is possibly Gilbertus Angelicus who was a physician and medic of the early thirteenth century.

44. G.E. Gask, 'The Medical Staff of King Edward III', *Proceedings of the Royal Society of Medicine*, 18 February 1925.

45. Ibid.

46. R. Sharpe (ed.), *Calendar of Wills in the Court of Hustings*, Pt 2, p. 275.

47. *CPR*, 15 Richard II, 1392.

48. *CPR*, 6 Henry IV, 1405.

49. G.E. Gask, 'The Medical Services of Henry V's Campaign', *Proceedings of the Royal Society of Medicine*, Vol. XVI, 1923.

50. Ibid., note 31.

51. Rymer and Sanderson, *Foedera*, Vol. X.

52. *Proceedings of the Privy Council*, Vol. VI. By this time one Michael Belwell had been added to the king's bank of surgeons, but he was not included in this new commission. *CPR*, 21 Henry VI, 1443.

53. Rymer and Sanderson, *Foedera*, Vol. II, p. 366.

54. Ronald Knox and Shane Leslie (eds), *The Miracles of King Henry VI*.

55. *CPR*, 1 Edward IV, 1461. Other rolls verify the several grants of land and money to Fryse.

56. *Ordinances of the Royal Household (ORH)*, pp. 15–86.

57. Ibid., note 55.

58. *CPR*, 1485–94.

CHAPTER ONE

1. Agatha Young, *Scalpel: Men Who Made Surgery*, pp. 32–51.

2. Ibid., p. 37.

3. William Munk, *Roll of the Royal College of Physicians*, 1. 21–2.

4. Rossell Hope Robbins, *The Encyclopedia of Witchcraft & Demonology*, p. 120.

5. Christopher Hibbert, *The Virgin Queen*, pp. 72–3.

6. Douglas Guthrie, *A History of Medicine*, p. 152.

7. Ibid., p. 176.

8. *A Trial of Witches at the Assizes Held at Bury St Edmunds*.

9. D. Harris Willson, *King James VI & I*, p. 446.

10. Robert Harley, *Harleian Miscellany*, 1714.

11. Antonia Fraser, *King James VI of Scotland and I of England*, p. 211.

12. J. Aikin, *Biographical Memoirs of Medicine in Great Britain*, p. 290.

13. J. Timbs, *Doctors and Patients*, Vol. 1, p. 37.

14. *Pipe Roll*, 1207. *See* Leslie G. Matthews, *The Royal Apothecaries*, pp. 3–4 (and note).

15. Matthews, *Royal Apothecaries*, p. 4.

16. Ibid., p. 47.

17. Rymer and Sanderson, *Foedera*, Vol. XI, 1727 edition, p. 347.

18. Broadsheet, 1685: *A True Relation of the late King's Death*, p. 1.

19. T.B. Macaulay, *History*.

20. Walter Harris, *Observations on Certain Grievous Diseases*, 1742.

21. Gila Curtis, *The Life and Times of Queen Anne*, p. 86.

22. P. Roberts (ed.), *The Diary of Sir David Hamilton 1704–14*.

23. Ibid. A very good summary of Queen Anne's health is to be found in Professor H.E. Emson, 'For the want of an heir: the obstetrical history of Queen Anne', *British Medical Journal*, Vol. 304, 23 May 1992, pp. 1365–6.

CHAPTER TWO

1. Joyce Marlow, *The Life and Times of George I*, p. 208.

2. The church suffered war damage and George's

cadaver was moved to the mausoleum at Herrenhausen.

3. Christopher Sinclair-Stevenson, *Blood Royal: The Illustrious House of Hanover*, p. 75.

4. David M. Wilson, *Awful Ends: The British Museum Book of Epitaphs*, pp. 82–3.

5. Harold Ellis, *Operations that made History*, Ch. 11, pt 3, p. 8.

6. Ibid., pp. 81, 83.

7. Ibid., p. 83.

8. Ibid., p. 85.

9. *See also* D'A. Power, 'A Case of Strangulated Hernia: Queen Caroline of Ansbach', *British Journal of Surgery*, 20:1, 1932.

10. Horace Walpole, *Memoires of the last ten years of the reign of George II*, ed. Lord Holland, Vol. II.

CHAPTER THREE

1. Robert Burns, *To Robert Graham, Esq, of Fintry*, *c.* 1790. Verse 2, line 11; Verse 4, line 3.

2. Michael Scott's magic dexterity was also mentioned in Dante Alighieri's *Divina Comedia* (1307): . . . Michael Scott
Practised in every slight of magic wile.

3. J.W. Brown, *The Life and Legend of Michael Scott. Pilulae* . . . British Library. Add. MS 24068 (22), fol. 97.

4. Guthrie, *History of Medicine*, pp. 102ff.

5. G.C. Coulton, *Scottish*

Abbeys and Social Life, p. 203.

6. *The Brus, an epic poem by John Barbour*, trans. and ed. Archibald A.H. Douglas. John Barbour (*c.* 1320–95) was Archdeacon of Aberdeen in 1372: his 13,000-line poem *The Brus* appeared in 1376.

7. Ibid.

8. Ibid.

9. G.W.S. Barrow, *Robert Bruce: and the Community of the Realm of Scotland*, pp. 444–5.

10. This diagnosis was corroborated by Dr J.A. Morris Rennie and Professor W.W. Watson Buchanan in the article 'The Bruce – Post-Mortem on the Warrior King', in *Practitioner Journal of Post-Graduate Medicine*, 1998.

11. *Rotuli Scaccarii Regum Scotorum*, 1264–1359, pp. 176, 213, 238.

12. Ibid., p. 562; 1359–79, p. 6.

13. F. Devon (ed.). *Extracts from the Issue Rolls of the Exchequer*, 1837, p. 166.

14. A. Leitch, 'Farquhar Leiche: Medicus Regis', *Proceedings of the Royal Society of Medicine*, Vol. XIII, pp. 17–18.

15. Coulton, *Scottish Abbeys*, p. 205.

16. *Rotuli Scaccarii Regum Scotorum*, p. 169.

17. Ibid., 1406–36, p. 679.

18. Wickersheimer, *Les Médecines de la Nation Anglaise*, p. 44.

19. *Rotuli Scaccarii Regum Scotorum*, 1455–60, pp. 3, 12 *et passim*.

20. Ibid., 1470–79, pp. lxviii, 11.
21. J. Maitland Thomson, *Dowden's The Bishops of Scotland*, pp. 33–5.
22. R.L. Mackie, *King James IV of Scotland*, p. 167.
23. E.J. Holmyard, *Alchemy*, pp. 219–20.
24. Mackie, *James IV*, pp. 167–8.
25. John D. Comrie, *History of Scottish Medicine to 1860*, p. 54.
26. Laing, J. (ed.), *Sir David Lyndsay's Works*, p. 125.
27. Rosalind K. Marshall, *Mary of Guise*, p. 239.
28. Marguerite Wood (ed.), *Foreign Correspondence with Marie de Lorraine, Queen of Scotland, from the Originals in the Balcarres Papers*, pp. 79–80.
29. Gladys Dickinson, *Two Missions of Jacques de la Brosse*, pp. 178–9.
30. W.K. Boyd (ed.), *Calendar of State Papers relating to Scotland and Mary Queen of Scots 1547–1603*, Vol. 3, p. 441.
31. Samuel Cowan, *Mary Queen of Scots*, pp. 345–56.
32. Ibid., pp. 374–5, in the household list for her captivity at Sheffield, 4 May 1571.
    Note: The data in the remaining part of this chapter is built up from entries in the records of the Privy Seal (Warrants), Great Seal, MS *Reg. Secreti Sigilii*, Secretary's Warrants, Calendar of State Papers (Domestic), Minute Book of Signatures, and relevant entries in the *Dictionary of National Biography* or as specified below.
33. This practice lapsed in 1847. *See* G.N. Clark, 'Royal Physicians in Scotland', *Medical History*, Vol. II, October 1967, p. 402.
34. William Forbes Skene, Bannatyne Club, 1860.
35. R.C. Buist, 'David Kinloch (Kynalochus) 1559–1617', *British Medical Journal* (1926), i, p. 793.
36. Although he held a prominent position as First Librarian and Second Treasurer of the Royal College of Physicians of Edinburgh, Dr Stevenson's name disappears from the College records because he became a Covenanter.
37. Robert Chambers, *A Biographical Dictionary of Eminent Scotsmen*, rev. Thomas Thomson, Vol. III pp. 349–50.
38. Clark, 'Royal Physicians', p. 405.
39. Chambers, *Biographical Dictionary*, Vol. II, pp. 339–41.

CHAPTER FOUR

Note: Both in contemporary diaries and in the Stuart Papers, physicians and surgeons who served the exiled Stuarts and in the Jacobite armies were termed 'royal doctors'.
1. Matthews, *Royal Apothecaries*, p. 178. *See*

citation, *Calendar of State Papers* (*Domestic*), 1685–8, p. 252.

2. Peter Earle, *The Life & Times of James II*, p. 168.
3. Matthews, *Royal Apothecaries*, p. 120.
4. Ibid., p. 121.
5. Chambers, *Biographical Dictionary*, Vol. III, pp. 248–9.
6. R.P. Ritchie, *The Early Days of the Royal College of Physitians, Edinburgh* p. 12. The Jereboam was consumed at the 148th anniversary of Archibald Pitcairne's death (1800) on the refurbishment of his tombstone at Greyfriars Churchyard, Edinburgh.
7. Ibid., p. 184.
8. R. Forbes, *The Lyon in the Morning*, Vol. I, p. 348.
9. W.A. Macnaughtan, 'The Medical Heroes of the "Forty-five"', *Caledonian Medical Journal*, no. 15, 1932, pp. 113–19.
10. Ibid., p. 114. *See also* entry in Index.
11. Ibid., p. 61.
12. John Prebble, *Culloden*, p. 149.
13. Ibid., p. 244.
14. Ibid., p. 236.
15. Ibid., p. 237.

CHAPTER FIVE

1. Duke of Buckingham (ed.), *Memoirs of the Court and Cabinets of George III*, Vol. II, pp. 6–7.
2. Lord Waldegrave, *Memoirs*, ed. Lord Holland, p. 9.
3. Sinclair-Stevenson, *Blood Royal*, p. 131.
4. Macalpine and Hunter, *George III and the Mad-Business*, p. 16.
5. John Baker Holroyd, *Memoirs*. For *Don Quixote*, *see* Miguel de Cervantes Saavedra (1547–1616), *Don Quixote*.
6. Robert Fulke Greville, *Diaries*, pp. 118–19. Francis Willis was to be the highest paid physician of mental illness of his day. He charged patients £25 a week for their treatment and in 1792 his fee to treat Queen Marie I of Portugal was £10,000.
7. Christopher Hibbert, *George III: A Personal History*, p. 278.
8. Ibid., p. 279.
9. Ibid., p. 300. The cost of George III's illness increased each year, with many visits being deemed unnecessary by his secretary Col. (Sir) Henry Taylor (1775–1839). From 1812 to 1818 the cost of treating the king was set at £271,691 18*s*. (Royal Archives. Ref: 50449–50452.)
10. Hibbert, *George III*, p. 405.
11. Ibid., pp. 408–9.
12. Vivian Green, *The Madness of Kings*, p. 200.
13. John Fergusson, *Notes on the Character and Health of His Majesty King George III*, 1857. Disbound papers.
14. Runyan McKinley, *Journal of Personality*, Vol. LVI, 1988, pp. 295–326.

CHAPTER SIX

1. Both Halford and Phipps changed their names, the former from Vaughan, while the latter became Sir Jonathan Wathen Waller.
2. Katherine Hudson, *A Royal Conflict: Sir John Conroy and the Young Victoria*, p. 40.
3. G.M. Willis, *Ernest Augustus: Duke of Cumberland, King of Hanover*, p. 40.
4. Ibid., pp. 422–3.
5. John H. Jesse, *Memoirs of the Life and Reign of King George III*.
6. Ibid., description of scene.
7. Lady Anne Hamilton, *Secret History of the Court of England*, p. 89.
8. Willis, *Ernest Augustus*, p. 80.
9. Raymond Lamont-Brown, *Royal Murder Mysteries*, p. 64.
10. *Calendar of State Papers*. According to *Statute 28, Henry VIII, 12, 1537* the inquest jury should have consisted of twelve 'Yeomen Officers of the King's Household'. Adams chose a jury he is purported to have deemed independent of royal court influence.
11. Willis, *Ernest Augustus*, p. 82. He identifies Place as a 'notorious Radical'.
12. Lamont-Brown, *Royal Murder Mysteries*, p. 67.
13. Willis, *Ernest Augustus*, p. 81.
14. Ibid., p. 83, note 1.
15. Ibid., p. 86.
16. Ibid., p. 86.
17. *The Times*, 2 July 1810.
18. Willis, *Ernest Augustus*, p. 87.

CHAPTER SEVEN

1. Percy Bysshe Shelley, Sonnet: *England in 1819*.
2. *The Times*, 1816.
3. J.B. Priestley, *The Prince of Pleasure and his Regency 1811–20*, p. 213.
4. Ibid., p. 288.
5. *See* R.C. Brock, *The Life and Work of Astley Cooper*.
6. Ellis, *Operations that made History*, p. 93.
7. Ibid., p. 95.
8. D'A. Power, 'The removal of a Sebaceous cyst from King George IV', *British Journal of Surgery*, 20:311, 1933.
9. Priestley, *Prince of Pleasure*, p. 58.
10. Robert Huish, *Memoirs of George the Fourth*.
11. Ibid.
12. Ibid.
13. B. Bransby Cooper, *The Life of Sir Ashley Cooper*. For a more detailed record of the post-mortem see the *Lancet*, July 1830.

CHAPTER EIGHT

1. Dorothy Jordan had thirteen children by three different men.
2. Philip Ziegler, *King William IV*, pp. 270–1.
3. Letter: John Fidge to Captain Elphinstone, 18 February 1788. *Royal Archives*: RA 44818.
4. Letter: Prince William

Henry to George, Prince of Wales, 20 May 1787. *Royal Archives*: RA 44769.

5. Lord Ilchester (ed.), *The Journal of the Hon Henry Edward Fox*, p. 50.

6. Letter: Sir Herbert Taylor to Lord Melbourne, 26 May 1837. *Royal Archives*: Melbourne Papers collection.

7. Benjamin Disraeli, Lord Beaconsfield. *Correspondence with his Sister*. Letter: 19 January 1837, p. 60.

CHAPTER NINE

1. Matthews, *Royal Apothecaries*, p. 165.

2. John W. Dodds, *The Age of Paradox*, p. 280.

3. Clifford Brewer, *The Death of Kings*, pp. 241–2.

4. Elizabeth Longford, *Victoria R.I.*, p. 26.

CHAPTER TEN

1. P.J. Anderson, *Roll of Alumni in Arts of the University and King's College Aberdeen*, p. 113.

2. *Writer to the Signet*: formerly a law-agent exclusively preparing Crown writs for the Scottish Supreme Court of Justice; 'writer' was a general term in Scotland for lawyer.

3. Robert Gittings, *John Keats*, pp. 420ff.

4. Ibid., p. 433.

5. Amy Lowell, *John Keats*, Vol. II, p. 501.

6. For a general biographical overview of Sir James Clark see *Dictionary of National Biography*, Vol. IV, pp. 401–2.

7. Hudson, *Royal Conflict*, p. 103.

8. Ibid., p. 104.

9. *Royal Archives*, Letter from Baroness Lehzen to King Leopold, undated, in German, ref: Add/A/11/22.

10. Ibid., Dr Clark's Memoranda for 21 and 29 January 1836, ref: M5/81 and 86.

11. Ibid., Letter: Duchess of Kent to Lord Melbourne, 12 July 1836, ref: MP115/73.

12. Clark remained physician to the Duchess of Kent.

13. Oliver Millar, *The Victorian Pictures of her Majesty the Queen*, pp. 194–5. Sir James Clark appears in two royal group portraits: Sir Henry Hayter's 'The Christening of the Prince of Wales, 25 January 1842', and William Powell Frith's 'The Marriage of the Prince of Wales, 18 March 1863'.

14. Queen Victoria, *Journal*, 18 April 1828.

15. Longford, *Victoria R.I.*, p. 117.

16. Ibid., p. 118.

17. *The Times*, 9 October 1839.

18. Queen Victoria, *Journal*, 2 February 1839.

19. Ibid., 18 and 21 January 1839.

20. Longford, *Victoria R.I.*, p. 119.

21. Queen Victoria, *Journal*, 2 February 1839.

22. Ibid.

23. Longford, *Victoria R.I.*, p. 121.

24. *Royal Archives*: Sir James Clark's *Diaries*.

25. Monica Charlot, *Victoria: The Young Queen*, p. 130.
26. *Royal Archives*, ref: MS Z486/1.
27. Ibid., Letter: Queen Victoria to the Duchess of Kent, undated, ref: MS Z486.
28. Ibid., ref: MS 286/15.
29. *The Times*, 12 August 1839; Letter from Lady Flora to Hamilton Fitzgerald (dated 8 March 1839).
30. Lytton Strachey and Roger Fulford, *The Greville Memoirs 1814–1860*, Vol. IV, pp. 152–3, 180–1.
31. Lady Florence Hastings, *Poems*.
32. Queen Victoria, *Journal*, 26 June 1839.
33. Strachey and Fulford, *Greville Memoirs*.
34. Queen Victoria, *Journal*, 27 June 1839.
35. Ibid., 5 July 1839.
36. In those days friends and acquaintances would send their (empty) carriages to society funerals as a mark of respect.
37. The *Lancet*, Vol. 1839–40, 1, p. 124.
38. Giles St Aubyn, *Queen Victoria*, p. 105.
39. Longford, *Victoria R.I.*, p. 207.
40. Ibid., p. 199.
41. *Memoirs of Ernest II of Saxe-Coburg-Gotha*, Vol. I, p. 97.
42. The Duchess of York with Benita Stoney, *Victoria & Albert at Osborne House*, p. 27.
43. A.G.W. Whitfield, 'The Scholar Prince', *Journal of the Royal College of Physicians of London*, Vol. 18, no. 3 (July 1984), p. 185.
44. Longford, *Victoria R.I.*, p. 291.
45. *Royal Archives*, ref: Z294/9, April 1853.
46. Ibid., ref: Z266/3, Dr Jenner to Queen Victoria, 6 October 1881.
47. Charlotte Zeepvat, *Prince Leopold: The Untold Story of Queen Victoria's Youngest Son*, p. 3.
48. *Royal Archives*, ref: Y206. Sir James Clark's *Diaries*, 5 February 1856.
49. Ibid., ref: Y203. Sir James Clark's *Diaries* 15 February 1856.
50. Longford, *Victoria R.I.*, p. 345.
51. Giles St Aubyn, *Edward VII*, p. 41.
52. *Royal Archives*, ref: Z63/117. Sir James Clark to Queen Victoria, 31 January 1859.
53. Lucius von Ballhausen, *Bismarck's Erinnerungen*, p. 74.

CHAPTER ELEVEN

1. Queen Victoria, *Journal*, 20 December 1873.
2. Francis, Duke of Saxe-Coburg, and his wife Augusta of Reuss-Ebersdorf were Queen Victoria's *maternal* grandparents and Prince Albert's *paternal* grandparents.
3. Godfrey and Margaret Scheele, *The World and the Age of Prince Albert, The Prince Consort: Man of Many Facets*, p. 24.

4. *See* J.A. Shephard, *Simpson and Syme of Edinburgh*, pp. 1–17.
5. Hamilton Bailey and W.J. Bishop, *Notable Names in Medicine and Surgery*, p. 67.
6. Queen Victoria, Letter to Princess Victoria, Crown Princess of Germany, from Osborne House, 24 August 1859.
7. Queen Victoria, *Journal*, 1 October 1860.
8. Longford, *Victoria R.I.*, pp. 360–1.
9. Stanley Weintraub, *Uncrowned King: The Life of Prince Albert*, pp. 378–9.
10. Longford, *Victoria R.I.*, p. 370.
11. H. Maxwell, *Life and Letters of the Fourth Earl of Clarendon*.
12. Longford, *Victoria R.I.*, p. 375.
13. Ibid., p. 376.
14. Queen Victoria, *Journal*, 14 December 1861.
15. Weintraub, *Uncrowned King*, p. 435.
16. Ibid.
17. Brewer, *Death of Kings*, p. 249.
18. Weintraub, *Uncrowned King*, p. 435.

CHAPTER TWELVE

1. A.C. Benson and Viscount Esher, *The Letters of Queen Victoria*, Vol. III, pp. 473–4.
2. Queen Victoria, *Leaves*, 7 September 1858, p. 149.
3. Ibid., 13 September 1850, pp. 125–6.
4. Richard B. Fisher, *Joseph Lister 1827–1912*, p. 58.

5. Ibid., p. 193.
6. Ibid.
7. Ibid., p. 194.
8. Ibid.
9. Obituary, *Aberdeen Journal*, 28 January 1897.
10. *Officers and Graduates of University & King's College, Aberdeen*, Vol. 1860, p. 307.
11. *Records*, Royal College of Surgeons of Edinburgh. Profeit qualified before the Medical Act of 1858 formally stipulated what a practising doctor's qualifications had to be.
12. Raymond Lamont-Brown. *John Brown: Queen Victoria's Highland Servant*, p. 145.
13. Obituary, *Aberdeen Journal*. Profeit's obituary in the *British Medical Journal* (January 1897 pp. 435–6) notes that he had 'a quite unique acquaintance amongst royal personages'.
14. Giles St Aubyn, *Queen Victoria*, p. 577.
15. Michaela Reid, *Ask Sir James*, pp. 227–8.

CHAPTER THIRTEEN

1. The personal details in this chapter are extracted from the biography of Sir James Reid, *Ask Sir James*, by his granddaughter-in-law, Michaela, Lady Reid.
2. Ibid., p. 31.
3. From the Papers of Sir James Reid. *See* Reid, *Ask Sir James*, pp. 37–8.
4. Princess Marie Louise, *My Memories of Six Reigns*, p. 146.

5. Reid Papers; Reid, *Ask Sir James*, p. 46.
6. Reid Papers; Reid, *Ask Sir James*, pp. 49–50.
7. Reid, *Ask Sir James*, p. 113.
8. Ibid., p. 114.
9. Ibid., p. 111.
10. Ibid., p. 166.
11. Ibid., p. 170.
12. Ibid., p. 184. The memo is written in the hand of Queen Victoria's personal private secretary the Hon. Harriet Phipps.
13. Reid, *Ask Sir James*, pp. 212–13.
14. The 'Instructions' were dated 9 December 1897 and had to be carried by Queen Victoria's chief dresser on duty at all times.
15. Lamont-Brown. *John Brown*, p. 162.

CHAPTER FOURTEEN

1. The number of 'Jack the Ripper murders' varies from four to eleven depending on the histories of the cases consulted. Today most writers agree to the five cited in the unpublished notes of Sir Melville Macnaughten (1853–1921), Assistant Chief Constable, Criminal Investigation Department, Scotland Yard. *Metropolitan Police Report: Mepo 3, 141, fols 177–83*. Public Record Office.
2. Fairclough, *The Ripper and The Royals*, p. 248. Letter to a Mrs James from Gull's home at Brook Street, London; Mrs James was in royal employ as a child carer; she died in royal service in 1881.
3. Ibid.
4. Georgina Battiscombe, *Queen Alexandra*, p. 113.
5. Dr T.E.A. Stowell, *The Criminologist*, Vol. 5, no. 18, November 1970, pp. 40–51.
6. *The Times*, 9 November 1970. Letter dated 5 November. Dr Stowell, b. 1885, died on 8 November 1970.
7. Fairclough, *The Ripper and The Royals*, p. ix.
8. Ibid., pp. 4–5, & 7.
9. Ibid., p. 10.
10. Ibid., pp. 8–9.
11. Ibid., p. 12.
12. Ibid., p. 14.
13. All cases, Sir Melville Macnaughten. For medical comments in coroner's reports, *see* Stowell, *The Criminologist*, at note 5.
14. Fairclough, *The Ripper and The Royals*, pp. 179–80 and Appendix 9, pp. 245–6.
15. Peregrine Churchill and Julian Mitchell, *Jenny: Lady Randolph Churchill*, p. 112.
16. Fairclough, *The Ripper and The Royals*, p. 36. On his visits to Fitzrovia it seems that Prince Eddy changed, *en route* from Marlborough House, from a liveried royal coach from the royal mews to a privately hired coach driven by John Charles Netley.
17. Ibid., p. 148.
18. Ibid., p. 153.
19. Ibid., quoting Thomas Dyke Acland *In Memoriam: Sir William Gull*, p. xxvix.

20. Stowell, *The Criminologist*, p. 46.
21. Fairclough, *The Ripper and The Royals*, p. 137.
22. Ronald Rumbelow, *The Complete Jack the Ripper*, p. 189.
23. William D. Rubinstein, 'The Hunt for Jack the Ripper', *History Today*, Vol. 50 (5), May 2000.
24. Stowell, *The Criminologist*, p. 50.
25. Kevin O'Donnell, *The Jack the Ripper Whitechapel Murders*, pp. 170–80.
26. Ibid., p. 177.

CHAPTER FIFTEEN

1. Christopher Hibbert, *Edward VII: A Portrait*, p. 112.
2. Ibid., p. 113.
3. Henry C. Burdett, *Prince, Princess and People*, p. 336.
4. Raymond Lamont-Brown, *Edward VII's Last Loves, Alice Keppel and Agnes Keyser*, pp. 13–14.
5. Ibid., Index entries for King Edward VII's Hospital for Officers.
6. Ibid., p. 194.
7. Procedure taken from: Ellis, *Operations that made History*, p. 111.

CHAPTER SIXTEEN

1. Stephen Trombley, *Sir Frederick Treves*, p. 11.
2. Francis Watson, *Dawson of Penn*, p. 71.
3. Trombley, *Treves*, p. 37.
4. Frederick Treves, *The Elephant Man and Other Reminiscences.*
5. Both Treves and Crocker overlooked the research of the German pathologist Frederich Daniell von Recklinghausen (1833–1910) – 'Recklinghausen's disease – neurofibromatosis.
6. Trombley, *Treves*, p. 49.
7. Treves, *The Elephant Man.*
8. Trombley, *Treves*, p. 80.
9. Victor G. Plarr, *Plarr's Lives*, entry for Frederick Treves.
10. Battiscombe, *Queen Alexandra*, p. 247.
11. Lamont-Brown, *Edward VII's Last Loves*, p. 128.
12. Ibid.
13. Reid, *Ask Sir James*, p. 240.

CHAPTER SEVENTEEN

1. Rose, *King George V*, p. 78.
2. Reid, *Ask Sir James*, p. 248.
3. Watson, *Dawson of Penn*, p. 9.
4. Ibid., p. 105.
5. Rose, *King George V*, p. 70.
6. Watson, *Dawson of Penn*, pp. 138–9.
7. Rose, *King George V*, p. 182.
8. Watson, *Dawson of Penn*, p. 159. Purists might like to note that Dr Sir B.W. Foster (d. 1913), Professor of Medicine at Queen's College, Birmingham, sat in the Lords (1910–13) as the 1st Lord Ilkeston. He was there because of his political services as a Member of Parliament and not as a medical man.
9. Ibid., p. 159.
10. R. Scott Stevenson, *Famous Illnesses in History*, p. 14.

11. Watson, *Dawson of Penn*, pp. 20–1.
12. Ibid., p. 215.
13. Ibid., p. 15.
14. *British Medical Journal*, 7 December 1928, Vol. ii, p. 15.
15. Scott Stevenson, *Famous Illnesses*, p. 16.
16. The Duke of Windsor, *A King's Story*, pp. 210–11.
17. Rose, *King George V*, pp. 35ff.
18. Ellis, *Operations that made History*, pp. 121–2.
19. Ibid., p. 122.
20. Scott Stevenson, *Famous Illnesses*, p. 21.
21. Ibid., pp. 21–2.
22. Watson, *Dawson of Penn*, p. 212.
23. Ibid., p. 273.
24. Ibid., pp. 278–9.
25. J.G. Lockhart, *Cosmo Gordon Lang*, p. 392.
26. Channel 5 Television, 18 July 2000. Programme: 'I'm not as nice as people think I am.'

CHAPTER EIGHTEEN

1. Frances Donaldson, *Edward VIII: The Road to Abdication*, p. 50.
2. Ibid., pp. 184–5.
3. Ibid., p. 50. The king made a formal request for Prince Edward to desist from racing in a letter from Buckingham Palace, 30 March 1924.
4. The Duke of Windsor, *King's Story*, p. 78.
5. Philip Ziegler, *Edward VIII*, p. 31.
6. *Royal Archives*, Prince of Wales's diary, 13 April 1912.
7. *Papers of Godfrey Thomas*, 5 March 1943.
8. Charles Higham, *Wallis: Secret Lives of the Duchess of Windsor*, p. 257.
9. Ibid., p. 198.
10. Ibid., p. 313.
11. Ibid., p. 500.
12. J. Bryan III and Charles J. Murphy, *The Windsor Story*, p. 675.
13. Dr Thin's words are quoted by Michael Bloch, *The Secret File on the Duke of Windsor*, p. 302.

CHAPTER NINETEEN

1. James Pope-Hennessy, *Queen Mary 1867–1953*, pp. 390–1.
2. *British Medical Journal*, Obituary, ii, p. 674, 1925; the *Lancet*, i, p. 785, 1925.
3. Ziegler, *Edward VIII*, p. 538.
4. Jennifer Ellis (ed.), *Thatched with Gold: The memoirs of Mabell, Countess of Airlie*, p. 113.
5. Anne Edwards, *Matriarch: Queen Mary & The House of Windsor*, p. 154.
6. Ziegler, *Edward VIII*, p. 80.
7. Edwards, *Matriarch*, p. 193.
8. Ross Benson, *Daily Mail*, 12 February 1998, p. 28.
9. Battiscombe, *Queen Alexandra*, p. 279.
10. David Williamson, *Brewer's British Royalty*, p. 228.
11. Pope-Hennessy, *Queen Mary*, p. 510.
12. Ibid., p. 511.
13. Ziegler, *Edward VIII*, p. 80.
14. Battiscombe, *Queen Alexandra*, p. 280.

CHAPTER TWENTY

1. For Dawson and Lloyd George *see* Watson, *Dawson of Penn*, Index entries.
2. Ibid., p. 325.
3. Roy Kenneth (ed.), *Dictionary of Scottish Biography*, Vol. 1: 1971–5, p. 168.
4. King George VI's Military Service Records, *Public Record Office*. Released 16 September 2000.
5. David Sinclair, *Two Georges: The Making of Modern Monarchy*, p. 180.
6. Ibid.
7. Ibid., note 4.
8. Ibid., pp. 176–7.
9. Sir John W. Wheeler-Bennett, *King George VI: His Life and Reign*.
10. Mabell, Countess of Airlie, *Thatched with Gold*, pp. 113–14.
11. Sinclair, *Two Georges*, p. 240.
12. Wheeler-Bennett, *King George VI*, p. 280.
13. Sir Philip Magnus-Allcroft, *King Edward VIII*, p. 333.
14. Ellis, *Operations that made History*, p. 120.
15. For this and succeeding bulletins *see British Medical Journal*, 2:793, 1951.
16. Ellis, *Operations that made History*, p. 129.
17. Quoted by *Sunday Times* medical correspondent Oliver Gillie.
18. Ellis, *Operations that made History*, p. 127.

EPILOGUE

1. The queen's household lists, the Lord Chamberlain's Office, Buckingham Palace, January 2001.
2. Ibid.
3. Richard Hough, *Sister Agnes: The History of King Edward VII's Hospital for Officers*, p. 156.
4. Ibid., pp. 97n, 123, 146, 157.
5. Michael Thornton, *Royal Feud*, pp. 109–10.
6. *The Times*, Wednesday, 29 November 2000, pp. 3–4.
7. Ibid.
8. Ibid.
9. Obituary, 28 November 1987. *British Medical Journal*.
10. 'When the President is the Patient'. http://www.collphyphil.org/presphyn.htn. Feb 2001.

APPENDIX

1. Gulielmus Malmesburiensis (William of Malmesbury), *Gesta Regum Anglorum*, ed. W. Stubbs, Rolls Series, 1887–9.
2. Matthew Paris, *Chronica Maiora*, ed. H.R. Luard, Rolls Series, 1872–84.
3. William of Malmesbury, *Gesta Regum Anglorum*.
4. Lamont-Brown, *Royal Murder Mysteries*, pp. 7–15.
5. Henry of Huntingdon, *Historia Anglorum*, ed. T. Arnold, 1879.
6. Gervase of Canterbury, *Chronica*, ed. W. Stubbs, Rolls Series, 1879–80.
7. Mattaeus Westmonasteriensis (Matthew of Westminster),

Flores Historicum, ed.
H.R. Luard, 1890.

8. William of Newburg, *Historia Rerum Anglicarum*.

9. Roger de Hovedene, *Chronica*, ed. W. Stubbs, Rolls Series, 1868–71.

10. Matthew Paris, *Chronica Maiora*.

11. Raphael Holinshed, *Chronicles of England, Scotland and Ireland*, ed. J. Johnston, 1807–8.

12. Thomas Walsingham, *Chronicon Angliae*, ed. E.M. Thompson, Rolls Series, 1874.

13. Cited by John Capgrave, *Chronicle of England of John Capgrave*, ed. F.C. Hingeston, 1858.

14. Joseph Rawson Lumby, *Polychronicon Ranulphi Higden, Monachi Cantrensis*, Rolls Series, 1882.

15. Walsingham, *Chronicon Angliae*.

16. Ibid. *See also La Chronique de la Traison et Mort de Richard Deux, roy Dengleterre*.

17. Capgrave, *Chronicle of England*.

18. See the description of the opening of his coffin in *Archaeologia*, vol. XXVI, 1832, pp. 444ff.

19. Walsingham, *Chronicon Angliae*.

20. W.F. Skene (ed.), *Scotichronicon*, Historians of Scotland Series, 1871–2. *St Fiacres III*: condition suffered by Abbot St Fiacre, an Irish saint of the Abbey of St Breuil, St Faro of Meaux, France. His healing shrine is still extant. He died *c.* 670.

21. *See* post-mortem assessment by Professor MacAlister, 4 November 1910. *The Times*, 12 November 1910.

22. Croyland Continuator, *Croyland Chronicle*.

23. Holinshed, *Chronicles*.

24. Thomas Goodwin, *Annals of England*.

25. Holinshed, *Chronicles*.

26. Sir Richard Baker, *The Chronicles of the Kings of England*, 1843.

27. Ibid.

28. Remark in 1690 by court lady: 'Piety makes people outrageously stupid.' Peter Earle, *The Life and Times of James II*.

29. Walter Harris, *Observations on Certain Grievous Diseases*, 1742.

30. Lord Holland, *Memoirs of the Reign of George II*, 1847.

31. Post-mortem report, the *Lancet*, 1830.

32. Extract: *The Post-Mortem Examination of his Late Majesty*, Windsor Castle, 20 June 1837.

33. These can be consulted at the General Register Office, Southport, Merseyside PR5 2JD.

BIBLIOGRAPHY

Ordinances, Rolls, Charters, Cartularies and Calendars
Public Record Office
Calendar of Patent Rolls
Calendar of Close Rolls
Calendar of Charter Rolls
Calendar of Documents Relating to Ireland
Calendar of Documents Relating to Scotland
Chancery Miscellanea
Close Rolls
Proceedings of the Privy Council

National Library of Scotland
R. Sharpe (ed.), *Calendar of Wills in the Court of Hustings*, London, n.d.
*Ordinances and Regulations of the Royal Household from Edward III to
    William and Mary*, Society of Antiquaries, 1790.
F. Devon (ed.), *Extracts from the Issue Rolls of the Exchequer*, London,
    1837.
Exchequer Rolls of Scotland, 1264–1359 and 1470–9.
Rotuli Scaccarii Regum Scotorum
Calendar of State Papers Relating to Scotland and Mary, Queen of Scots.
Theiner, A. *Vetera monumenta Hibernorum et Scotorum, 1216–1547*.

Chronicles:
Arnold, T. (ed.). Henry of Huntingdon, *Historia Anglorum*, London, 1879.
Croyland Continuator. *Croyland Chronicle*.
Gaddesden, John of. *Praxis medica seu Rosa anglica dicta*, London, n.d.
Goodwin, Thomas. *Annals of England*.
Hingeston, F.C. (ed.). John Capgrave, *Chronicle of England of John
    Capgrave*, 1858.
Holinshed, Raphael. *Chronicles of England, Scotland and Ireland*, ed. J.
    Johnston, 1807–9.
Luard, H.R. (ed.). Matthew Paris, *Chronica Majora*, London, Rolls Series,
    1872.
—— (ed.). Matthew of Westminster, *Flores Historicum*, London, 1890.
Lumby, Joseph Rawson. *Polychronicon Ranulphi Higden, Monachi
    Cantrensis*, London, Rolls Series, 1882.
Paget, Julius Leopold (ed.). Henri de Mandeville, *Chirurgia*, Berlin, 1892.
Rymer, Thomas and Sanderson, Robert. *Foedera, Conventiones et
    Cujuscunque generis Acta Publica* (to 1654), London, 1704–35.
Skene, W.F. (ed.). *Scotichronicon*. Historians of Scotland Series, 1871–2.
Stevenson, J. (ed.). *Chronica Monasterii de Abingdon*, London, Rolls Series,
    1855.
Stubbs, W. (ed.). *The Historical Works of Gervase of Canterbury*.
——. (ed.). Roger de Hovedene, *Chronica*, London, Rolls Series, 1868–71.

— —. (ed.). William of Malmesbury, *Gesta Regum Anglorum*, London, Rolls
    Series, 1887–9.
Thompson, E.M. (ed.). Thomas Walsingham, *Chronicon Angliae*, London,
    Rolls Series, 1874.
William of Newburg. *Historia Rerum Anglicarum*.

Private and Learned Papers, Series:
'A Trial of Witches at the Assizes Held at Bury St Edmunds.'
'A True Relation of the King's Death.' Broadsheet, 1685.
Annals of Medical History. Various issues.
Archaeologia. Relevant issues.
Balcarres Papers.
British Medical Journal. Relevant issues.
British Journal of Surgery.
Caledonian Medical Journal. Relevant issues.
Criminologist.
Gentleman's Magazine.
Journal of the Royal College of Physicians of London. Relevant issues.
Lancet. Relevant issues.
Papers of Godfrey Thomas.
Practitioner Journal of Post-Graduate Medicine. Relevant issues.
Proceedings of the Royal Society of Medicine. Various issues.
Royal College of Physicians. 'The Harveian Oration: Royal Physicians', George
    Whitfield, 1986.

Letters, Memoirs, Diaries and Journals:
Acland, Theodore Dyke (ed.). *A Collection of Published Writings of William
    Withey Gull*, London, 1894.
Anon. *A Minute Detail of Attempts to Assassinate HRH the Duke of
    Cumberland*, London, 1810.
Aspinall, A. *The Correspondence of George, Prince of Wales 1770–1812*,
    Cassell, 1967.
— —. *Letters of King George IV*, Cassell, 1938.
Benson, A.C. and Esher, Viscount. *The Letters of Queen Victoria*. Murray,
    1908.
Buckingham, Duke of (ed.). *Memoirs of the Court and Cabinets of George III*,
    London, 1853.
Clark, Sir James. *Diaries*, Private Collection.
The Diary of Thomas Cartwright, Bishop of Chester, Camden Society, 1843.
Disraeli, Benjamin, Lord Beaconsfield. *Correspondence with His Sister*,
    London, 1886.
Douglas, Archibald A.H. (trans. and ed.). *The Brus, an epic poem by John
    Barbour*, William MacLellan, 1964.
Ernest II of Saxe-Coburg Gotha. *Memoirs*.
Greville, Robert Fulke. *Diaries*, London, n.d.
Holland, Lord (ed.). *Horace Walpole: Memoirs of the last ten years of the
    Reign of George II*, London, 1822.
— — (ed.). *Lord Waldegrave, Memoirs*, London, 1829.
Holroyd, John Baker. *Memoirs*, London, n.d.

Huish, Robert. *Memoirs of George IV*, London, 1830.

Ilchester, Lord (ed.). *The Journal of the Hon. Henry Edward Fox*, London, n.d.

Jesse, John Heneage. *Memoirs of the Life and Reign of King George III*, London, 1867.

HH Marie Louise. *My Memories of Six Reigns*, Evans, 1956.

Maxwell, H. *The Life and Letters of the Fourth Earl of Clarendon*, Arnold, 1913.

Roberts, P. (ed.). *The Diary of Sir David Hamilton 1709–14*, Oxford University Press, 1975.

Strachey, Lytton and Fulford, Roger. *The Greville Memoirs 1814–1860*, Macmillan, 1938.

Victoria, Queen. *Journal*. Various extract editions available.

Wood, Marguerite (ed.). *Foreign Correspondence with Marie de Lorraine, Queen of Scotland, from the Originals in the Balcarres Papers*, Scottish History Society, 1923–5.

Biographical Dictionaries and Biographies of Individual Medical Practitioners: The Concise Dictionary of National Biography, Oxford University Press, 1992.

Dictionary of National Biography, Smith Elder, 1908.

Anderson, P.J. *Roll of Alumni in Arts of the University and King's College Aberdeen*, University of Aberdeen. Current.

Bailey, Hamilton and Bishop, W.J. *Notable Names in Medicine & Surgery*, H.K. Lewis, 1944.

Macmichael, W. *Lives of British Physicians*, London, 1830.

Matthews, Leslie G. *The Royal Apothecaries*, Wellcome Historical Medical Library, 1967.

Munk, William. *Roll of Physicians of the Royal College of Physicians of London*, London, 1878.

Pettigrew, T.J. *Medical Portrait Gallery*, London, 1840.

Plarr, Victor G. *et al. Lives of the Fellows of the Royal College of Surgeons of England*, Bristol, John Wright & Sons, 1930.

Roy, Kenneth (ed.). *Dictionary of Scottish Biography*, Carrick Media, 1999.

Thomson, Revd Thomas (ed.). *Robert Chambers: A Biographical Dictionary of Eminent Scotsmen*, Edinburgh, 1870.

Acland, Theodore Dyke. *William Withey Gull: A Biographical Sketch*, London, 1896.

Aiken, J. *Biographical Memoirs of Medicine in Great Britain*, London, 1780.

Atlay, J.B. *Henry Acland – A Memoir*, Smith Elder, 1903.

Fisher, Richard B. *Joseph Lister 1827–1912*, Macdonald & Jane's, 1977.

Hone, C.R. *The Life of John Radcliffe*, Faber & Faber, 1950.

Hurry, Jameson B. *Imhotep: The Vizier and Physician to King Zoser*, Oxford University Press, 1928.

Reid, Michaela. *Ask Sir James*, Hodder & Stoughton, 1987.

Shephard, J.A. *Simpson and Syme at Edinburgh*, Edinburgh, 1969.

Timbs, J. *Doctors and Patients*, London, 1873.

Trombley, Stephen. *Sir Frederick Treves: The Extra-Ordinary Edwardian*, Routledge, 1989.

Watson, Francis. *Lord Dawson of Penn*, Chatto & Windus, 1986.
Wickersheimer. *Les Médecins de la Nation Anglaise*, Paris, 1913.
Young, Agatha. *Scalpel: Men who Made Surgery*, Robert Hale, 1957.

Medical Histories:
Bloch, Marc. *The Royal Touch: Monarchy and Miracles in France & England*, Routledge Kegan Paul/Dorset Press, 1989.
Breasted, James Henry. *The Edwin Smith Surgical Papyrus*, University of Chicago Press, 1930.
Brewer, Clifford. *The Death of Kings*, Abson, 2000.
Browne, E.G. *Arabian Medicine*, London, 1921.
Chi Min Wang and Lien-Teh Wu. *History of Chinese Medicine*, Tientsin, 1932.
Comrie, John D. *History of Scottish Medicine*, London, 1932.
Ellis, Harold. *Operations that made History*, Greenwich Medical Media, 1996.
Guthrie, Douglas. *A History of Medicine*, Thomas Nelson, 1945.
Hamilton, David. *The Healers: A History of Medicine in Scotland*, Canongate, 1981.
Kealey, Edward J. *Medieval Medicus: A Social History of Anglo-Norman Medicine*, The Johns Hopkins University Press, 1981.
Mould, Richard F. *Mould's Medical Anecdotes*, London, n.d.
Nunn, John F. *Ancient Egyptian Medicine*, British Museum, 1996.
Ritchie, R.P. *The Early Days of the Royall Colledge of Physitions, Edinburgh*, G.P. Johnston, 1899.
Rubin, Stanley. *Medieval English Medicine*, David & Charles, 1974.
Stevenson, R.S. *Famous Illnesses in History*, Eyre & Spottiswoode, 1912.
Talbot, C.H. and Hammond, E.A. *The Medical Practitioners in Medieval England*, Wellcome Historical Medical Library, 1965.
Withington, Dr E.T. *Medical History from the Earliest Times*, London, 1894.

General Titles
Airlie, Mabell, Countess of. *Thatched with Gold*, Hutchinson, 1962.
Barrow, G.W.S. *Robert Bruce: And the Community of the Realm of Scotland*, Edinburgh University Press, 1976.
Battiscombe, Georgina. *Queen Alexandra*, Sphere Books, 1972.
Block, Michael. *The Secret File of the Duke of Windsor*, Bantam Press, 1988.
Brock, R.C. *The Life and Work of Astley Cooper*, E.S. Livingstone, 1952.
Brougham, Lord. *The Life and Times of Henry Lord Brougham By Himself*, London, 1871.
Brown, J. Wood. *An Enquiry into the Life and Legend of Michael Scott*, David Douglas, Edinburgh, 1897.
Bryan, J. III and Murphy, Charles J.V. *The Windsor Story*, Granada, 1979.
Chadwick, Nora. *The Celts*, Pelican, 1970.
Charlot, Monica. *Victoria: The Young Queen*, Blackwell, 1991.
Churchill, Peregrine and Mitchell, Julian. *Jennie: Lady Randolph Churchill*, Collins, 1974.
Cooper, B. Bransby. *Life of Sir Astley Cooper*, London, 1843.
Coulton, G.C. *Scottish Abbeys and Social Life*, Cambridge University Press, 1933.
Cowan, Samuel. *Mary Queen of Scots*, Sampson Low, Marston, 1901.

Curtis, Gila. *The Life & Times of Queen Anne*, Weidenfeld & Nicolson, 1972.

Dickinson, Gladys. *Two Missions of Jaques de la Brosse*, Scottish History Record, 1942.

Dodds, John W. *The Age of Paradox*, Gollancz, 1953.

Donaldson, Francis. *Edward VIII: The road to Abdication*, Weidenfeld & Nicolson, 1978.

Earle, Peter. *The Life & Times of James II*, Weidenfeld & Nicolson, 1972.

Edwards, Anne. *Matriarch: Queen Mary & the House of Windsor*, Hodder & Stoughton, 1984.

Fairclough, Melvyn. *The Ripper and the Royals*, Duckworth, 1991.

Fergusson, John. *Notes on the Character and Health of HM King George III*, London, 1857.

Forbes, R. *The Lyon in Mourning*, Scottish History Society, 1895.

Fraser, Antonia. *King James VI of Scotland, I of England*, Weidenfeld & Nicolson, 1974.

Gittings, Robert. *John Keats*, Heinemann, 1968.

Green, Vivian. *The Madness of Kings*, Alan Sutton, 1993.

Hamilton, Lady Anne. *Secret History of the Court of England*, Stevenson, 1832.

Hennessey, James Pope. *Queen Mary 1867–1953*, Allen & Unwin, 1959.

Hibbert, C. *The Virgin Queen*, Viking-Penguin, 1992.

Higham, Charles. *Wallis: Secret Lives of the Duchess of Windsor*, Sidgwick & Jackson, 1988.

Holmyard, E.J. *Alchemy*, Penguin, 1957.

Hough, Richard. *Sister Agnes*, Murray, 1998.

Hudson, Katherine. *A Royal Conflict: Sir John Conroy and the Young Victoria*, Hodder & Stoughton, 1994.

Iskander, Z. and Badawy, A. *Brief History of Ancient Egypt*, Madkour Press, 1960.

Keevil, J.J. *The Stranger's Son*, Geoffrey Bles, 1953.

Knox, Ronald and Leslie, Shane (eds). *The Miracles of King Henry VI*. London, n.d.

Lamont-Brown, Raymond. *Royal Murder Mysteries*, Weidenfeld & Nicolson, 1990.

— —. *Edward VII's Last Loves: Alice Keppel & Agnes Keyser*, Sutton, 1998.

— —. *John Brown: Queen Victoria's Highland Servant*, Sutton, 2000.

Laing, D. (ed.). *Sir David Lyndsay's Works*, Edinburgh, 1879.

Lockhart, J.G. *Cosmo Gordon Lang*, Hodder & Stoughton, 1949.

Longford, Elizabeth. *Victoria R.I.*, World Books, 1967.

Lowell, Amy. *John Keats*, Jonathan Cape, 1925.

Macalpine, Ida and Hunter, Richard. *George III and the Mad-Business*, Pimlico, 1995.

Macaulay, Thomas Babbington, Lord. *History of England*, London, 1849–55.

Mackie, R.L. *King James IV*, Oliver & Boyd, 1958.

McKinley, Runyan. *Journals of Personality*, London, 1988.

Magnus-Allcroft, Sir Philip. *King Edward VII*, Penguin, 1967.

Marlow, Joyce. *The Life and Times of George I*, Weidenfeld & Nicolson, 1973.

Marshall, Rosalind K. *Mary of Guise*, Collins, 1977.

Meyer, E. *Geschichte des alten Aegyptens*, Berlin, 1885.

Millar, Oliver. *The Victorian Pictures*, Cambridge University Press, 1992.

O'Donnell, Kevin. *The Jack the Ripper Whitechapel Murders*, Ten Bells Publishing, 1997.

Prebble, John. *Culloden*, Penguin, 1967.

Priestley, J.B. *The Prince of Pleasure and his Regency 1811–20*, Heinemann, 1969.

Robbins, Rossell Hope. *The Encyclopaedia of Witchcraft and Demonology*, Crown Publishing, New York, 1959.

Rose, Kenneth. *King George V*, Weidenfeld & Nicolson, 1983.

——. *Kings, Queens & Courtiers*, Weidenfeld & Nicolson, 1985.

Rumbelow, Donald. *The Complete Jack the Ripper*, W.H. Allen, 1975.

St Aubyn, Giles. *Queen Victoria*, Sinclair-Stevenson, 1991.

——. *Edward VII*, Collins, 1979.

Scheele, Godfrey and Scheele, Margaret. *The Prince Consort*, Oresko Books, 1977.

Sinclair, David. *Two Georges*, Hodder & Stoughton, 1988.

Sinclair-Stevenson, Christopher. *Blood Royal: The Illustrious House of Hanover*, Jonathan Cape, 1959.

Stirton, John. *Glamis Castle. Its Origins and History*, Shepherd, 1938.

Stockmar, Baron E. von. *Memoirs of Baron Stockmar*, Longmans Green, 1872.

Thomson, J. Maitland. *John Dowden: The Bishops of Scotland*, Maclehose, 1912.

Thornton, Michael. *Royal Feud*, Joseph 1985.

Treves, Sir Francis. *The Elephant Man and Other Reminiscences*, Cassell, 1923.

Van Thal, Herbert. *Ernest Augustus, Duke of Cumberland, King of Hanover*, Arthur Barker, 1936.

Von Ballhausen, Lucius. *Bismarcks Erinnerungen*, Stuttgart, 1920.

Weigall, A.E. *Guide to the Antiquities of Upper Egypt*, London, 1913.

Weintraub, Stanley. *Uncrowned King: The Life of Prince Albert*, The Free Press, New York, 1997.

Williamson, David. *Brewer's British Royalty*, Cassell, 1996.

Willis, G.W. *Ernest Augustus Duke of Cumberland King of Hanover*, Arthur Barker, 1936.

Willson, D. Harris. *King James VI and I*, Jonathan Cape, 1956.

Wilson, David M. *Awful Ends: The British Museum Book of Epitaphs*, 1992.

Windsor, HRH, The Duke of. *A King's Story*, Cassell–RS, 1953.

York, HRH the Duchess of and Stoney, Benita. *Victoria and Albert at Osborne House*, Weidenfeld & Nicolson, 1991.

Zeepvat, Charlotte. *Prince Leopold*. Sutton, 1998.

Ziegler, Philip. *King William IV*, Fontana, 1973.

Ziegler, Philip. *Edward VIII*, Collins, 1990.

ACKNOWLEDGEMENTS

Text

For this general overview of the medical practitioners in royal service many sources have been consulted; the main texts are listed in the bibliography. Throughout, the textual emphasis has been anecdotal rather than historical to make the medical personnel mentioned live rather than be reflected in a general history of medicine. In bringing out the flavour of individual biographies, and the interplay of physicians, surgeons and apothecaries with monarchs and their families, the author is grateful to the following.

Mr Clifford Brewer FRCS has supplied comment on various topics and has generously allowed quotes on the 'probable causes of death of the Kings and Queens of England' from his volume *The Death of Kings* (Abson, 2000). The author acknowledges too, with gratitude, permission to quote from Michaela Reid's *Ask Sir James* (Hodder & Stoughton, 1987), and from the literary estate of Lord Dawson of Penn. Useful comment was also garnered from the works of the late Professor G.E. Gask on royal surgeons, Professor George Whitfield on royal physicians and John F. Nunn on Ancient Egyptian court medical practice.

Every effort has been made to trace literary heirs of copyright material – all duly acknowledged in text – and valuable advice on tracing these heirs has been given by Ruth Sloss, David Higham Associates and Catherine Trippett, The Random House Group. Esteemed advice, comment and information has been supplied by the following: Dr R.P.H. Thompson, Head of the Medical Household to the Queen; Jonathan Spencer, Secretary, Lord Chamberlain's Office, Buckingham Palace; Mrs Gill Pattinson, Public Enterprises Manager, Sandringham Estate; Dr John Burton, Coroner to the Queen's Household; Kevin Flude, The Old Operating Theatre, Museum & Herb Garret; Debbie Parsons, Search Services, The Royal Society of Medicine; Cathy

Fowler, Archivist, Royal College of Physicians, London; Jonathan Evans, Trust Archivist, The Royal London Hospital; Patricia Allderidge, Archivist and Curator, Bethlem Royal Hospital Archives & Museum; Dee Cook, Archivist, Worshipful Society of Apothecaries of London; Joy Pitman, The Royal College of Surgeons, Edinburgh; Carol Parry, The Royal College of Physicians and Surgeons of Glasgow; Clare Jackson, Archivist, The Royal College of Surgeons of Edinburgh; and Christine Butler, Archives, Corpus Christi College. The author would also like to add a special thank you to his wife Dr E. Moira Lamont-Brown for advice, help and support during the compilation of the book. While all of the above have contributed to the book's content the author wishes to emphasise that he takes full responsibility for the historical interpretation and conclusions drawn.

Photographs
Each photograph is individually acknowledged for source and ownership. Particular thanks are due to the following for help in tracing some illustrations: Evan York and Tania Watkins, British Museum; Ms K.M. Firkin, Bodleian Library; and Cathy Fowler, Royal College of Physicians.

INDEX

Note: Not all royal court medical practitioners mentioned in the text appear in this index. See court lists on relevant pages for all other name entries, and cross-reference with monarch's entries below.